INTERPRETATION AND USES OF
MEDICAL STATISTICS

Gerry Banks
Castlebar '86

INTERPRETATION AND USES OF MEDICAL STATISTICS

Geoffrey J. Bourke
MA, MD, FRCPI, FFCM, FFCMI
Professor of Community Medicine and Epidemiology
University College, Dublin
Consultant in Epidemiology and Preventive Medicine
St. Vincent's Hospital, Elm Park, Dublin

Leslie E. Daly
MSc, PhD
Lecturer in Community Medicine and Epidemiology
University College, Dublin

James McGilvray
MA, MLitt
Director of the Fraser of Allander Institute
University of Strathclyde

THIRD EDITION

Blackwell Scientific Publications
OXFORD · LONDON · EDINBURGH
BOSTON · PALO ALTO · MELBOURNE

© 1969, 1975, 1985 by
Blackwell Scientific Publications
Editorial offices:
Osney Mead, Oxford, OX2 0EL
8 John Street, London, WC1N 2ES
23 Ainslie Place, Edinburgh, EH3 6AJ
52 Beacon Street, Boston
  Massachusetts 02108, USA
667 Lytton Avenue, Palo Alto
  California 94301, USA
107 Barry Street, Carlton
  Victoria 3053, Australia

First published 1969
Second edition 1975
Reprinted 1978
Third Edition 1985

DISTRIBUTORS
USA
  Blackwell Mosby Book Distributors
  11830 Westline Industrial Drive
  St Louis, Missouri 63141

Canada
  Blackwell Mosby Book Distributors
  120 Melford Drive, Scarborough
  Ontario M1B 2X4

Australia
  Blackwell Scientific Book Distributors
  31 Advantage Road, Highett
  Victoria 3190

British Library
Cataloguing in Publication Data

Bourke, Geoffrey J.
  Interpretation and uses of medical
  statistics. — 3rd ed.
  1. Medical statistics
  I. Title   II. Daly, Leslie E.
  III. McGilvray, J. W.
  610'.212   RA407

ISBN 0-632-00864-4

Typeset printed and bound by
H Charlesworth and Co Ltd, Huddersfield

PREFACE

The first edition of this book, published in 1969, was designed to introduce basic concepts of statistics, and their application to medicine, to readers who had no formal training in statistical theory or methods. The book emphasized interpretation rather than techniques of calculation, and sought to make readers familiar with the expressions and methods commonly employed in the analysis and presentation of data in journal articles and other medical research publications. Its success demonstrated the need for such a book, and a second edition, incorporating a number of minor revisions and extensions, was published in 1975.

While retaining its basic aim of interpretation, this new edition entails a comprehensive revision to the scope and content of the book. In the past decade, there have been significant developments in the range and sophistication of statistical techniques in medical research, and there is wider recognition of the need for an understanding of statistical methods in undergraduate and graduate training in medicine. This need has been underlined by the widespread establishment of faculties or departments of community medicine in the medical schools of many universities. As a consequence of these developments, graduates in medicine and allied subjects generally have, and need to have, a greater awareness of statistical concepts and methods, and this is recognized in the range and content of the new edition of this book. The material on sampling distributions and hypothesis testing has been greatly extended and the book now includes illustrations of and computational details for a fair range of statistical tests. Particular emphasis is given to non-parametric approaches. The choice of statistical procedures covered in the book was dictated by two main factors. Firstly, only those procedures commonly encountered in the medical literature were included and secondly, computational details were given only if they were practicable using a pocket calculator. In particular, computational details are not presented for either analysis of variance or multiple regression.

Totally new chapters on study design and methodology emphasize the need for careful planning and execution of research projects, though it was decided that certain topics (experimental design and the analysis of dose response curves) were best left to more advanced textbooks. 'Vital Statistics' and 'Computers in Medicine' are now separate chapters which are included as basic introductions to subject areas which are worthy of book-length texts in their own right.

Despite this expansion in content and methodological rigour, it is hoped that the book will continue to appeal to those who, while less interested in the methods of statistical calculation, seek a basic understanding of statistical concepts and their role in medicine. Parts of the book may be skipped over by the inidivudal who only wants a simple introduction, while enough detail is also given to enable the researcher to actually analyse some results. Thus, this book should be a useful text for the undergraduate who may only require broad principles, for the qualified doctor sitting a membership or other postgraduate examination (especially in community medicine, public health or epidemiology) or for researchers who require more detailed knowledge of statistics and study design.

To assist the reader, a brief guide to the structure and contents of the book is included in the following pages. It is not attempted however to outline a course structure in statistics and research methodology based on this book since everyone has his/her own ideas on what should and should not be included and how much time would be necessary to cover the material.

We are grateful to many people who offered advice and suggestions: to Mrs Christine Delaney, who undertook the daunting task of preparing the typed manuscript with patience, dedication and humour; to Mr Guido Haas who helped modify the word processing program used for the preparation of the manuscript, and to Blackwell Scientific Publications, for their support, encouragement and efficiency.

Geoffrey J. Bourke
Leslie Daly
James McGilvray

STRUCTURE OF THE BOOK

Chapter 1 introduces the reader to the different types of data, to tables, bar charts, histograms and polygons. The section on drawing histograms is somewhat technical and can be omitted without loss of continuity. The second chapter introduces the mean, median and mode together with percentile indices and the standard deviation.

Chapter 3 introduces the notion of probability and chance at a basic level and describes sample surveys in detail. The normal distribution is introduced. Chapter 4 describes the process of statistical estimation and explains the calculation and interpretation of confidence intervals for means and proportions. The Student's *t* distribution is introduced. Without doubt this chapter requires somewhat greater concentration than the previous chapters but it is the corner-stone on which much of the rest of the book is based.

Chapter 5 contains a simple, non-mathematical introduction to statistical tests of significance, and gives the reader a broad overview of the subject. In Chapter 6 the general principles of significance tests are explained and the concept of power calculations introduced. Applications of one-sample tests for means and proportions are considered. Again, this chapter is not necessarily easy, but if the principles enumerated are grasped a major hurdle has been overcome.

Chapter 7 concentrates on the comparisons of two or more groups. The reader is introduced to independent and paired comparisons and to parametric and non-parametric tests. The main body of the chapter describes the application of, and computational formulae for, the common parametric and non-parametric two-group tests. The chapter concludes with a brief description of analysis of variance and the problems of confounding in group comparisons.

Chapter 8 considers regression and correlation in some detail. For the reader who wishes to gain a broad overview the sections detailing computations can be skipped. The interpretation and use of non-linear, multiple and logistic regression are considered without computational formulae.

The remainder of the book concerns itself more with research methodology and study design than pure statistics. Chapter 9 describes cross-sectional, prospective and case-control studies and details some of the risk measures encountered in epidemiological research. The chapter also includes a description of the clinical life table and details its calculation. Chapter 10 devotes itself entirely to the randomized controlled trial in medicine, outlining its advantages and disadvantages.

Chapter 11 considers the use of vital statistics data in medical research, and outlines some of the common techniques in this area. Chapter 12 discusses the use of the computer in medical research. The concluding chapter of the book examines the sources of bias present in many studies and comments on relevant points. Some brief guidelines are presented for critical reading of the medical literature and the setting up of a research project.

Four appendices are included for the benefit of those who wish to perform their own analyses. Appendix A details short-cut computational methods for some of the techniques discussed in the text. Appendix B contains a set of statistical tables and Appendix C outlines, in step-by-step form, the computational procedures for all the statistical tests described in the body of the book. The final appendix gives some simple sample size formulae that may help in determining the number of subjects required for a particular study.

CONTENTS

CHAPTER 1
Descriptive Statistics: Data Presentation

1.1 Introduction

A first step in the description and analysis of statistical data is usually to
present the data in the form of a table, graph or diagram. This is a convenient
way of summarizing the statistics, and also serves to demonstrate to the
reader the principal characteristics of the data. In effect, it presents the reader
with a compact view of what would otherwise be a jumbled mass of statistics.
The exact form in which the data are presented will naturally depend upon
the subject matter as well as upon the methods and aims of the statistical
analysis. Most readers will already be familiar with the use of tables and
diagrams for these purposes. It is not intended here to give a detailed account
of the numerous ways in which data can be presented but by means of
examples some general types and features of tables and diagrams will be
explained.

   It is important to distinguish between descriptive and inferential statistics.
Descriptive statistics embody the techniques used to organize, summarize
and describe data in a scientific manner. This chapter and the following one
introduce the topic. The other area of statistical analysis involves generalizing
from a sample of observations to a larger group and is referred to as
inferential statistics. The remainder of the book is chiefly concerned with this
topic.

1.2 Types of data

Suppose that it is necessary to study certain characteristics in a group of
medical students such as age, sex, city of birth, socio-economic group and
number of brothers/sisters. Each of these characteristics may vary from
person to person and is referred to as a *variable* and the values taken by these
variables (e.g. eighteen years of age; male; born in Dublin etc.) are referred to as
data. Data and the variables that give rise to them can be divided into two
broad categories — qualitative and quantitative.

   Qualitative data are not numerical and the values taken by a qualitative
variable are usually names. For example, the variable 'sex' has the values male
and female, and the variable 'city of birth' values such as London or Dublin.

characteristics → variables → data

Qualitative :- nominal
- categorical
- attribute
ORDINAL   QUANTITATIVE - discrete
- continuous

(BINARY)

Socio-economic group is also, essentially, a qualitative variable although often people may talk of socio-economic group I or II. The numerical unit is not a unit of measurement however, but merely a tag or label. Qualitative variables are also called *nominal, categorical* or *attribute* variables. In the special case where a variable assumes two values only (e.g. alive/dead) it is called a *binary variable.* Some qualitative variables also have an intrinsic order (e.g. socio-economic group I is, in some sense, higher than or above socio-economic group II) and are referred to as *ordinal* variables.

The variables 'age' and 'number of brothers/sisters' are examples of quantitative variables. They assume numerical values which are a result of measurement. In essence, qualitative data refer to qualities and quantitative data to quantities.

A *discrete* (quantitative) variable is one whose values vary by finite specific steps. The variable 'number of brothers/sisters' takes integral values only; numbers such as 2·6 or 4·5 cannot occur. A *continuous* variable, on the other hand, can take any value. Given any two values, however close together, an intermediate value can always be found. Examples of continuous variables are 'birth weight', 'age', 'time', and 'body temperature', while examples of discrete variables are 'number of children per family', 'number of hospital admissions' or 'number of tablets in bottles of different sizes'. In practice, variables which are continuous are measured in discrete units and data may be collected accurate to the nearest kg (for weight) or cm (for height) for example. The distinction between continuous and discrete variables is important however.

1.3   Tables and bar charts

Obviously, it is necessary to have some way of presenting data other than by means of a long list of the values for each variable looked at, in each individual studied. The basic rule for displaying qualitative data is to count the number of observations in each category of the variable and present the numbers and percentages in a table. The object of a table is to organize data in a compact and readily comprehensible form. A fault which is fairly common is to attempt to show too much in a table or diagram. In general, a table should be self-explanatory without the need for over-elaborate explanations including 'keys' or notes. Examples have often been seen in which it is more difficult to interpret a table or diagram than to read the accompanying text, and this defeats the whole purpose of the presentation.

In Table 1.1 the results of a study of smoking in 2724 persons are presented. The smoking variable has three categories, non-, ex- and current smokers, and the number of persons falling into each category was counted. The table also presents the results separately for each sex. The figures which appear in the body of the table are referred to as the *frequencies* and record the total

Table 1.1 Smoking status of the Irish population, based on a study of 2724 persons. O'Connor & Daly (1983) with permission.

	Male No. %	Female No. %	Total No. %
Current smokers	669 (49·5%)	499 (36·4%)	1168 (42·9%)
Ex-smokers	328 (24·2%)	215 (15·7%)	543 (19·9%)
Non-smokers	356 (26·3%)	657 (47·9%)	1013 (37·2%)
	1353 (100·0%)	1371 (100·0%)	2724 (100·0%)

number of observations in each group or class; the sum of the frequencies in each column makes up the *total frequency* or the total number of observations.

It will be seen that the percentage frequencies are also shown. *Percentage* or *relative* frequencies are quite often used in tables and are advantageous for comparative purposes. In the example, the percentage distributions facilitate a comparison of smoking habits between males and females.

Qualitative data can also be presented in a diagrammatic form such as a *bar chart* (Fig. 1.1). The categories of the variable are shown on the horizontal axis (abscissa) and the frequency, or if required the relative frequency, is measured on the vertical axis (ordinate). (Sometimes, the variable is shown on the vertical axis and the frequencies on the horizontal.) Bars are constructed to show the frequency, or relative frequency, for each class of the attribute. Usually the bars are equal in width although this is not always the case, as will be explained later. Fig. 1.1 is a simple bar chart illustrating the data relating to females in Table 1.1. The height of the bar shows the frequency of each group and gives a useful 'picture' of the distribution. When bar charts are being constructed it is important that the scale should start at zero, otherwise the heights of the bars are not proportional to the frequencies, which is the essential thing. They could then be very misleading as a source of information.

Another method for displaying qualitative data is by means of a *pie chart* or *pie diagram*. Essentially, a circle is drawn whose total area represents the total frequency. The circle is then divided into segments (like the slices of a pie) with the area of each proportional to the observed frequency in each category of the variable under examination. While the pie diagram has its uses, in most cases the pictorial representation of a qualitative variable given by the bar chart is preferred. Moreover, the bar chart is easier to construct and with slight adaptations extends to the display of quantitative data as discussed in the following section.

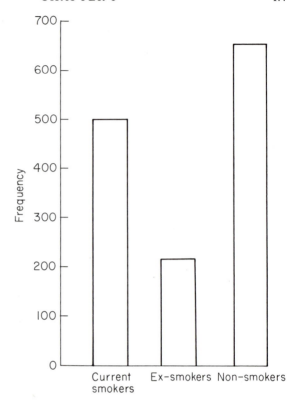

Fig. 1.1. Bar chart of data (females only) in Table 1.1. Distribution of 1371 females by smoking status.

1.4   Frequency distributions, histograms and polygons

It was explained in the previous section that the basic rule for displaying qualitative data was to count the number of observations or units in each category of the variable and to display these frequencies in a table or bar chart. The same rule can also be used for quantitative data but categories may have to be created by grouping the values of the variable.

Tables 1.2 and 1.3 show what are called the *frequency distributions* for two quantitative variables. Family size in Table 1.2 is a discrete variable and birth weight in Table 1.3 is a continuous variable. Since family size is a discrete variable and there are not too many different values, no grouping is required for the tabular presentation in Table 1.2 apart from the last category which includes all families sized seven and over. The birth weight data however, being continuous, had to be grouped for tabular presentation. Fourteen classes were created: the first is from 1·76–2·00 kg, the second is 2·01–2·25 kg and so on as shown in Table 1.3. The limits for these classes (1·76, 2·00, 2·01, 2·25 etc.) are referred to as the *tabulated class limits* and must take account of

Table 1.2   Distribution of family size in 20 coronary heart disease patients who had at least one sibling.

Family size	Frequency (numbers)
2	2
3	2
4	2
5	3
6	4
7 and over	7
Total	20

Table 1.3   Birth weight distribution of 1260 female infants at 40 weeks gestation. Original data from Hayes, Daly, O'Brien & MacDonald (1983) with permission.

Birth weight (kg)	No. of births
1·76–2·00	4
2·01–2·25	3
2·26–2·50	12
2·51–2·75	34
2·76–3·00	115
3·01–3·25	175
3·26–3·50	281
3·51–3·75	261
3·76–4·00	212
4·01–4·25	94
4·26–4·50	47
4·51–4·75	14
4·76–5·00	6
5·01–5·25	2
Total births	1260

the accuracy to which the data were recorded. The birth weight data in this study were recorded to the nearest 0·01 kg. Thus, a value of 1·764 kg would have been recorded as 1·76 kg and a value of 2·008 kg would have been recorded as 2·01 kg. Values like 2·255 kg would have been recorded as 2·26 or 2·25 kg according to the judgement of the person taking the measurements. (The sensitivity of the weighing scales would, in practice, probably not allow for a reading of exactly 2·255 anyway.) The upper tabulated limit of one class, 2·00 kg say, is just 0·01 kg (the recorded accuracy of the data) below the lower tabulated limit, 2·01 kg, of the next class. All recorded values must fit into one of the tabulated classes.

The *true class limits* on the other hand are the limits that correspond to the actual birth weights included in each class. Thus, all weights from 1·755 to 2·005 kg (ignoring weights of exactly these values) are included in the class 1·76 to 2·00 kg; weights between 2·005 and 2·255 kg are included in the class 2·01 to 2·25 kg etc. The tabulated limits depend on the accuracy to which the data are recorded, while the true limits are those that would have been employed if it was possible to measure with exact precision. The true class limits are the more important for later applications, although it must be remembered that these depend on the tabulated limits chosen, which in turn depend on the degree of accuracy in the recorded data (see Table 1.4).

The *class interval* is the difference between the true upper class limit and the true lower class limit. Thus, the class 1·76 kg to 2·00 kg has true upper and lower limits of 2·005 and 1·755 and a class interval of 2·005−1·755 = 0·25 kg. In the birth weight example all the class intervals are equal.

Another important concept is the *class midpoint,* the use of which will be referred to later. This is the value of the variable midway between the lower class limit and upper class limit. It can be calculated by adding together these upper and lower limits, then dividing by 2. The midpoint for the first class in Table 1.3 is, thus, (1·755 + 2·005)/2 = 1·88 kg. The midpoint for the second class is 2·13, for the third 2·38, and so on (see Table 1.4).

Usually, measurements are rounded up or down, to give a particular degree of accuracy, and the true class limits are determined as described

Table 1.4 Tabulated limits, true class limits, class intervals and class midpoints for the birth weight data (kg).

Tabulated limits	True class limits	Class interval	Class midpoint
1·76−2·00	1·755−2·005	0·25	1·88
2·01−2·25	2·005−2·255	0·25	2·13
2·26−2·50	2·255−2·505	0·25	2·38
2·51−2·75	2·505−2·755	0·25	2·63
2·76−3·00	2·755−3·005	0·25	2·88
3·01−3·25	3·005−3·255	0·25	3·13
3·26−3·50	3·255−3·505	0·25	3·38
3·51−3·75	3·505−3·755	0·25	3·63
3·76−4·00	3·755−4·005	0·25	3·88
4·01−4·25	4·005−4·255	0·25	4·13
4·26−4·50	4·255−4·505	0·25	4·38
4·51−4·75	4·505−4·755	0·25	4·63
4·76−5·00	4·755−5·005	0·25	4·88
5·01−5·25	5·005−5·255	0·25	5·13

above, midway between the upper and lower tabulated limits of two adjacent classes. In medical applications however, age is often measured as 'age last birthday'. In this case, tabulated limits of 20–24 years, 25–29 years etc. correspond to true limits of 20–25, 25–30 etc. and class midpoints of 22·5 and 27·5 years respectively. The difference between the method for dealing with age compared to that used for most other variables often causes confusion, but it is still most important to understand how the accuracy to which data are recorded affects calculation of the true class limits and midpoints.

The notion of class intervals cannot be applied in quite the same way to discrete frequency distributions. Thus, in Table 1.2 the values 2, 3 and 4 cannot be interpreted as 1·5–2·5, 2·5–3·5, 3·5–4·5... The variable takes only the integral values 2·0, 3·0 and 4·0, and there are no class intervals as such.

Quantitative data can be represented diagrammatically by means of a *histogram*. A histogram is a 'bar chart' for quantitative data. Fig. 1.2 shows the histogram for the birth weight data. For equal class intervals (0·25 kg in the example) the heights of the bars correspond to the frequency in each class but, in general (see below), it is the area of the bars that is more important. With equal class intervals, the area is of course proportional to the height. The total area of all the bars is proportional to the total frequency.

The main differences between a histogram and a bar chart are that in the latter there are usually spaces between the bars (see Fig. 1.1) and the order in

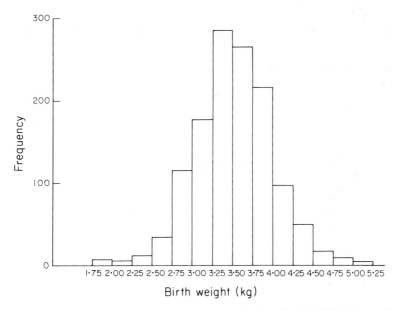

FIG. 1.2. Histogram of data in Table 1.3. Birth weight distribution of 1260 female infants at 40 weeks gestation.

which the bars are drawn is irrelevant, except for the case of an ordered qualitative variable.

The histogram gives a good picture of the shape of the distribution, showing it to rise to a peak between 3·25 and 3·50 kg and to decline thereafter. An alternative method of presenting a frequency distribution is by means of a *frequency polygon* which in Fig. 1.3 has been superimposed on the histogram of Fig. 1.2. The frequency polygon is constructed by joining the midpoints of the top of each bar by straight lines and by joining the top of the first bar to the horizontal axis at the midpoint of the empty class before it, with a similar construction for the last bar. The area under the frequency polygon is then equal to the area of the bars in the histogram. Earlier it was mentioned that the area of the bars of the histogram was proportional to the total frequency. It follows that the area enclosed by the frequency polygon is also proportional to the total frequency. Fig. 1.4 shows the frequency polygon for the birth weight data with the histogram removed.

Quantitative data are sometimes presented in the form of a *composite bar chart*. In Fig. 1.5 two frequency distributions have been superimposed on the same diagram. By means of this, a visual comparison can be made between the total number of patients at each age and the mortality at six months in relation to age, among patients with infective endocarditis.

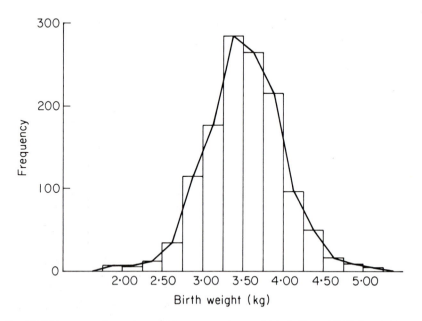

Fig. 1.3. Histogram and superimposed frequency polygon of data in Table 1.3. Birth weight distribution of 1260 female infants at 40 weeks gestation.

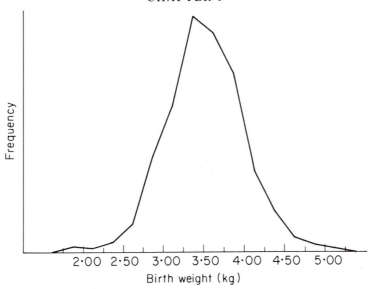

FIG. 1.4. Frequency polygon. Birth weight distribution of 1260 female infants at 40 weeks gestation.

FIG. 1.5. Mortality in relation to age in 60 patients with infective endocarditis. Lowes, Hamer, Williams, Houang, Tabaqchali, Shaw, Hill & Rees (1980) with permission.

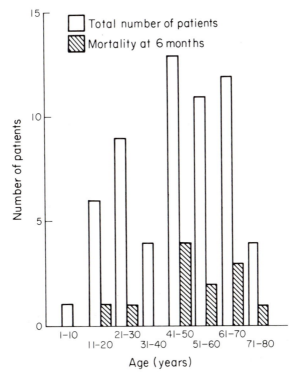

Although such diagrams are common, it is the frequency distribution of a single variable such as birth weight which is mostly considered in the remainder of the book.

1.5   Drawing histograms

This section considers some of the points that must be observed when constructing frequency histograms in practice, and can be omitted at a first reading.

When preparing quantitative data for presentation, the chosen class intervals should not overlap each other and should cover the full range of the data. Depending on the total number of persons or units studied, the data should be divided into somewhere between five and twenty intervals. If too many intervals are employed the resulting histogram may have too many peaks and valleys instead of rising to a maximum and falling off as in Fig. 1.2. This is most often due to small frequencies in each class and when it occurs a larger class interval should be employed. If too few intervals or classes are used, too much information may be lost. Creating appropriate classes is often a trial and error procedure. Sometimes the number of persons or units in a study may be too small for a histogram to be drawn.

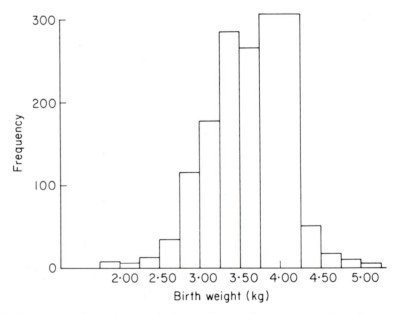

Fig. 1.6. Incorrectly drawn histogram due to non-allowance for unequal class intervals.

The edges of the bars in the histogram should, ideally, be drawn on the true class limits, but for presentation purposes, to give 'nice' units on the horizontal axis, the bars are sometimes shifted over slightly. This should only be done however if the class intervals are much larger than the accuracy to which the data were recorded. In the birth weight example the accuracy, 0·01 kg, is 4·0% of the class interval of 0·25 kg and the bars are drawn at 1·75, 2·00 ... instead of at the true class limits of 1·755, 2·005 ... These differences could not be detected by the naked eye, but in other situations the true class limits may have to be employed.

In this example too, equal class intervals of 0·25 kg were used throughout and such a practice is to be strongly encouraged. If class intervals are unequal, problems can arise in drawing the histogram correctly. Note too, that open-ended intervals such as ⩾ (greater than or equal to) 4·76 kg will also lead to problems and should be avoided if possible.

Suppose, for example, that the two classes 3·76–4·00 and 4·01–4·25 were combined. From Table 1.3, the frequencies in these classes were 212 and 94 persons, so there are 306 persons in the new combined class of 3·76–4·25. If the histogram was drawn with the height of the bar over this class as 306, Fig. 1.6 would be obtained. Something seems very wrong here and it is due to the fact, already noted, that the *area* of each bar should be proportional to the frequency, not its height. Since the class interval for this class at 0·5 kg is twice that for the other classes, the bar should only be drawn to a height of 306

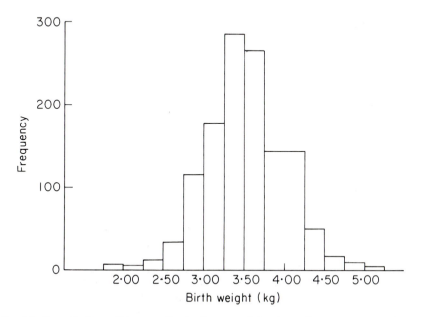

FIG. 1.7. Correctly drawn histogram allowing for unequal class intervals.

divided by 2, which equals 153. If this is done, the areas of each bar will be proportional to the frequencies in their corresponding classes and Fig. 1.7 is obtained. This is similarly shaped to the histogram obtained with equal class intervals, which shows that unequal class intervals do not distort the picture of the data. It is much easier however to draw histograms with equal class intervals.

If one has a histogram — or its corresponding polygon — created from data broken into many different sized class intervals, it can be difficult to interpret the scale on the vertical axis. In fact, it is difficult to interpret the scale for any polygon without first knowing the class interval on which the original histogram was based. As has been said, it is area that is important and for this reason the frequency scale is often omitted from frequency polygons.

1.6   Frequency curves

The main importance of a frequency polygon is that it gives a picture of the shape of a variable's distribution. As is seen in later chapters, the shape of such a distribution can materially affect the type of statistical analysis that can be employed.

As opposed to a frequency polygon (made up of segments of straight lines),

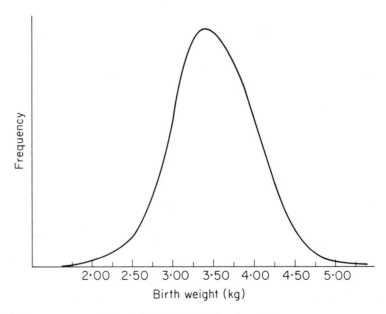

FIG. 1.8. Frequency curve for female birth weight at 40 weeks gestation.

reference is often made to a variable's *frequency curve*. This is the frequency polygon that would be obtained if a very large number of units were studied. Suppose that 20 000 female births had been studied, instead of the 1260 in the example, and that a histogram with class intervals of 0·05 kg instead of 0·25 kg were constructed. The histogram of this distribution would, in all likelihood, be similar in shape to the earlier one and although there would be many more bars, each bar would be much narrower in width, in fact, one-fifth as wide. In the same way as before, a frequency polygon could be drawn. However, because the midpoints of each class are much closer together, the frequency polygon would approximate much more closely to a smooth curve. In appearance it might resemble Fig. 1.8.

By studying larger and larger groups, and by continually reducing the class interval, the frequency polygon will approximate more and more closely to a smooth curve. Thus, when frequency curves are mentioned it is usually the distribution of a variable based on a very large (infinite) number of observations which is being considered. In describing the shapes of distri-

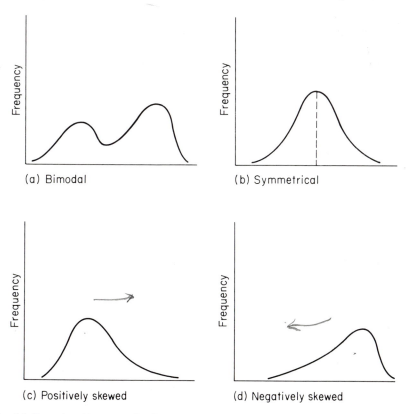

(a) Bimodal

(b) Symmetrical

(c) Positively skewed

(d) Negatively skewed

Fig. 1.9. Examples of frequency distributions.

butions, frequency curves rather than polygons are often referred to.

There are three important concepts in describing the shape of a frequency distribution. The first question to ask is whether the distribution has one 'hump' or two 'humps'. Fig. 1.9a shows a 'two-humped' frequency curve for a variable. The technical term for this is a *bimodal* distribution and although such distributions do occur the *unimodal* ('one-humped') distribution is much more common. In a unimodal distribution the frequency of observations rises to a maximum and then decreases again.

Unimodal distributions can be subdivided into *symmetrical and skewed* distributions. Symmetrical distributions can be divided into two halves by the perpendicular drawn from the peak of the distribution and each half is a mirror image of the other half. (Fig. 1.9b)

Figs. 1.9c and 1.9d are skewed distributions. Such asymmetrical distributions are said to be positively or negatively skewed depending upon the direction of the 'tail' of the curve. Fig. 1.9c is a *positively skewed* distribution with a long tail at the upper end. Fig. 1.9d is *negatively skewed*; there is a long tail at the lower end of the distribution. Since the curves shown on p. 13 are smooth continuous curves, the variable which is plotted along the horizontal scale must also be assumed to be continuous. Curves of frequency distributions may assume any particular shape, of which the four illustrated are special cases.

1.7   Cumulated frequency polygons

A further way of presenting quantitative data is by means of the *cumulated* (or *cumulative*) *frequency polygon* or *ogive*. In Table 1.5 the birth weight data have been rearranged by a process of successive cumulation of the frequencies in Table 1.3. Thus, 4 infants weigh less than or equal to 2·0 kg, 7 (4 + 3) weigh less than or equal to 2·25 kg, 19 (7 + 12) weigh less than or equal to 2·5 kg, 53 (19 + 34) weigh less than or equal to 2·75 kg, and so on. These are the cumulated frequencies. The cumulated frequencies in Table 1.5 are given for values less than the upper tabulated limit for each class. This is done for convenience of presentation and the values in the first column should be more correctly given as the true upper class limits which are 0·005 kg above the tabulated limits (see discussion in last section). In Fig. 1.10 the cumulated frequencies have been plotted in the form of a cumulated frequency polygon or ogive. When the points have been plotted, successive points are joined by straight lines. In principle, the ogive can be used to estimate the number of female babies weighing less than or equal to a certain number of kilograms, by interpolation. Suppose that it is necessary to estimate the number of babies weighing less than or equal to 4·1 kg. By drawing a vertical line from the relevant point on the horizontal scale, noting where it meets the polygon

Table 1.5 Cumulated frequencies for the birth weight data of Table 1.3. (The weights given should theoretically be increased by 0·005 kg — see text.)

Birth weight less than or equal to (kg)	Cumulated frequency
2·00	4
2·25	7
2·50	19
2·75	53
3·00	168
3·25	343
3·50	624
3·75	885
4·00	1097
4·25	1191
4·50	1238
4·75	1252
5·00	1258
5·25	1260

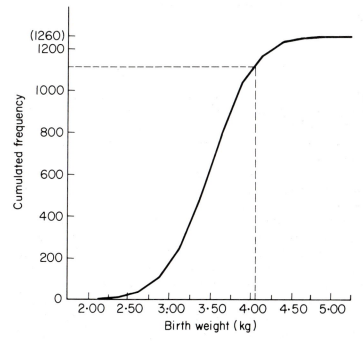

FIG. 1.10. Cumulated frequency polygon (ogive) for birth weight of 1260 female infants at 40 weeks gestation.

and moving horizontally across to the vertical scale, it can be estimated that about 1133 infants weigh less than or equal to 4·1 kg (see Fig. 1.10). Obviously, it would be possible to give a mathematical formula for estimating this number but the graphical method is sufficient for most practical applications. If the original (ungrouped) measurements were available this calculation could, of course, be performed by direct counting.

1.8   Graphs and scattergrams

Graphs and scattergrams are often a very effective means of presenting data and can be a considerable help to the reader. A fault which is fairly common is to attempt to show too much material in a graph. In general, it should be self-explanatory, avoid excessive information and detail, and be self-contained in the sense that it should present the essential points without the reader having to search the text for explanations. The lines of the graph should be capable of being easily followed to observe a change in the value of the ordinate (vertical scale) for a given change in the value of the abscissa (horizontal scale). The choice of scales is of vital importance since the same material can be made to look very different by this choice. When observing graphs, the scales should be examined to determine if a *relative* or *absolute* scale has been used. Relative scales and logarithmic scales are synonymous, and require to be interpreted with caution, otherwise they can create spurious impressions. The arithmetic or natural number corresponding to a logarithm value 1·0 is 10, the natural number 1·0 corresponds to the log value zero and so on. Why use a logarithmic rather than an arithmetic scale? To understand this, the following property of a logarithmic scale may be noted: equal vertical distances on a logarithmic scale measure equal *proportionate distances*, whereas equal vertical distances on an arithmetic or absolute scale measure equal *absolute differences*. The use of a logarithmic scale implies that what is of interest is the relationship between one characteristic and proportionate changes in another. As a further illustration of this point consider the example in Table 1.6.

Table 1.6   Subjects in a screening programme recorded over 4 years.

Year	No. of subjects in screening programme
1980	5 000
1981	10 000
1982	20 000
1983	40 000

The absolute change in the number of subjects in the screening programme increases rapidly from year to year. The proportionate change from year to year is, however, constant at 100%. If two graphs of these data are drawn, one using an arithmetic scale and the other a logarithmic scale, and the two graphs superimposed, a marked difference in the appearance of the graphs will be seen (Fig. 1.11). Note that the log scale in Fig. 1.11 records the natural numbers corresponding to the log values on the scale, rather than the log values themselves. Comparison of the two scales in the figure also shows how the use of a log scale enables a much greater range of values to be recorded on a given size of graph. In general, logarithmic scales are used when there is interest in proportionate changes, or the *rate* of change in a variable, rather than in the absolute amount of change. There is nothing esoteric or complex about logarithmic charts, but they must be carefully interpreted. The important point to bear in mind is that a logarithmic scale measures proportionate or percentage changes in a variable.

Misleading impressions can also be created if the ordinate (vertical scale) does not start at zero. The title of the graph should contain the complete information and the scales should be adequately designated also. Fig. 1.12 represents another important type of diagram called a *scattergram*. Like the graph, it displays a relationship between two variables (a bivariate relationship). Typically however, graphs display how one variable may change over time with a line joining the corresponding points, while a scattergram is designed more to show the association, or lack of association, between two variables. For each subject, or whatever the unit of observation might be, a pair of readings is taken for each variable and a point is then plotted in relation to the two readings.

Fig. 1.12 shows a scattergram relating 'age at first urinary tract infection' and 'age at development of first renal stone' among a sample of women with two or more stone-associated urinary tract infections. For example, one extreme point can be seen in the upper right-hand corner of the diagram. This point corresponds to an age, at first urinary tract infection in a female, of 68 years and an age at first renal stone which is approximately the same. On the

FIG. 1.11. Arithmetic and logarithmic scales.

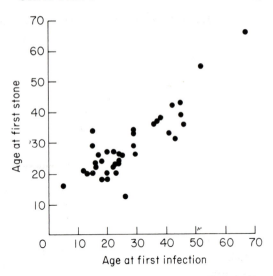

FIG. 1.12. Relation between age at first stone and age at first infection in 38 women with two or more stone-associated urinary tract infections. Abbreviated from Parks, Coe & Strauss (1982) with permission.

other hand, another isolated point will be seen corresponding to an age at first urinary tract infection of about 25 years, in a female whose age at first renal stone was approximately 12 years. The spread of points on the scattergram shows an upward trend to the right. This indicates that there is an association or relationship between the two variables considered and that the older the women are at first infection, the higher the age at first kidney stone.

In Chapter 8 various techniques for measuring associations of this kind are explained.

1.9   Summary

This chapter has concentrated on the presentation of data relating to descriptive statistics. Distinctions have been made between qualitative and quantitative data and some methods for the diagrammatic presentation of these data have been outlined. The importance of the histogram, frequency polygon and cumulated frequency polygon has been stressed.

The major pitfalls associated with graphical presentation are mentioned and the notion of bivariate analysis is introduced with an example of a scattergram which is a first step in demonstrating an association between two characteristics.

CHAPTER 2
Descriptive Statistics: Summarizing Data

[handwritten: Measure of Location]
[handwritten: Dispersion]

2.1   Introduction

In the previous chapter it was seen how a collection of quantitative data may be presented in the form of a frequency distribution, such as a histogram, which gives a useful picture of the 'shape' of the distribution. In this chapter the process of presentation and description is carried one stage further.

A variety of descriptive measures may be used to describe the same collection of data. Most readers are probably familiar with the idea of an 'average', which is used to describe the general level of magnitude of a particular variable. For example, it is common to refer to the average number of days spent in hospital by a given group of patients. There are a number of different ways in which the 'average' may be defined and measured and such measures are called *measures of central value* or *central location*. A measure of central value, as its name suggests, 'locates' the middle or centre of a collection of values; sometimes, however, as will be seen, extreme values may also be of interest. A measure of central value may be used to divide observations into two equal groups, so that it may be said, for example, half of a number of patients spent X days or less in hospital, and the remaining half spend X days or more in hospital. Other measures of location may be used to divide observations into two unequal groups.

[handwritten margin note: avg: Measure central value]

Another type of measure frequently used in conjunction with a measure of central value is a *measure of dispersion*. The purpose of this measure will be explained more fully later in this and in subsequent chapters; suffice it to say here that it is an extremely important measure which is used to describe the dispersion or variability of values in a distribution around their central value.

2.2   Measures of central value

The most common measure of central value is the *arithmetic mean*; generally, this is what is meant by the 'average' of a collection of values. The arithmetic mean of a number of observations is calculated by adding up the values of all the observations and dividing this total by the number of observations. The purpose of the arithmetic mean is to summarize a collection of data by means of a representative value — an average value.

19

Table 2.1 shows the ages of 15 patients. The sum of all the ages is $4+5$ $+5$ ... which equals 139. Since there are 15 observations, the arithmetic mean is obtained by dividing 139 by 15, obtaining 9·3 years. If X represents the value of any variable measured on an individual, the mean is calculated by adding up all the Xs and dividing by the number of persons studied which is denoted n. A special symbol Σ (sigma — the capital Greek 's') is used as a shorthand for 'add up all the' so that the arithmetic mean ($\bar{X}$; pronounced 'X-bar') of a variable is expressed as:

$$\bar{X} = \frac{\Sigma X}{n} \tag{2.1}$$

In the example above, $\Sigma X = 139$, $n = 15$ and therefore $\bar{X} = 9·3$ years. Σ is also called the summation sign. When ambiguity can be avoided the term 'mean' is often employed for the arithmetic mean.

It is particularly easy to calculate the arithmetic mean from data such as those in Table 2.1. The actual age of each patient is known and it is a simple matter to add up all the individual ages and divide by 15. It has been pointed out however, that quantitative data are often presented in a frequency distribution, and the exact value the variable takes for each person is not then known, but only the class into which each person falls. Table 2.2 repeats the frequency distribution of birth weight presented in the last chapter. An

Table 2.1 Ages of 15 patients. Abbreviated from Lagos, Lagona, Kattamis & Matsaniotis (1980) with permission.

Patient	Age (years)
1	4
2	5
3	5
4	6
5	6
6	6
7	6
8	7
9	8
10	10
11	12
12	12
13	16
14	18
15	18

Table 2.2 Birth weight distribution of 1260 female infants at 40 weeks gestation.

Birth weight (kg)	Class midpoint (kg)	No. of births
1·76–2·00	1·88	4
2·01–2·25	2·13	3
2·26–2·50	2·38	12
2·51–2·75	2·63	34
2·76–3·00	2·88	115
3·01–3·25	3·13	175
3·26–3·50	3·38	281
3·51–3·75	3·63	261
3·76–4·00	3·88	212
4·01–4·25	4·13	94
4·26–4·50	4·38	47
4·51–4·75	4·63	14
4·76–5·00	4·88	6
5·01–5·25	5·13	2
Total Births		1260

estimate of the arithmetic mean birth weight can still be made by making a few assumptions.

1. Assume that the infants in each class all have a birth weight corresponding to the class midpoint. Thus, the 4 infants in the class 1·76–2·00 kg are assumed to have a birth weight of 1·88 kg, and the 3 infants in the next class are assumed to weigh 2·13 kg, and so on. Thus, the midpoint of each class is taken as being representative of all the values within that class. In doing this, it is not suggested that the 4 infants in the class 1·76–2·00 kg have an exact weight of 1·88 kg; it is suggested only that the *average* weight of these 4 infants will be about 1·88 kg, and since this is midway along the range of possible weights in this class it seems to be a reasonable assumption to make.

Using this approach, the mean birth weight of the 1260 infants is estimated by adding up the 4 weights of 1·88 kg, the 3 weights of 2·13 kg, the 12 weights of 2·38 kg and so on, up to the final 2 weights of 5·13 kg. The sum of these weights is 4429·05 kg. Dividing by the total number studied, $n = 1260$, the mean birth weight of these infants is obtained as 3·52 kg. Of course, since the actual birth weight of each infant is not given this is only an estimate, but unless there is something peculiar about the distribution this estimated mean should be very close to the true mean which would have been obtained if all the actual weights were known.

The interpretation and use of the arithmetic mean requires little comment, since the concept of the 'average' is widely used and understood. The mean provides a useful summary measure for a particular collection of data, as in the example above, and it is also useful for purposes of comparison. If, for instance, it is wished to compare the ages of two groups of patients, the most convenient form of comparison is in terms of the mean age of the two groups. Comparisons of this kind are very important in statistical analysis, and they are discussed at greater length in a subsequent chapter.

Although the arithmetic mean is the most common measure of central value, there are several other measures which are widely used. One of these is the *median*. The median is the value of that observation which, when the observations are arranged in ascending (or descending) order of magnitude, divides them into two equal sized groups. Consider the age data shown in Table 2.1. The 15 observations are already arranged in ascending order of magnitude, so the middle observation or median is the 8th one, which has the value of 7 years. This can be obtained either by counting up from the bottom until the 8th highest observation is reached, or counting down from the top until the 8th lowest observation is reached. Had the data not been in ascending order of magnitude it would have been necessary to order them.

The median can also be calculated for data where there is an even number of observations by taking the arithmetic mean of the two middle observations. The median would exceed in value not more than half the observations and be exceeded in value by not more than half the observations.*

A more complex method must be employed to calculate the median if only a frequency distribution of the variable is available. Although a mathematical formula can be derived, the easiest approach is to construct the cumulated frequency polygon for the observations. Fig. 2.1 gives this for the birth weight data. (This was already presented in Fig. 1.10.) The vertical scale can be given as a percentage of all the observations (i.e. 1260 corresponds to 100%) or, as previously, in terms of the number of observations. The median is the birth weight below which half or 50% of the values lie. Given the construction of the frequency polygon this is obtained by drawing a horizontal line from the 50% point (or at $1260/2 = 630$ observations)† to the polygon. The value where the vertical line dropped from this point meets the bottom axis gives the median of the distribution. From Fig. 2.1, the median birth weight can be estimated as 3·51 kg. Thus, half the infants have birth weights below 3·51 kg and half have birth weights above this figure. The assumption underlying this approach for estimation of the median is that observations are distributed evenly within each class. In terms of a frequency curve or polygon, a vertical line from the median divides the area under the curve in half. Fifty per cent of the

---

* If there are n observations, the median is the value of the $[(n+1)/2]$th observation. If n is odd, $(n+1)/2$ will be an integer. If n is even, $(n+1)/2$ will involve the fraction $\frac{1}{2}$.

† Note that with this approach the point on the axis corresponding to $n/2$ will define the median rather than $(n+1)/2$ used with ungrouped data.

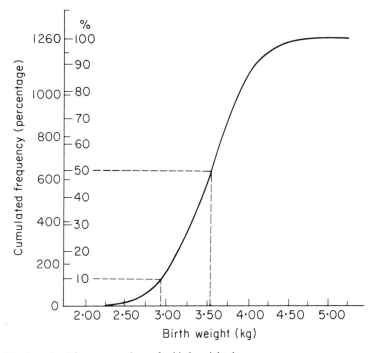

Fɪɢ. 2.1. Cumulated frequency polygon for birth weight data.

area lies below the median, representing 50% of the total frequency (see Fig. 2.2).

To summarize then, the median is calculated by arranging the observations in ascending (or descending) order of magnitude and the middle value of the series is selected as being representative of the average level of magnitude of the variable. Thus, the median is an alternative to the arithmetic mean as a measure of the average value for a given group of observations.

Although the median is quite simple to calculate and commonly used as a measure of central value, the arithmetic mean is generally preferred. The reasons for this are dealt with later, but at this stage it should be noted that, in general, the arithmetic mean and the median will be different in value. In the example of the ages of 15 patients (Table 2.1), the arithmetic mean is 9·3 years and the median is 7·0 years. In the birth weight example, the mean is 3·52 kg while the median is 3·51 kg. Whether the median is less than, greater than, or in rare cases equal to the mean depends upon the general shape and characteristics of the particular distribution concerned, a point which is discussed later in this chapter. However, for many types of distribution the mean and the median will be fairly close in value, and the median is also a useful measure of central value.

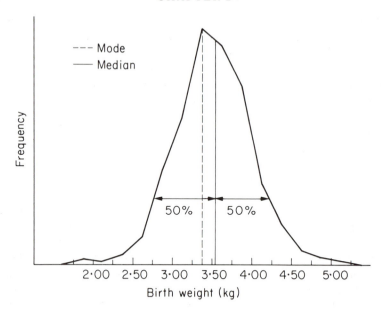

Fig. 2.2. Frequency polygon for birth weight data showing the position of the median and mode.

A third measure of central value is the *mode*. The mode may be defined as the most commonly occurring value, or as the value of the variable which occurs with the greatest frequency. Among the 15 patients in Table 2.1, four were aged 6 years. This can also be considered a representative value for these data since it occurs in 4/15 or 26·7% of the observations and is the most commonly occurring value. Six years is the modal value for this distribution.

The mode can also be calculated for data arranged in a frequency distribution. It may be remembered that in the previous chapter it was explained how a frequency distribution may be illustrated by means of a histogram or a frequency polygon. It was explained also, that as the number of observations is increased and the class intervals are reduced, the frequency polygon approximates more and more closely to a smooth unbroken curve. The point at which this curve reaches a peak represents the maximum frequency, and the value which corresponds to this maximum frequency is the mode.

In a histogram, the group into which most observations fall is the *modal group*, or more generally, the *modal class*. In the birth weight histogram the modal class is seen to be 3·26–3·50 kg which has a total of 281 observations (see Fig. 1.2). The value at which a frequency polygon reaches its maximum gives a single estimate of the mode, though a more precise estimate of exactly where the mode is within the modal class can be derived algebraically. In the birth weight data, the mode occurs at 3·38 kg — the midpoint of the modal class (see Fig. 2.2). In the sense that the mode is the most frequently occurring value, it may be said to be a representative or average value, and may also be used as a measure of central value like the mean or the median. The mode is usually different in value from both the mean and the median.

As a measure of central value the mode is less commonly used than either the arithmetic mean or the median. Moreover, some distributions do not have a modal value, while other distributions may have more than one such value. A 'one-humped' distribution with one mode is called unimodal while a 'two-humped' distribution is generally referred to as bimodal even if one of the 'humps' is higher than the other.

There is one further measure of cental value which is sometimes used. This is the *geometric mean*. As explained, the arithmetic mean is calculated by adding up all the values in the distribution and dividing the resulting total by the number of observations. The geometric mean is calculated by adding up all the logarithm values of the variable, dividing the total by the number of observations and taking the antilogarithm of the answer. This is equivalent to taking the nth root of the product of all the observations where n is the number of observations. Thus, the geometric mean of 2, 3 and 5 is the cube root of 30 or 3·107.

$$\bar{X} = \left[\frac{\sum \log X}{n} \right]$$

antis

This may be thought a rather peculiar method of calculating an average. However, the geometric mean is sometimes a more appropriate measure to use than the arithmetic mean, for instance in averaging ratios or for distributions which are markedly skewed. Since the geometric mean is the average of the logarithm values of a series of observations, it is also appropriate to use it in cases where data are transformed logarithmically. The geometric mean is always less than the arithmetic mean in value.

It is necessary to be careful in statistical calculations not to blindly employ techniques in situations where they may not be appropriate. One example of this is the use of the ordinary arithmetic mean when a *weighted mean* should be used. Table 2.3 shows the average length of stay observed in three wards of a hospital. It would be incorrect to calculate the overall average length of stay

Table 2.3   Average length of stay of patients in different hospital wards.

Ward	No. of patients	Average length of stay (days)
A	30	9·0
B	20	12·0
C	5	20·0

for all three wards by taking the mean of the three lengths of stay $(9\cdot0 + 12\cdot0 + 20\cdot0)/3 = 13\cdot7$ days.

The overall average length of stay should, in some manner, take account of the number of patients in each ward for which an individual length of stay was calculated. To calculate an overall representative value, each component length of stay in the average must be 'weighted' by the number of patients in the ward. The weighted average length of stay is then

$$\frac{(30 \times 9\cdot0) + (20 \times 12\cdot0) + (5 \times 20\cdot0)}{30 + 20 + 5} = 11\cdot1 \text{ days}$$

where one divides by the sum of the weights (patients). In notational form a weighted mean can be expressed by

$$\bar{X} = \frac{\Sigma W X}{\Sigma W} \tag{2.2}$$

where W represents the weights for each observation. Generally, it is incorrect to take an unweighted average of a series of means, and the approach outlined above should be used.

Four different measures of central value have now been described. At this stage it may occur to the reader that the concept of an 'average' or 'central value' is not at all precise, and this is in fact the case. Each of the measures described may be claimed to be an 'average' in some sense, and yet they will generally be different in value when used to describe the same data. Yet this is less confusing than it may seem, because the same ambiguities occur when the word 'average' is used in normal conversation, even though one may be quite clear what is meant when the term is used. If, for instance, it is said that the 'average' number of children per family in Ireland is 4, this does not mean that it is the precise arithmetic mean, which may be $3\cdot7$ or $5\cdot6$. What is probably meant is that 4 is the most commonly occurring family size — that more families have 4 children than have one, two or three, for example. In this case, the mode is being used as the 'average' value. In contrast, if it is said that the average age of the Irish male population is $32\cdot4$ years, probably the arithmetic mean age is being referred to. Or again, if it was decided to say something about the average income of medical practitioners, the median might be preferred, for this will indicate that half the doctors earn the median income or less and half earn the median income or more. In general, no hard and fast rules can be laid down about which measure to use — any one of the measures may be the most suitable in a particular instance. The mean, median and mode may be close together in value, or they may differ considerably in value; this depends upon the shape of the distribution.

In symmetrical distributions, the mean, median and mode all coincide; in asymmetrical or skewed distributions the values of these measures will generally differ. The arithmetic mean is sensitive to extreme values while the median and mode are not. For example, the mean of the following series of observations

4   5   5   5   5   5   75

is 14·9 which seems a poor representative value. The extreme value of 75 increases the mean, which uses all the observations in its calculation. The median, on the other hand, is not affected by the value of 75 and is seen to be 5. The median seems more appropriate as a central measure in this situation, although if it is necessary to take account of extreme values the mean should be used. In most practical situations, the mode is not a useful representative value. In the example above, the mode has the same value as the median (5) but many sets of data may have more than one mode (e.g. 1, 2, 2, 4, 4, 9 has modes of 2 and 4) or no mode (e.g. 1, 2, 4, 5, 9). Data with more than one mode are called *multimodal* or, as has been said, in the case of the two modes only, *bimodal*.

The example above with the extreme value of 75 is, in some sense, a very skewed distribution. If now, the mean, median and mode are examined in terms of their positions in a skewed frequency curve, what is happening can be seen more clearly. Fig. 2.3 shows a positively skewed frequency distribution with some values far away from its 'centre' in the right-hand tail. The position of the mode at the peak of the distribution is easily found. Obviously, there is now a larger area to the right of the mode than to the left, so that the median, which divides the total area into halves, must be greater than the mode. Finally, the arithmetic mean is larger than either of the other measures because it is influenced by the extreme values in the upper tail of the distribution. (In a negatively skewed distribution the order of magnitude will, of course, be reversed to mean, median, mode — in alphabetical order!)

Looking at Fig. 2.3 it can be seen that in highly skewed distributions the median or mode may well be a more appropriate measure of central value

FIG. 2.3. A positively skewed distribution.

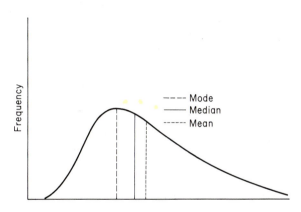

than the arithmetic mean, and it has already been pointed out that the geometric mean is also a good measure for such distributions. The arithmetic mean, however, remains the most commonly used measure of central value, partly because it is very amenable to further mathematical manipulations. Whatever measure is used however, its purpose is the same — to describe or summarize a collection of data by means of an average or representative value.

2.3   Other measures of location — quantiles

All the measures discussed so far are measures of central value; that is, they are designed to 'locate' the centre or middle of a distribution. However, it may also be of interest to locate other points in the distribution. Consider the polygon for the birth weight data shown in Fig. 2.4. The vertical lines divide up its total area in certain proportions and the values (of birth weight) at which the lines are drawn are given special names — *percentiles*. Ten per cent of the area of the polygon lies below 2·91 kg and 2·91 kg is called the 10th percentile of the distribution. (It is seen later how to actually estimate these percentiles.) Since area is proportional to frequency, this can be interpreted to mean that in the example 10% of female infants at 40 weeks gestation weigh

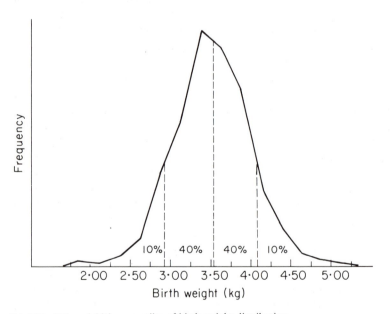

FIG. 2.4. 10th, 50th and 90th percentiles of birth weight distribution.

less than (or equal to) 2·91 kg and 90% have birth weights above this figure.*

It has already been pointed out that the median divides a distribution in two halves so that 50% of infants weigh less than the median — 3·51 kg. For this reason, the median is often called the *50th percentile*. It is drawn in as the middle line in Fig. 2.4. Other percentiles are similarly interpreted. The 90th percentile of the birth weight distribution is, for instance, 4·10 kg. Ninety per cent of infants weigh less than 4·10 kg and 10% weigh more. The 90th percentile is sometimes called the 'upper 10th percentile'. Like the 50th percentile (the median), the 25th and 75th percentiles are sometimes given special names — the *lower quartile* and *upper quartile* respectively.

The percentiles divide the distribution into 100ths but sometimes it is more convenient to refer to a different set of divisions. Thus, quartiles divide the distribution into quarters, quintiles divide the distribution into fifths and deciles divide it into tenths. For example, the 3rd quintile is the same as the 60th percentile and the 9th decile is the 90th percentile. Note that some people refer to percentiles as plain 'centiles' and that the general term for all such divisions is *quantiles*.

Percentile values are calculated in a manner similar to that used for the calculation of the median described in the last section. The cumulated frequency polygon with the vertical scale marked in percentage terms should be used. To estimate the 10th percentile of the birth weight distribution, for instance, find the 10% point of Fig. 2.1, move horizontally across to the polygon, drop a vertical line from this intersection and read off the corresponding birth weight. It is, as already noted, approximately 2·91 kg. This graphical method is quite adequate for percentile calculations.

The measures included in the example and their interpretation should illustrate, without requiring formal definitions, the meaning and purpose of percentiles. They are used to divide a distribution into convenient groups. The median or 50th percentile locates the middle of a distribution. The other percentiles similarly locate other points or values in the distribution. All these measures are called measures of location. The median, like the mean and the mode, is a special (i.e. particularly important) measure of location and is called a measure of central value or central location. Whilst measures of central location are the most important, other measures of location assist in describing a distribution more fully. In certain circumstances, measures like the 5th and 95th percentiles may be of greater interest than the median. By using the median in conjunction with these other measures, a compact description of a distribution can be made.

The ability of percentile measures to summarize a frequency distribution is

---

* The question of whether an individual with the exact value given by a particular percentile should be included in the upper or lower group is, for all practical purposes, immaterial in continuous distributions.

the basis of the *centile chart*. Fig. 2.5 shows such a chart for the birth weight of female infants by gestational age. The chart displays the 5th, 10th, 50th, 90th and 95th percentiles of birth weight at each gestational age from 34 to 43 weeks. The chart is used to make a judgement if a newborn infant is heavier or lighter than would be expected. Suppose, for example, a female is born at 38 weeks weighing 2·9 kg. It can be seen from the chart that this weight is below the median (below 'average') but is well above the 10th percentile (about 2·68 kg) for this gestational age. Thus, the birth weight is not exceptionally unusual. On the other hand, a birth weight below the 5th percentile for a particular gestational age would suggest that an infant was much lighter than expected and would probably result in further investigation. Centile charts for height and weight by chronological age are also used to detect any growth retardation in children.

The centile chart in Fig. 2.5 was constructed by forming, for each gestational age (in completed weeks), the birth weight distribution of a large number of female infants. The percentiles of each separate distribution were then calculated and plotted on the chart.*

FIG. 2.5. Centile chart of birth weight for gestational age. Hayes, Daly, O'Brien & McDonald (1983) with permission.

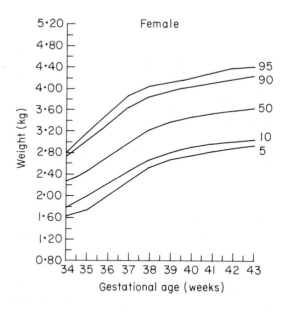

---

* The birth weight distribution at 40 weeks is based on the data discussed in this text (Table 1.3). The percentile values on the chart may, however, differ slightly from those obtained from these data; this is because a statistical 'smoothing' technique was employed to 'even out' the plotted percentile lines.

2.4   Measures of dispersion

When looking at a set of values or a frequency distribution it can be easily seen if the observations are widely dispersed from the measure of central value or are scattered fairly closely around it, but it may often be desirable to describe the dispersion in a single summary figure. One method of doing this is to calculate the *range* of the values, which is the difference between the highest and lowest values in the set. Although this measure may be of interest, it has the major disadvantage that it is based only on extreme values (i.e. highest and lowest) and ignores all the other values. For this reason, some further measure of dispersion is required, which will include all the values in its calculation and which will, in addition, be subject to further mathematical manipulation.

Table 2.4 shows two sets of data, each with the same mean of $\bar{X} = 13\cdot5$. The first set of data is far less spread out than the second, as can be seen by comparing the ranges. Concentrating on the second set of data, an intuitive approach to defining a measure of dispersion or spread might be to first see how far each individual observation is away from the (arithmetic) mean. The deviations of the four observations from the mean are

$$10\cdot0 - 13\cdot5, \quad 11\cdot0 - 13\cdot5, \quad 15\cdot0 - 13\cdot5, \quad 18\cdot0 - 13\cdot5$$
or $\qquad -3\cdot5, \qquad -2\cdot5, \qquad +1\cdot5, \qquad +4\cdot5$

Now try taking an average of these deviations using the arithmetic mean. At this point an important property of the arithmetic mean will be noted. This is that the sum of deviations from the arithmetic mean is always zero. The minus deviations cancel out the plus deviations; a measure of variation cannot be calculated algebraically as the average of the deviations, since their sum is always zero. In calculating the dispersion of values around the arithmetic mean, however, it is immaterial whether the deviations are plus or minus; only the numerical magnitude of the deviation is of interest. Hence, to avoid

Table 2.4   The variance and standard deviation.

Observations	12 13 14 15	10 11 15 18
Mean $(\bar{X})$	13·5	13·5
Range	15 − 12 = 3	18 − 10 = 8
Squared deviations from the mean $(X - \bar{X})^2$	$(12\cdot0 - 13\cdot5)^2 (13\cdot0 - 13\cdot5)^2$ $(14\cdot0 - 13\cdot5)^2 (15\cdot0 - 13\cdot5)^2$	$(10\cdot0 - 13\cdot5)^2 (11\cdot0 - 13\cdot5)^2$ $(15\cdot0 - 13\cdot5)^2 (18\cdot0 - 13\cdot5)^2$
Sum of squared deviations $\Sigma(X - \bar{X})^2$	5·0	41·0
Variance $S^2 = \dfrac{\Sigma(X - \bar{X})^2}{n-1}$	5·0/3 = 1·66	41·0/3 = 13·66
Standard deviation S	$\sqrt{1\cdot66} = 1\cdot29$	$\sqrt{13\cdot66} = 3\cdot69$

getting zero when the deviations are added together, try squaring these deviations. The squared deviations are

$$(-3.5)^2, \quad (-2.5)^2, \quad (1.5)^2, \quad (4.5)^2$$
or $12.25, \quad 6.25, \quad 2.25, \quad 20.25$

An average of these squared deviations would now appear to be a reasonable definition of variability. For reasons that are not considered here, the average value is determined by summing the squared deviations and dividing by one less than the total number of deviations. The resulting measure is called the *variance*. The sum of the squared deviations in the example is 41, so that the variance is $41/3 = 13.66$. To avoid working with 'squared' units, the square root of the variance can be taken and this is called the *standard deviation*. The square root of 13.66 is 3.69 which is the standard deviation of the four observations 10, 11, 15, and 18. The standard deviation can be defined in mathematical notation as

$$S = \sqrt{\frac{\Sigma(X - \bar{X})^2}{n-1}} \tag{2.3}$$

where S represents the standard deviation (S^2 is the variance), X is an individual observation, $\bar{X}$ is the arithmetic mean and n is the number of observations. The mean ($\bar{X}$) is subtracted from each observation or value (X), and the resulting deviation is squared. This is done for each of the values. Finally, the sum of the squares of the individual deviations from the mean is divided by the total number of observations less one ($n-1$), and the square root of the result gives S. Appendix A details an equivalent computational method for determining the standard deviation which is easier to use in practice. The standard deviation is sometimes called the *root mean square deviation*.

Table 2.4 shows the standard deviations and variances for the example just considered and for the four observations 12, 13, 14, 15, which have the same arithmetic mean, but are less spread out. Their standard deviation is 1.29 compared to the value of 3.69 obtained for the observations 10, 11, 15, and 18. The standard deviation then can be interpreted as a measure of the average dispersion of values around their central value. The arithmetic mean and the standard deviation are complementary measures. The arithmetic mean measures the general level of magnitude of the distribution, or its central value; the standard deviation shows how closely the individual values in the distribution are dispersed around the central value. The greater the range of values in a particular distribution, the greater the value of the standard deviation.

Frequent references to the standard deviation and its properties are made in subsequent chapters of this book, and the reader should make a special effort to grasp the meaning of this measure. The variance and standard deviation may also be calculated for a grouped frequency distribution. As for the mean, the calculation is somewhat longer and is presented in Appendix A.

If it is necessary to compare the variability of some measurement in two groups the standard deviation can be used. However, if the two groups have very different means, the direct comparison of their standard deviations could be misleading in cases when more variability in the group with the larger mean might inherently be expected. For instance, the standard deviation of doctors' salaries is likely to be greater than the total income of a grant-dependent medical student! Suppose that the annual mean income of a group of doctors is found to be £35 000 with a standard deviation of £4000, and that the mean income for medical students is £3500 with a standard deviation of £600. To compare the relative amount of variation, the *coefficient of variation* can be employed. This is simply the standard deviation expressed as a percentage of the mean.

$$CV = \frac{S}{\bar{X}} \times 100 \qquad\qquad (2.4)$$

This is independent of the unit of measurement and is expressed as a percentage. The coefficients of variation of doctors' and students' incomes are 11·4 and 17·4% respectively, showing that the income of a medical student is *relatively* more variable than that of a qualified practioner, though it is of course less variable in absolute terms.

Other measures of dispersion are available. The *mean deviation* is calculated similarly to the standard deviation, by ignoring the minus signs in the individual deviations from the mean (rather than squaring them), adding the deviations together and taking the average. The *quartile deviation* (or *semi-interquartile* range) is calculated as half the difference between the upper and lower quartiles, and is the appropriate measure of dispersion to use if the median is used as the measure of central value.

In essence, measures of dispersion are designed to show how closely the values in a distribution are grouped around their central value. If there is a considerable variation or range of values in a distribution, a relatively high value for the measure of dispersion would be expected. At the other extreme, if all the values in a distribution were equal, then the measure of dispersion would be zero.

2.5   Summary

In the foregoing sections of this chapter, and in the previous chapter, methods which may be used to describe and summarize a collection of data have been discussed and illustrated. In the previous chapter it was explained how the data might be organized and presented. In this chapter it has been explained how the important characteristics of a distribution might be summarized by means of measures of location and measures of dispersion.

CHAPTER 3
Probability, Populations and Samples

3.1 Introduction

Having read the first two chapters of this book, it should now be understood how data collected in a particular study might be organized, summarized and presented. Descriptive statistics, however, form only one part of statistical analysis and the remainder of this book, for the most part, deals with what is called inferential statistics. In this chapter some of the groundwork is laid for the material that is to follow.

Essentially, statistical inference embodies a methodology which enables something about a large population to be discovered on the basis of observing a subgroup or sample from that population. This chapter starts with a brief foray into the notion of probability and then considers the properties required of a good sample. Sample survey techniques are considered and the normal distribution, one of the most important in statistics, is introduced. An understanding of the meaning of a variable's frequency distribution is needed for this chapter.

3.2 Definition of probability

Central to all statistical analysis is the mathematical theory of probability or chance. Interest in this area arose during the 17th century in the context of gambling, and since then the subject has been studied in depth and is a field of investigation in its own right. Although some purists might disagree, a fairly sound grasp of statistical concepts is possible with an understanding of only some of the aspects of probability theory. In line with the origins of the theory of probability, examples in this section tend to be from games of chance such as cards or dice.

Intuitively, everyone has an idea of what probability is. The probability of a coin landing heads is 1/2; the probability of getting a 3 on the roll of a die is 1/6; the probability of drawing an ace from a pack of cards is 4/52. The truth of such probability statements will depend on whether the coin or die is unbiased (not a two-headed coin or a loaded die) or whether all the aces are actually in the pack and that it is well shuffled.

What can be deduced about probability from the above examples? Firstly, a probability is measured on a numerical scale ranging from 0 to 1. An event with the probability of 0, for all practical purposes, cannot occur; an event with a probability of 1 is a certainty (e.g. death). Between these two extremes, a probability can take any value from 0 to 1 and can be expressed as a fraction (1/6) or a decimal (0·1667). Probabilities can also be expressed in terms of percentages; e.g., a probability of 16·67%. The second point about a probability of an event is that it can be calculated if it is known how many times the event can occur out of all possible outcomes, if each outcome is equally likely. Thus, there are six equally likely outcomes to the throw of a die; one of these is the appearance of a 3 on the upper face so that the probability of a 3 is 1/6. In a pack of cards, there are 4 aces in 52 cards. Of the 52 possible outcomes, all equally likely, 4 are favourable so that the probability of an ace is 4/52. The caveat that each outcome must be equally likely is important. For instance, to determine the probability of obtaining two heads after tossing a 10p coin and a 50p coin, it would be incorrect to conclude, because there are three possible outcomes (2 heads, 1 head and 0 heads) and only one is favourable, that the answer is 1/3. In fact, there are four *equally likely* outcomes for the 50p and 10p coin respectively; these are H/T, T/H, H/H and T/T, where H/T means a head on the 50p coin and a tail on the 10p coin. Of these four equally likely outcomes, only one is favourable so that the probability of 2 heads is 1/4.

The probabilities discussed above were all defined from outside the particular experiment (drawing of a card, tossing of a coin) and can, thus, be called *a priori* probabilities. Such probabilities have the property that if the experiment was repeated a large number of times, the proportion of times the event would be observed would approach the *a priori* probability. If a coin was tossed 3 times, 3 heads might be obtained, but if it was tossed a million times or more the proportion of heads should be very close to 0·5 or 50%.

This gives rise to the frequency definition of probability, which is an event's relative frequency in a very large number of trials or experiments performed under similar conditions. This suggests that a probability could be estimated on the basis of a large number of experiments. For instance, to determine the probability of a live-born child being a male, one could examine a large series of births and count how many males resulted (ignoring the problem of hermaphrodites!). In Ireland in 1982 there were 70 933 live births of which 36 328 were male. Thus, the best estimate of the probability of a male, on the assumption that the same underlying process in sex determination is appropriate, is 51·2% or 0·512.

There is another type of probability which does not fit into the framework discussed above. A person may say, for instance, that the probability of their getting an honours in the first year medical examination is 0·6 or 60%. There is no way that such a probability may be interpreted as an event's long-term relative frequency as described above, and such a probability is referred to as a subjective probability. Such definitions are not considered in this book, although subjective probability can provide an alternative framework within which to view statistical inference.

3.3 Probability and frequency distributions

Having defined a probability in terms of an event's long-term relative frequency in repeated trials, it is now necessary to examine the relationship of probability to statistical calculations. A simple example will illustrate most of the concepts, and no mathematical rigour is attempted. Consider a bag of 10 coloured marbles, 5 red, 3 green and 2 blue (Fig. 3.1), from which one marble is drawn. The *a priori* probability that this marble will be red is $5/10 = 0.5$, that it will be green is $3/10 = 0.3$ and that it will be blue is $2/10 = 0.2$. If now it was not known either how many marbles were in the bag or what colours they were, the proportions of each colour could be estimated by drawing one marble, noting its colour, replacing it and continuing in the same manner for a large number of trials. If a bar chart was drawn for the number of different

Fig. 3.1. A bag of coloured marbles.

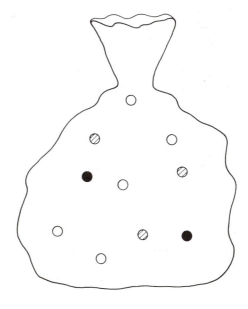

○ Red (5)

⊘ Green (3)

● Blue (2)

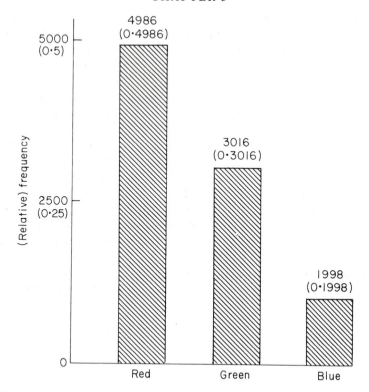

FIG. 3.2. A bar chart showing the colours obtained in 10 000 draws of a single marble (with replacement) from the bag in Fig. 3.1. Relative frequencies are given in parenthesis.

times each colour was obtained, the results might be similar to those shown in Fig. 3.2 which is based on the results of 10 000 such draws: 4986 of the draws were of a red marble, 3016 were of a green marble and 1998 were of a blue marble. If each of these figures is divided by the total number of trials (10 000) relative frequencies for red, green and blue of 0·4986, 0·3016 and 0·1998 respectively are obtained. These relative frequencies are nearly identical to the actual *a priori* probabilities, as would be expected, given the original definition. When the number of observations on the bar chart is replaced by the relative frequency, a relative frequency diagram is obtained as also illustrated in Fig. 3.2. Note that the relative frequencies must sum to 1·0.

The experiment described then, gives rise to a relative frequency diagram showing the distribution of colours in the bag of marbles. From the opposite point of view however, given the relative frequency diagram in Fig. 3.2, the probability of obtaining a specific result in one draw of a marble from that particular bag could be known to a high degree of accuracy.

This example serves to illustrate the close connection between probability and frequency distributions. Instead of working with a bar chart, the frequency distribution of a quantitative variable such as birth weight at gestational age 40 weeks might be given, as in the last chapter. This may easily be transformed into a relative frequency distribution when, instead of the total area under the curve representing the 1260 births studied, it represents the total frequency of all observations, which is given a value of 1. Whereas in the bar chart example the relative frequencies of a particular colour were represented by the height of the bar, in a relative frequency distribution it is the area under the curve above a certain range of values that represents their relative frequency. (Remember — it was pointed out that it was the area of a bar that was important in frequency distributions of quantitative data, rather than its height.)

Fig. 3.3 shows the relative frequency polygon for the birth weight data. Note that the vertical axis is not given a scale since it is relative areas under the curve that are of interest. As an illustration, the relative frequency of birth weights between 2·50 and 3·00 kg* is about 0·12 or 12%. Given this frequency distribution, it can be deduced that the probability of any one child in the study (female, 40 weeks gestation) having a birth weight within these limits is 0·12 or 12%.

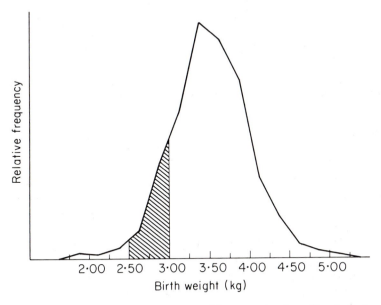

Fɪɢ. 3.3. A relative frequency distribution of birth weight at gestational age 40 weeks for females. The shaded area is 12% of the total area.

---

* Actually 2·505 to 3·005 kg. See discussion in Section 1.5.

Thus, the relative frequency distribution for a variable provides information on the probability of an individual being within any given range of values for that variable. It should be noted that with a continuous distribution such as weight, a probability cannot be ascribed to an exact weight of, say, 2·4 kg; such an exact weight would really signify a value of exactly 2·40 kg — the zeros continuing indefinitely — and the area over such a value is actually zero. However, the probability of an individual having a value, for instance between 2·395 and 2·405 kg, can be established, which is in the example as accurate as the original measures were in the first place.

3.4 Combining probabilities

Going back to the example of the bag of marbles, some simple rules of combining probabilities can be illustrated. Suppose that it is necessary to determine the probability of obtaining, in one draw from the bag, either a red marble *or* a green marble. Of the 10 possible outcomes 8 are favourable, therefore the probability of a red or green marble is 8/10 or 0·8. This result could, however, have also been obtained by adding together the separate probabilities of a red marble (0·5) and a green marble (0·3). This gives rise to the general addition rule of probability; the probability of the occurrence of two *mutually exclusive* events is obtained by adding together the probability of each event. If A and B are two such events,

$$P(A \text{ or } B) = P(A) + P(B) \tag{3.1}$$

where P(event) means the probability of an event. Mutually exclusive means that if one event occurs, the other event cannot occur, and the additive rule only holds under this condition. If a marble is red, it cannot be green at the same time. On the other hand, to determine the probability of an ace or a diamond in a pack of cards, the additive principle would not hold, since the existence of the ace of diamonds makes the two events not mutually exclusive.

Suppose now that a marble is drawn, returned to the bag and then a second marble drawn. What is the probability of obtaining a red marble first, and then a green one? In this situation, the multiplicative rule of probability holds and the probability of the joint occurrence of two *independent events* is given by the multiplication of the separate probabilities.

$$P(A \text{ and } B) = P(A) \times P(B) \tag{3.2}$$

Thus, the probability of a red and a green marble is $0·5 \times 0·3 = 0·15$. The requirement of independence means that the occurrence of the first event does not affect the probability of the second event, and this is required for the multiplicative rule. Since in the example the marbles were replaced, the result of the first draw could have no influence on the result of the subsequent draw.

If the events are not independent, a different rule must be used. This is:

$$P(A \text{ and } B) = P(A) \times P(B \text{ given } A) \tag{3.3}$$

where $P(B \text{ given } A)$ means the probability of the event B given that the event A has already occurred. An example of this more general rule follows. Suppose that the first marble was not replaced. What now is the probability of a red marble and a green marble? The probability of a red marble is 0·5, but if a red marble is drawn from the bag and not replaced, the probability of a green marble is not now 0·3. There are only 9 marbles left after a red marble has been drawn: 4 red, 3 green, and 2 blue, and the probability of a green marble is, thus, 3/9 or 0·3333 if a red marble was drawn already. Thus, in this instance the probability of a red and a green marble is $0·5 \times 0·333 = 0·1666$. Examples of the use of this rule in its application to the calculation of survival rates are seen in Chapter 9. $P(B \text{ given } A)$ is referred to as a *conditional probability* and the independence of two events A and B requires in probability terms that

$$P(B \text{ given } A) = P(B) \tag{3.4}$$

3.5 Populations and samples

When medical researchers collect a set of data, their interest usually goes beyond the actual persons or items studied. For instance, in the study of birth weights in the previous chapters, the purpose was to construct centile charts that would be applicable to future births. Because of this desire to generalize, describing the results of a particular study is only a first step in a statistical analysis. The second step involves what is known as statistical inference. In technical terms, a statistical inference is an attempt to reach a conclusion about a large number of items or events on the basis of observations made on only a portion of them. The opinion poll, which studies a small number of persons to estimate attitudes or opinions in a large population, is a good example of this. In the medical field, a doctor may prescribe a particular drug because prior experience leads him/her to believe that it may be of value to a particular patient. A surgeon too may use a particular operative technique because in previous operations it seemed to give good results. As is seen in Chapter 10, however, such inferences may be erroneous, and the controlled clinical trial provides a method to test such subjective inferences in a scientific manner.

In statistical terminology, it is usual to speak of *populations* and *samples*. The term population is used to describe all the possible observations of a particular variable or all the units on which the observation could have been made. Reference may be made to a population of doctors, a population of ages of Irishmen at death, or a population of readings on a thermometer. What is to be understood as the 'population' varies according to the context in which it is used. Thus, the population of doctors in Dublin and the population of doctors in the whole of Ireland are quite distinct populations. It is, then, important to understand that the term 'population' has a precise meaning in any given context.

A population may be finite or infinite. The population of hospital patients in Ireland at or over any particular period of time is finite. On the other hand, the population of readings on a thermometer is infinite since, in principle, an infinite number of such readings can be taken. Many populations are so large that they may be regarded as infinite — for example, the number (population) of red blood cells in the human body.

In its broadest sense, a sample refers to any specific collection of observations drawn from a parent population. It is possible to have a sample of doctors, a sample of temperature readings, and so on. The two properties required of any sample are that it be of reasonable size and that it be representative of the population from which it was taken. At one extreme, a sample may include all of the units in the parent population in which case it is referred to as a census. In many countries a census of the full population is taken at regular intervals. A census is, by definition, completely representative of the population. At the other extreme, a sample may consist of only one unit selected from the population. Although it is of theoretical interest, such a sample cannot in practice reveal very much about a parent population unless many assumptions are made. In this sense, a reasonably sized sample is somewhere between two units and all the population. Intuitively, however, it would be felt that sample sizes of two or three are also inadequate, and that the larger the sample, the more reliance can be placed on any inference made from it. Exactly what is an adequately sized sample depends on the precise nature of the study being carried out, and on many other factors which are considered at a later stage.

Why study samples at all? Why not always examine the full population, as in a census? There are two basic reasons which may be put forward. Firstly, it is usually too expensive and time-consuming to study an entire population and in fact it may not even be possible to define the population precisely. What for instance is the population of patients with coronary heart disease? The second reason, just as important, is that a sufficiently sized representative sample can give information concerning a population to whatever degree of accuracy is required. Thus, a census is, in many instances, a waste of resources and effort, although it is only with a census that the number of persons in a population can be determined.

A large sample does not by itself, however, make for a representative sample. One of the best examples of this is taken from the early days of the opinion poll. In 1936, an American magazine, *The Literary Digest*, sampled telephone subscribers and its own readers to forecast the result of the forthcoming American presidential election. They received 2·4 million replies and predicted as a consequence that one of the candidates, Landon, would have a landslide victory over Roosevelt. Few people have ever heard of Landon, so what went wrong? A little thought might suggest that telephone subscribers and readers of a particular magazine could be of a different social class than the entire voting population, and that voting preferences may indeed depend on this factor. Such was the case, since few of the sampled groups were to have been found on the breadline or in the soup queues of those depression years. The voting preferences of the sample were not representative of the entire population, and so an erroneous inference was drawn. The large sample size could not alter the inherent *bias* of the sample. (A bias can be broadly defined as a factor which will tend to lead to an erroneous conclusion.)

How then, is it possible to ensure that a representative sample is selected? An intuitive approach might be to uniquely identify all the units in a (finite) population and 'put all the names in a hat', mix well, and draw out enough names to give a sample of whatever size is required. This is the principle used in the selection of wining tickets in a raffle or lottery, and it has many desirable properties. Every unit of the population has the same chance of being included in the sample, and biases such as in the opinion poll discussed above do not arise. Samples chosen in such a way are called *simple random samples* and form the theoretical basis for most statistical inference. Such samples are representative of the population insofar as no particular block of the population is more likely to be represented than any other. The definition of a simple random sample given above will suffice here, noting that the more general term 'random sampling' refers to the situation when each member of the population has a known (non-zero, but not necessarily the same) probability of selection. Random is thus a term that describes how the sample is chosen, rather than the sample itself.

When certain data are to be studied, it must always be remembered that they are (usually) a sample from a far larger population of observations and that the purpose of the study is to make inferences about the population on the basis of the sample. Any time a frequency polygon for a variable is constructed, it is being used to estimate the underlying distribution of that variable. Although, in practice, it is never known precisely what this distribution looks like, one could imagine taking a measurement on everyone in the population and forming a population frequency curve. With such a large number of observations, and using very small class intervals, a curve rather than a polygon would be obtained. For the population of all female births at 40 weeks gestation, for example, a curve similar to that in Fig. 3.4 for birth weight might be obtained.

Now, considering only quantitative variables, the frequency distribution in

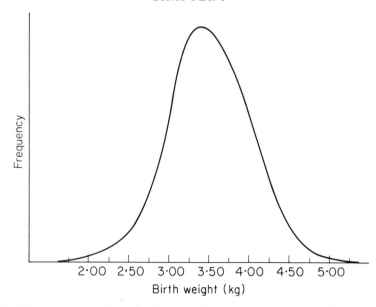

FIG. 3.4. The underlying frequency distribution of birth weight for females at 40 weeks gestation.

the population will have a mean and standard deviation. These are given special symbols: μ (mu — the Greek letter 'm') refers to the population mean and σ (sigma — the lower case Greek letter 's') refers to a population standard deviation. Any such measures, when applied to a population, are called 'population parameters'. When, on the other hand, the mean and standard deviation refer to samples, they are often symbolized $\bar{X}$ and S respectively, and such measures in a sample are called 'sample statistics'. (A good way of remembering this is that populations have parameters with a 'P' and samples have statistics with an 'S'.) With this terminology, it can be said that the purpose of sampling is to estimate population parameters on the basis of sample statistics.

3.6   Sample surveys

To draw a simple random sample from a given population, it is necessary to have some list of all the units in the population. Such lists are referred to as the sampling frame. Obviously, to put 'all the names in a hat' and draw a sample would be, in practice, a very tedious operation and fraught with potential biases, due to lack of mixing for example. An alternative and equivalent method is, however, available. This requires the use of a table of random numbers. One page from such a table is given in Appendix B (Table B.1). Essentially, a table of random numbers can be thought of as being produced by a little man sitting down in front of a hat containing the numbers 0 to 9 on ten separate pieces of paper. He draws a number, notes it down, replaces it in the hat, mixes well and draws another number, repeating the process millions of times. Tables of random numbers are not, of course, produced by little men but are now generated by computers. They have the important property that every digit has a one in ten chance of being present at any particular position in the table. Thus, such tables can be used to simulate the physical drawing of a sample from a hat. Suppose that a sample of size 5 is required, from a population of 80 individuals. First, number the 80 units in the population from 01 to 80. Start at an arbitrary point (use a pin) in a table of random numbers and read down the nearest column. Since two digits are sufficient to identify any member of the population, read the first 2 digits of a column and continue reading down the column until 5 different 2-digit numbers between 01 and 80 are obtained. Repeat numbers should be ignored, as should numbers outside this range. The numbers chosen in this way identify the particular members of a population who are in the sample. For example, start at the top of the sixth column in Table B.1. The first eight 2-digit numbers are 72, 12, 90, 86, 15, 28, 28, 36; ignoring 90, 86 and the second 28 for the reasons stated, the remaining numbers identify the members of the sample.

A refinement of the simple random sample is the *stratified random sample*. The population is divided into groups, or strata, on the basis of certain characteristics, for example age and sex. A simple random sample is then selected from each stratum and the results for each stratum are combined to give the results for the total sample. The object of this type of sample design is to ensure that each stratum in the population is represented in the sample in certain fixed proportions which are determined in advance. For example, in determining the smoking habits of the national population, age and sex are obviously important factors, and it might be desirable to select a sample whose age and sex composition exactly reflects the age and sex composition of the whole population. With a simple random sample, it is unlikely that the age and sex composition of the sample would achieve this. However, by dividing the population into age/sex groups and selecting a random sample within each group it can be ensured that the proportions in each age/sex group in the sample will be identical with these proportions in the total population. Although the sample proportions may reflect exactly the proportions in the population, not all stratified random samples are selected in this way. Certain strata may be deliberately 'over-represented' in the sample, while others are 'under-represented'. The important point is that the sample proportions are predetermined. For this reason, stratified random samples are often preferred to simple random samples.

A sampling method similar to the stratified random sample, and commonly used in opinion polls and market research, is the *quota sample*. This, however, is not a random sample in the true sense of the word and the method should be avoided. In quota sampling, the main objective is to fill certain quotas of individuals in well-defined groups, such as males aged 25 to 34 years. The quotas are arranged so that the final sample mirrors the population exactly in relation to, say, age and sex groups, and to that extent a quota sample is similar to the stratified sample. However, one is free to choose anyone who will fit the requirements of the quotas, and obviously only co-operative individuals and easily contactable persons would be included. There is no guarantee that the persons chosen within a particular group are representative of the population in that group as regards the factors being studied, and large unquantifiable biases may occur. In a stratified random sample however, every person in a particular stratum has the same probability of inclusion in the sample, and this ensures, in a probability sense, representativeness in terms of other variables.

The *multistage random sample* is another sampling technique, which has the advantage that a full list of the population to be surveyed is not required. Suppose that primary school children in a certain area are to be sampled. Rather than obtaining (with great difficulty) a full list of all such children and taking a simple random sample of these, a list of the different schools in the area could be obtained, and a simple random sample taken of the schools. From a list of the children in these schools only (much smaller than the full list of children in the population) a simple random sample could then be taken. The sampling would, thus, be accomplished in two stages with a large reduction in the practical work involved. There are potential difficulties in multistage samples however, and a statistician should be consulted before undertaking such a task. A variant on the multistage sample is the *cluster sample*, where a simple random sample of groups (e.g. schools) is taken, and everyone in the chosen group is studied. This method too should be used only with professional advice.

An approximation to the simple random sample which, though requiring a list of the population is much easier in practice, is the *systematic sample*. In such a sample every *n*th person is chosen, where *n* depends on the required sample size and the size of the population. One starts at random in the list, somewhere among the first *n* members; thus, if every 10th member of a population is to be chosen, one would start by choosing a random number from 1 to 10 — say 7 — and include the 7th, 17th, 27th etc. persons on the list. Such a method could be used advantageously for sampling hospital charts, for instance, when a simple random sample might prove very difficult indeed.

Sample surveys of defined populations have an important part to play in medical research, and should be characterized by the care taken in choosing the sample correctly. Random samples refer to very specific techniques and should not be confused with haphazard sampling, when anyone and everyone can be included in the sample on the researcher's whim. The importance of a random sample is threefold: it avoids bias, most standard statistical inferential methods assume such sampling and, as is seen in the next chapter, precise statements concerning the likely degree of accuracy of a sample result can be made.

Apart from bad sampling, there are two main sources of bias in any sample survey. The first is that of non-response. To conduct any survey of people, one must eventually contact the individuals actually sampled. If some are unco-operative or impossible to trace, these exclusions from the sample may affect its representativeness. Non-response rates higher than 10 to 15% may throw doubts on any conclusion drawn from a particular study. The second source of the bias in a sample survey relates to the inference actually made. It is very important not to draw conclusions about a different population from that actually sampled. It is always necessary to check the adequacy of the sampling frame (the population list) in terms of its coverage of the population, and care should be taken in not over-generalizing the results. For instance, a medical researcher may sample rheumatoid arthritis patients who attended a particular teaching hospital, but would be in error to generalize any of the results to a target population of all rheumatoid arthritis patients. Rheumatoid arthritis does not necessarily lead to hospitalization, and in a teaching hospital in particular, a more severe type of arthritis may be seen. At best, the results of such a study should be generalized to rheumatoid arthritis patients in hospital.

A major problem of medical research however, is that in many situations random sampling is impossible because the population of interest is not strictly definable. Many studies are performed on what are known as samples of convenience, or *presenting samples*. Typically, a doctor may decide to study 100 consecutive hospital admissions with a particular condition. There is no sense in which such individuals could be considered a random sample from a particular population, but it can be reasonably hoped that information on such patients migh provide insight into other similar patients who may be diagnosed some time in the future. The best approach is to ask from what population the patients actually in the study could be considered a random sample, and to make a statistical inference about that hypothetical, and possibly non-existent, population. There are large departures from the theoretical assumptions underlying statistical analysis with this approach, but it still seems the only solution to the problem of definite non-random samples often met with in the medical situation.

3.7 The normal distribution

In this section, one of the most important theoretical distributions in statistics — the *normal*, or as it is often called, the *Gaussian distribution* — is introduced. The importance of this distribution is seen in the next chapter, where its use in statistical estimation is examined but, for the moment, it is considered in its own right. The term 'normal' applied to this particular distribution should not be taken to mean that the distribution is common or typical. In fact, many variables in medical research are non-normal (not abnormal!) but there is nothing wrong with them. It should also be mentioned that a normal distribution for a variable is not a prerequisite for many forms of statistical analysis, although it can be a great help.

The normality of a distribution always refers to the distribution of a variable in a population, so that the mean and standard deviation of such distributions are denoted by μ and σ respectively. The normal distribution has certain definite features: it is unimodal, symmetrical, and bell-shaped, but this is not to say that all unimodal, symmetrical, bell-shaped distributions are normal. Since normal distributions are unimodal and symmetrical, the mean, median and mode are equal in value. A normal distribution is characterized completely by its mean and standard deviation; that is to say, two normal distributions with the same means and standard deviations are identical. Normal distributions can, of course, have different means and different standard deviations. Fig. 3.5 illustrates (a) normal curves with the same standard deviations but different means and (b) normal curves with the same means but different standard deviations. What distinguishes normal distributions from other unimodal, symmetrical, bell-shaped distributions are their area properties, or more precisely, specific relationships between their percentile values and their means and standard deviations.

What are some of these properties? Fig. 3.6 shows a typical normal distribution with a mean μ and standard deviation σ. Obviously, 50% of the

Fig. 3.5. Normal distributions: (a) same standard deviations, different means (b) same means, different standard deviations.

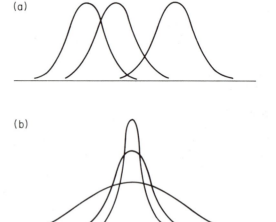

(a)

(b)

FIG. 3.6. Area properties of
the normal distribution.

area lies above the mean and 50% lies below the mean. Now, in a normal distribution it is also true that 68·27% (just over two-thirds) of the area lies between the values obtained by subtracting and adding the value of the standard deviation to the value of the mean i.e. between $\mu - \sigma$ and $\mu + \sigma$ or within $\mu \pm \sigma$. Also, 95% of the area of a normal curve lies within $\mu \pm 1\cdot96\,\sigma$. (The figures 68·27% and 1·96 in these relationships arise from the normality of the distribution and are specific to such distributions.) The area within which all (100%) of the area is contained cannot be stated since the two tails of the distribution continuously approach, but never reach, the horizontal axis.

Suppose, for example, systolic blood pressure is known to follow a normal distribution with a mean of 125 mm Hg and standard deviation of 12 mm Hg in males aged 35–39 years. Remembering that any area under a distribution curve can be interpreted as a proportion or percentage of the possible observations, it can be said that 68·27% of the blood pressures of the persons in this population will lie between $125 - 12$ and $125 + 12$ mm Hg, that is to say, between 113 and 137 mm Hg. Similarly, it could be said that 95% of the blood pressures will lie within $125 \pm 1\cdot96(12)$ or between 101·48 and 148·52 mm Hg (Fig. 3.7). These results can, of course, be taken to mean that if one

FIG. 3.7. Population
distribution of systolic
blood pressure in males
aged 35–39; a normal
distribution with mean 125
mm Hg and standard
deviation 12 mm Hg.
(Hypothetical example.)

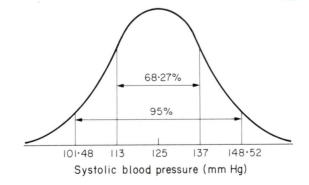

person in this population is randomly chosen, there is a 68·27% chance that the blood pressure of this person will lie between 113 and 137 mm Hg. These area properties are, of course, true for any normal distribution of a given mean and standard deviation, and essentially, are statements concerning percentiles of such distributions. For instance, $\mu + 1·96\sigma$ gives the $97\frac{1}{2}$th percentile of a normal distribution because 95% of the area is between $\mu \pm 1·96\sigma$, leaving 2·5% in each of the two tails. $\mu - 1·96\sigma$ gives the $2\frac{1}{2}$th percentile. In fact, any percentile of a normal distribution can be calculated by adding or subtracting a particular multiple of the standard deviation to or from the mean. Tables of these multiples are widely available, and a very abbreviated table is to be found in Appendix B (Table B.2). These properties, of course, are valid only for normal distributions.

Since the multiplying factors are independent of the mean and standard deviation of the distribution, the table conveniently gives the factors for a particular normal distribution of mean zero and standard deviation unity. This is called the *standard normal distribution*. For such a distribution, 68·27% of the observations lie between $\pm 1·0$; 95% are within $\pm 1·96$, and 99% are within $\pm 2·58$ (e.g. with $\mu = 0$, and $\sigma = 1$, $\mu \pm 1·96 \, \sigma$ becomes $\pm 1·96$). Table B.2 gives these factors (denoted Z_c) for specified areas in both tails and also in the upper tail of the standard normal distribution. The table is given in terms of areas in the tails for later application, and much more extensive tables are to be found in most statistical textbooks. (It is worthwhile becoming familiar with one particular table of the normal distribution, since the layout and notation tend to change from book to book.)

To find the Z value, which cuts off a particular area in both tails of a standard normal distribution, look at the areas in the top row. (Ignore for the moment the alternative description — two-sided significance level etc.) The area is given as a proportion rather than as a percentage, thus 0·05 means 5%. The Z value corresponding to each area is given in the last row. For example, in the standard normal curve, the values given by $\pm 2·326$ cut off a total area of 2% in the two tails. For a normal distribution of mean μ and standard deviation σ, the figures which encompass 98% of the area are $\mu \pm 2·326 \, \sigma$. Note that since the normal distribution is symmetrical, only the $+Z$ value is given in the table. The table also gives the Z values which cut off particular areas in the upper tail of the normal distribution; thus, for example, 0·5% or 0·005 of the area is above 2·576 in the standard normal curve, or in a normal distribution of mean μ and standard deviation σ, 0·5% of the values will lie above $\mu + 2·576 \, \sigma$.

The standard normal curve is obtained by a transformation of the observations in a general normal distribution. This is akin to changing the measurement unit, as for example, from inches to centimetres in measuring height, or from degrees Fahrenheit to degrees Centigrade in measuring temperature. If X has a normal distribution with mean μ and standard deviation σ, then $X - \mu$ has a normal distribution with mean zero and standard deviation σ, while $(X - \mu)/\sigma$ has the standard normal distribution of mean 0 and standard deviation 1. Often,

$$Z = \frac{X - \mu}{\sigma} \qquad (3.5)$$

is written as the equation for transforming a variable with a normal distribution to a variable with the standard normal distribution. $X - \mu$ measures how far the observation is from the mean and division by σ converts this to multiples of the standard deviation. Rather than being measured in the original units, each value is thus assigned a number which measures how many standard deviations it is away from the mean. Z is often referred to as a *standard normal deviate*.

3.8   Summary

In this chapter some background material, necessary for a complete grasp of the chapters to follow, has been introduced. A basic understanding of probability and its relationship to frequency distributions is central to most statistical inference. The distinction between populations and samples and the notion of making an inference about a population on the basis of a sample from that population is, of course, the core idea in statistical analysis, while from the practical point of view, the different techniques which can be used in actually taking a random sample from a population are important. The normal distribution was introduced here as a theoretical population distribution which will play a central role in many of the analytical techniques which are discussed in the remainder of the book.

CHAPTER 4
Statistical Inference: Estimation and Confidence Intervals in the One-Sample Situation

4.1 Introduction

The first two chapters of this book discussed various methods available to organize, present and summarize data obtained in a particular study, and as has been said, such descriptive statistics form the basis of any statistical analysis. The third chapter considered the notion of probability or chance, and discussed the various methods of choosing samples from a population, leading to the idea of statistical inference. The normal distribution was also discussed. This chapter considers statistical inference in the context of estimating population parameters on the basis of sample statistics. The estimate of a single population mean is discussed in detail, and the extension of the method to estimate population proportions is also indicated.

Prerequisites for this chapter are an understanding of frequency distributions and, in particular, the normal distribution.

4.2 Sampling variation

Some of the concepts are illustrated in this chapter using a simple example. The length of survival of 100 lung cancer patients on a particular new therapy is determined. Overall, these patients are observed to have a mean survival of 27·5 months with a standard deviation of 25·0 months. From these sample statistics, the researcher wants to estimate the true (population) mean survival of such patients. Assume for the moment that the standard deviation in the population, σ, is actually 25·0 months even though, in reality, this is only the sample estimate. Assume also (see discussion in the last chapter) that it is meaningful to talk about a population of all such lung cancer patients from which this particular random sample was taken.

The sample mean, $\bar{X} = 27·5$ months, could of course be used as an estimate of the population mean μ. This is called a point estimate and is the best single estimate available. It cannot be said that the population mean is exactly equal to this particular sample mean. Intuitively, however, it seems reasonable to assert that the true unknown mean is *fairly likely* to be *somewhere around* the sample mean, or that the true mean survival is

52

somewhere around 27·5 months. The theoretical considerations in the remainder of this chapter are purely to make it possible to quantify (put figures on) the vague terms 'fairly likely' and 'somewhere around'.

The problem is, however, that the sample obtained is one of many (an infinite number) possible samples; a different sample would, most probably, give a different sample mean. Thus, the sample mean itself, on which the estimate of the population mean is based, is one of many possible sample means. *Sampling variation* refers to the fact that the sample mean can vary with the particular sample chosen. Can then the single sample mean actually obtained reveal anything about the population mean, since another sample would have given a different result?

At this stage, it is necessary to do a 'thought' experiment, which is basically the consideration of a 'what if' situation. It is important to realize that this experiment is never carried out in reality — one sample only is taken to estimate a population parameter. What would happen though if very many different samples, all of the same size, were taken from the population? Many different sample means would be obtained. If these means were then considered as a collection of quantitative data, a frequency distribution of these means could be produced and a frequency polygon formed from the histogram in the usual manner. If a large enough number of samples (an infinite number) was taken, the frequency polygon would become a smooth frequency curve, and it would be possible to talk about the underlying frequency distribution of these means.

This is, perhaps, where most of the confusion in the interpretation of statistical results arises. To recap in the context of the example already mentioned: a particular sample of 100 lung cancer patients have survival times which may be formed into a frequency distribution whose mean, $\bar{X}$, happens to be 27·5 months. There is also the underlying distribution of survival times in the population of all such patients; it is not known what this distribution looks like and it is necessary to estimate its mean μ. The third distribution of interest is also a theoretical one, based on the 'thought' experiment. It is not, however, a distribution of survival times; it is a distribution of mean survivals, calculated from repeated samples sized 100, taken from the population of lung cancer patients. For obvious reasons, this distribution is called the *sampling distribution of the mean*. Again, it must be emphasized that the only distribution which can actually be formed is the distribution of survival times in the sample and that the sampling distribution of the mean, in particular, is a theoretical distribution which exists only in the mind of the statistician, but exists nonetheless. Fig. 4.1 summarizes the properties of these three distributions.

Original (underlying) distribution of a variable X in the population, with a mean μ and standard deviation σ (not necessarily normal).

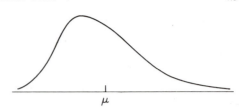

Distribution of the variable in a sample sized n from this population with a mean of $\bar{X}$.

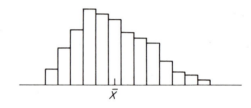

Distribution of all possible means from samples sized n — a normal distribution with mean μ and standard deviation $\sigma/\sqrt{n}$.

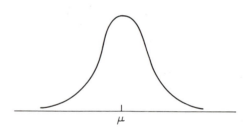

FIG. 4.1. The sampling distribution of the mean.

4.3   Properties of the sampling distribution of the mean

It was seen in Chapter 2 that any frequency distribution could be summarized by describing its shape, and giving its mean and standard deviation. Now, the theoretical sampling distribution of the mean also must have a shape, must itself have a mean and must also have a standard deviation. From studies in theoretical statistics, certain facts can be deduced about these quantities. Proofs are not given here.

Firstly, the sampling distribution of the mean turns out to be a normal distribution. This is always true if the underlying distribution of the variable (survival time in the example) is itself normal; but even more importantly, it is approximately true as long as the distribution of the original variable is not very skewed, and the approximation improves as the sample size (n) increases.

1. CENTRAL LIMIT THEOREM

This is called the *central limit theorem* and explains the important role of the normal distribution in statistics. Note that non-normality of the distribution of the variable under examination does not invalidate this very important result, except with small sample sizes. Unless the distribution of the variable is very skewed, sample sizes of over 30 are likely to be adequate for application of the central limit theorem.

The second result which is of concern relates to the mean of all the sample means in the sampling distribution of the mean. Fairly reasonably it turns out that the mean of all these means is nothing more than the mean (μ) of the population from which the samples were chosen (in the 'thought' experiment). Thus, sample means are distributed normally about the un-known population mean which is being estimated. This justifies the intuitive notion that most of the possible sample means should be fairly near this population value.

Finally, the question arises of how near is fairly near, which, of course, relates to the dispersion of the sample means around the population mean. It can be shown that the standard deviation of the sampling distribution of the mean is given by $\sigma/\sqrt{n}$,* where σ is the standard deviation of the original population, and n is the sample size. The standard deviation of the sampling distribution of the mean is, more usually, called the *standard error of the mean*, or, when there is no ambiguity, the standard error. It is often denoted SE or SE($\bar{X}$). This name arose from the historical context in which the parameter was introduced, and 'error' has nothing at all to do with a mistake.

$$SE(\bar{X}) = \sigma/\sqrt{n} \tag{4.1}$$

This formula for the standard error of the mean may seem strange, but it is possible to justify it if one is willing to take some liberty and not question the explanation too much. If, for instance, samples sized 1 were taken from the population, the mean of each of these would be nothing more than the value of the observation on the individual unit chosen in the sample. The distribution of all possible means from different samples sized 1 would then be identical to the distribution of the variable in the original population. Thus, with a sample size of 1, the standard deviation of the sampling distribution of the mean would be equal to the standard deviation in the population itself — σ. This agrees with Eqn. 4.1 when n is set equal to 1. If now it is imagined that samples are taken whose size is the size of the original population, the mean of each of these samples (all identical) would be necessarily equal to the population mean μ. In this case, there would be no spread of sample means around μ and the standard deviation of the sampling distribution of the mean, for sample sizes equal to the size of the population,

---

* For infinite populations; the finite population case is not considered.

would be zero. For an infinite population, the sample size n would be infinite also and Eqn. 4.1 would give the standard error as zero also. This serves to explain the reasonableness of Eqn. 4.1 as representing the standard deviation of the sampling distribution of the mean. The standard error increases with increasing variability in the original population and decreases with sample size. The fact that the divisor is the square root of n rather than n itself (or any other function of n) is best accepted on faith.

In this section then, it has been seen that the distribution of the means from all possible samples of a given size is normal, with a mean equal to the mean of the population from which the samples were taken, and a standard deviation (called the standard error of the mean) equal to the standard deviation of the population divided by the square root of the sample size. This result and variants on it form the basis of much of statistical inference.

4.4   Confidence intervals for a mean

Having looked at the theoretical properties of the sampling distribution of the mean, it is now possible to return to the practicable example of the 100 lung cancer patients whose mean survival is $\bar{X} = 27.5$ months and whose population standard deviation σ, as mentioned, is known to be 25.0 months. It can now be said that the sample mean actually obtained is one random observation from all the possible means which could have been obtained with different samples of 100 patients. These possible means have a normal distribution, whose mean is equal to the unknown population mean, μ, which is being estimated, and whose standard deviation (the standard error) is equal to $\sigma/\sqrt{n} = 25/\sqrt{100} = 2.5$.

From the properties of the normal distribution discussed in Chapter 3, it can be said that there is a 95% chance that

    27.5 is within $\mu \pm 1.96(2.5)$
or   27.5 is within $\mu \pm 4.9$

Note that 2.5 is the standard error of the mean, which is the standard deviation of the sampling distribution of the mean from which the observation of 27.5 was taken. This statement can now be switched around to say that the following expressions have a 95% chance of being correct:

    μ is within 27.5 ± 4.9
or μ is between 22.6 and 32.4

Alternatively, it could be said that the level of certainty or confidence about the truth of either of these statements is 95%. The range 22.6 to 32.4 is called a *95% confidence interval* for the unknown population mean μ, and the figures 22.6 and 32.4 are called the *confidence limits*.

It was stated earlier that, intuitively, the unknown population mean is fairly likely to be somewhere around the sample mean. In the example above, 'fairly likely' has been quantified as 95% likely and 'somewhere around' as ± 4.9. Note that the confidence interval is not a statement concerning the bounds within which a proportion of the survival times in a population can be found; rather, it is a statement which gives a range within which the unknown population mean survival is likely to be. The bounds for proportions of the population should be estimated using percentile indices.

In terms of a formula, a 95% confidence interval for an unknown population mean is given by

$$\bar{X} \pm 1.96 \; SE(\bar{X}) \tag{4.2}$$

or $\quad \bar{X} \pm 1.96 \; \sigma/\sqrt{n} \tag{4.3}$

What if a higher level of confidence is desired — say 99%? What you gain on the roundabout, you lose on the swings; a 99% level of confidence would mean that the width of the confidence interval would be wider than that for 95% confidence. In Eqns. 4.2 and 4.3 the value 1.96 would be replaced by 2.576 (in a normal distribution 99% of observations are within ± 2.576 standard deviations of the mean) obtaining for a 99% confidence interval

$$\bar{X} \pm 2.576 \; \sigma/\sqrt{n} \tag{4.4}$$

which, in the example, would give confidence limits of 21.06 and 33.94. Usually, only 99% or 95% confidence intervals are used, but with tables of the normal distribution it is obviously possible to calculate confidence limits for any specified level of confidence.

4.5 Standard deviations and standard errors

There is often much confusion between a standard deviation and a standard error in the medical literature. The standard deviation is a measure of the spread of a particular population, and is a descriptive statistic for a sample. If it is necessary to describe or summarize sample results, then the standard deviation should be presented. Often figures such as 44.3 ± 17.0 are seen where it may be stated in the text that this represents a mean plus or minus a standard deviation. If the distribution of the variable is normal, then it can be concluded that just over two-thirds of the observed values lie within these bounds. If the distribution is not normal, as will often be the case, there is no immediate interpretation which can be put on such an expression.

If, on the other hand, it is necessary to give an idea of how accurate a sample mean is as an estimate of a population mean, then the standard error is the more appropriate statistic to present. A mean $\pm$ a standard error

$(\bar{X} \pm SE)$ gives a 68·27% confidence interval for the population mean. (Remember the properties of the normal distribution.) To get a 95% confidence interval, it is then necessary to add and subtract about two standard errors* rather than the one standard error usually presented.

Whether standard deviations or standard errors are presented depends on the purpose of the presentation. Just because they are smaller and therefore look better is not a sufficient reason to present standard errors. It is also worthwhile noting, when reading the medical literature, how many times a mean ± something is presented with no statement as to what that something is. After all, it could be 1 standard deviation, 2 standard deviations, 1 standard error or 2 standard errors, and its interpretation is impossible without knowing which.

PSDev ← S.SDev

4.6 The Student's *t* distribution

So far in this chapter it has been assumed that the population standard deviation σ was known. This, of course, is an unrealistic assumption in most cases, and what happens when σ is replaced by the sample standard deviation, *S*, in the formula for the standard error is now examined. Remember that a 95% confidence interval for an unknown population mean was given by

$$\bar{X} \pm 1 \cdot 96 \, \sigma/\sqrt{n} \tag{4.3}$$

where $\bar{X}$ is the sample mean, σ is the population standard deviation, n is the sample size, and $\pm 1 \cdot 96$ are the values that include 95% of the area under the standard normal curve.

It was realized that the above formulation, based on the normal distribution, would be inaccurate whenever S, the sample standard deviation, was substituted for σ, the population value, and especially so for small sample sizes. It was not until 1908, however, that the solution to this problem was determined. In that year, a chemist-cum-mathematician, William Gosset, who was employed in the Guinness brewery in Dublin, published a paper under the pseudonym 'Student', detailing the corrections which must be made in this situation. (Arthur Guinness Son & Co. did not allow Gosset to publish under his own name — possibly because they did not wish their competitors to realize just how useful statistics could be in sampling the quality of the brew!) Gosset's work essentially was to introduce what is now called the *Student's t distribution*, or the *t* distribution for short, for use in place of the normal distribution in the situation just described. The *t*

---

* Usually, the standard error is not known exactly (see below) and 1·96 is a suitable multiplying factor only with an exact result. A value of 2 usually gives a good enough approximation.

distribution is, in fact, many different distributions, each of which has what is called a *degree of freedom (d.f.)*. Thus, there are *t* distributions with 1 *d.f.*, 2 *d.f.* etc. Like the normal distribution, the *t* distribution is symmetrical, unimodal and bell-shaped, but it is more spread out, and has different area properties. The fact that this distribution is more spread out allows for the increased variability introduced into the calculation of confidence intervals when only the sample value of the standard deviation is known. The precise meaning of degrees of freedom is not of concern here, except to note that they increase with sample size in the applications considered, and that the Student's *t* distribution with a large number of degrees of freedom is pretty well identical to the standard normal distribution (see below).

The *t* distribution with any particular number of degrees of freedom is akin to the standard normal distribution, and Appendix B (Table B.3) gives a table of this distribution for degrees of freedom from 1 to 30 and some higher values. The table is laid out similarly to that for the normal distribution in Table B.2. Take, for example, the Student's *t* distribution with 8 degrees of freedom. The values of *t*, t_c which cut off specified areas in the tail(s) of this distribution are found on the row marked with *d.f.* = 8. It is seen that, for instance, 2·5% of the area is above *t* = 2·306 while 1% of the area lies outside the limits defined by *t* = ±3·355. Fig. 4.2 illustrates these values for the *t* distribution with 8 degrees of freedom. In the normal distribution, the corresponding values would have been 1·960 and ±2·576 respectively, thus illustrating the extra spread of the *t* distribution. Looking at Table B.3 it can also be seen that as the degrees of freedom increase the *t* distribution becomes closer to the normal distribution, and that at about 60 degrees of freedom, for instance, the values tabulated are indeed fairly close to those given for the normal distribution. (The entry for degrees of freedom equal to ∞ refers to an infinite number of degrees of freedom when the *t* distribution and standard normal distribution coincide exactly.)

FIG. 4.2. The Student's *t* distribution with 8 degrees of freedom.

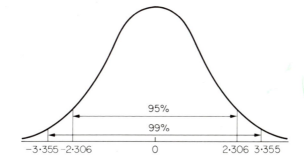

4.7 Confidence intervals using the t distribution

It was explained in the last section that when the population standard deviation is not available the sample standard deviation may be used in calculating confidence intervals provided that the t distribution is employed instead of the normal distribution. An alternative derivation of the confidence interval formulae (Eqns. 4.2 and 4.3) is to note that the standardized variable

$$Z = \frac{\bar{X} - \mu}{\sigma/\sqrt{n}} \qquad (4.5)$$

with the usual notation has a standard normal distribution. (See Eqn. 3.5 where the standard deviation of the sampling distribution of the mean is given by $\sigma/\sqrt{n}$.) Since 95% of the time Z lies between ± 1.96, this can be reformulated to give the 95% confidence interval for μ as

$$\bar{X} \pm 1.96\, \sigma/\sqrt{n} \qquad (4.3)$$

which is the equation obtained before. Now, Student showed that

$$t = \frac{\bar{X} - \mu}{S/\sqrt{n}} \qquad (4.6)$$

had a t distribution with $n-1$ degrees of freedom, where $\bar{X}$ is the sample mean, μ is the population mean, S is the sample standard deviation and n is the sample size. From this a 95% confidence interval for the mean can be calculated as

$$\bar{X} \pm t_c\, S/\sqrt{n} \qquad (4.7)$$

where t_c is the t value on $n-1$ degrees of freedom which cuts off 5% of the area in the two tails of the distribution (e.g. for $d.f. = 8$, $t_c = 2.306$). It can be seen that because the t distribution is more spread out the confidence interval is wider than would be obtained with normal theory when 1.96 would replace the 2.306 above. However, for large sample sizes ($n > 60$ is often suggested) the difference between the t value and that for the normal distribution is so small that the normal distribution can be used with very little loss of accuracy.

Take a simple example. A research group studied the age at which 9 children with a specific congenital heart disease began to walk. They obtained a mean figure of 12.8 months with a (sample) standard deviation of 2.4 months. What are the 95% and 99% confidence intervals for the mean age of starting to walk in all children affected with this disease? There are 8 degrees of freedom in this problem (one less than the sample size). The t value for a 95% confidence interval is, as noted above, 2.306. Thus, the researchers can be 95% sure that the mean age of walking for such children is

$$12.8 \pm 2.306(2.4/\sqrt{9})$$

or $12\cdot8 \pm 1\cdot84$

that is to say between $10\cdot96$ and $14\cdot64$ months. The 99% confidence interval is obtained by reading the t value corresponding to 1% of the area in both tails. For 8 degrees of freedom the t value is $3\cdot355$ so that the 99% confidence interval is

$$12\cdot8 \pm 3\cdot355(2\cdot4/\sqrt{9})$$

or $12\cdot8 \pm 2\cdot68$

This interval is, of course, wider than the 95% confidence interval. The quantity $S/\sqrt{n}$ is usually called the standard error, even although it is only an estimate of this quantity which is only known precisely when the population standard deviation σ is itself known. Section C.2 in Appendix C summarizes the calculations of confidence intervals for means in the one-sample situation.

4.8   Confidence intervals for proportions

In the previous sections the calculation of a confidence interval for an unknown population mean on the basis of sample statistics has been described. This method arose from a consideration of the sampling distribution of the mean, which was the frequency distribution of all possible means in samples of a particular size drawn from the parent or underlying population whose mean was being estimated. The standard error of the mean was defined as the standard deviation of this sampling distribution. In fact, any statistic calculated from a sample has a sampling distribution. The mean of this distribution is usually the population value of the specified statistic, and its standard deviation is called the standard error of the statistic and can be determined from theoretical considerations.

A parameter often of great interest in a population is the proportion of individuals with a given characteristic (e.g. the proportion of deaths due to coronary heart disease; the proportion of smokers among patients with a particular disease). As usual, the aim is to estimate a population proportion, denoted π (pi—the greek letter 'p'), on the basis of the proportion p observed in a sample sized n. As a practical example, suppose that from a sample of 200 death certificates 64 recorded coronary heart disease as the primary cause of death, and that it is necessary to estimate the proportion of all deaths due to this condition. The sample proportion p is, thus, $64/200 = 0\cdot32$. The remainder of the discussion is confined to calculations on the actual proportion of deaths, since only slight modifications are required to analyse the percentage instead, which in this case is 32%.

The exact approach to this problem requires the use of the *binomial distribution*, which is the sampling distribution of the number of units with a particular characteristic in repeated samples of a given size. The binomial distribution is not considered in this text, but instead the *normal approximation to the binomial distribution* is used, which holds so long as $n(\pi)$ and $n(1-\pi)$ are both greater than 5, where n is the sample size and π is the proportion of units in the population with the required characteristic. Under these conditions, the sampling distribution of the proportion of individuals with the characteristic, in repeated samples sized n, is normal, with mean equal to the population parameter π and standard deviation (called the *standard error of the proportion*) equal to $\sqrt{\pi(1-\pi)/n}$. Whereas with means

$$SE(\bar{X}) = \sigma/\sqrt{n} \tag{4.1}$$

for sample proportions

$$SE(p) = \sqrt{\pi(1-\pi)/n} \tag{4.8}$$

where $SE(p)$ is the standard error of a proportion. Using arguments similar to those in the last section, it can be said that

$$Z = \frac{p-\pi}{\sqrt{\pi(1-\pi)/n}} = \frac{p-\pi}{SE(p)} \tag{4.9}$$

has a standard normal distribution, where p is the proportion of individuals with the characteristic in the sample, π is the unknown proportion in the population which is to be estimated and n, as usual, is the sample size.*

In practice, of course, π is being estimated, so that the standard error of the proportion must be approximated by

$$SE(p) \approx \sqrt{\frac{p(1-p)}{n}} \tag{4.10}$$

where the symbol $\approx$ is interpreted as approximately equal to, and p is the proportion observed in the sample. Even though this approximation is used for the standard error of a proportion, tables of the normal distribution are still used for calculating confidence intervals.

A 95% confidence interval for a proportion is then given by (using the properties of the normal distribution)

$$p \pm 1 \cdot 96 \, SE(p) \tag{4.11}$$

$$\text{or} \quad p \pm 1 \cdot 96 \sqrt{\frac{p(1-p)}{n}} \tag{4.12}$$

---

* Some authors suggest that for $n\pi$ and $n(1-\pi)$ fairly close to 5 what is called the *continuity correction* should be employed in this formulation. This is, basically, a correction to allow for the fact that a discrete distribution (the binomial) is being approximated by a continuous distribution (the normal). The continuity correction is not used in this text.

and a 99% confidence interval is given by

$$p \pm 2 \cdot 576 \; SE(p) \qquad\qquad\qquad\qquad (4.13)$$

In the example, the proportion of death certificates giving coronary heart disease as the cause of death was $p = 0 \cdot 32$ with the standard error estimated as

$$\sqrt{\frac{(0 \cdot 32)(0 \cdot 68)}{200}} = 0 \cdot 033$$

The normal approximation holds in this case, since 200(0·32) and 200(0·68) are both very much greater than 5. A 95% confidence interval for the proportion of deaths due to coronary heart disease is then given by

$$0 \cdot 32 \pm 1 \cdot 96 \; (0 \cdot 033)$$

which is from 0·255 to 0·385 or from 25·5% to 38·5%. The 99% confidence interval for the proportion of coronary heart disease deaths is from 0·235 to 0·405 which is obtained from Eqn. 4.13. If, in practice, calculating a confidence interval for a percentage is preferred, it is suggested that confusion will be avoided if the steps outlined above are carried out using proportions, and translated back to percentages at the end of the calculation. Section C.3, Appendix C summarizes the calculation of confidence intervals for proportions in the one-sample situation.

4.9   Summary

This chapter concentrated on the estimation of population parameters using statistics calculated on a single sample from the population. It was explained how theoretical considerations led to the concept of a sampling distribution of a statistic, which was the distribution of that statistic in repeated samples from a particular population. The important distinction between the standard error of the mean and the standard deviation was emphasized and the Student's t distribution was introduced. The estimation of confidence intervals was explained for both means and proportions. The confidence interval is a range which, at a specified level of probability, is expected to contain the population parameter being estimated.

The following chapter presents a non-mathematical introduction to the second area of statistical inference, that of hypothesis testing which, although distinct from, is closely related to the estimation of population parameters by confidence intervals.

CHAPTER 5
Hypothesis Testing: Introduction to Statistical Tests of Significance

5.1 Introduction

In the previous chapter, the problems of estimating a population parameter using the information contained in a sample from that population were discussed. It was seen that confidence intervals provide a technique whereby it is possible to simultaneously express the degree of reliance and the degree of accuracy with which a sample result can be said to represent the true situation in a population. In medical applications however, statistical inference is more usually carried out by hypothesis tests (significance tests) rather than by estimation via confidence intervals. The basic situation is the same — discovering something about populations on the basis of sampling — but the approach, although complementary, is quite different. This chapter introduces some of the concepts underlying hypothesis testing in the context of a specific clinical example, but avoids mathematical manipulations. The succeeding chapters examine hypothesis tests in more detail, and flesh out the skeleton introduced here. The concepts underlying hypothesis tests are central to an understanding of the use of statistics in medicine, and the concept is far more general than the application of any specific test to a given set of data.

Prerequisites for this chapter include a knowledge of descriptive statistics and an acquaintance with the distinctions between samples and populations. A particular example will be taken to illustrate some of the ideas involved.

5.2 The example

A research group is interested in comparing the effects, on five-year survival in breast cancer patients, of two different drug preparations, drug B, which is the standard therapy, and drug A which is potentially useful. They decide to put 25 patients on each of the two treatments and to follow the patients for five years to determine their mortality.

As described, such a study would fit into the category of a clinical trial, and as is seen in Chapter 10, the proper setting up of a clinical trial is more complex than outlined above. Postponing more detailed discussion to that chapter,

Table 5.1 Five-year outcome in a trial comparing drugs A and B.

Treatment	Alive	Dead	Total
Drug A	17(68·0%)	8(32·0%)	25(100·0%)
Drug B	12(48·0%)	13(52·0%)	25(100·0%)

however, assume for the moment that the two groups of patients (25 on drug A and 25 on drug B) are similar as regards all factors which might affect overall mortality, such as age or the severity of their disease. The only factor which differentiates the two groups is assumed to be the particular treatment which they have been given. On this basis, a comparison between the two groups should be valid in determining the drug effects.

Suppose now, that at the end of the study the results shown in Table 5.1 are obtained. The five-year survival rate with drug A is 68% compared to only 48% with the standard therapy, drug B. What can be concluded about the effects of the two drugs?

5.3 Medical importance

The first step in a statistical analysis of a particular study is to examine the results. As already seen in the example, the absolute survival advantage of drug A-treated patients over drug B-treated patients was 20% (68% − 48%). Examining the results of any study requires, usually, only the application of the simple methods of descriptive statistics and is a task which may be carried out with an absolute minimum of specialist statistical knowledge. Amazing as it may seem however, this task is sometimes overlooked by a researcher who mistakenly thinks that a statistical analysis in the form of a hypothesis test (considered in the next section) is all that is required. This point cannot be emphasized too strongly; examination of results, in terms of means, proportions, percentages or whatever, is a prerequisite for any formal statistical analysis.

In examining the results, the researcher must ask a question akin to 'Are my results medically important?' By this is meant — 'Do the results as they stand suggest that an important new finding has emerged that will perhaps change medical practice, or alter one's view of a disease process, or have a major impact of some sort?' Certainly a difference in mortality of 20%, as in the example above, would seem to be an important finding. On the other hand, if the two mortality rates had been 48% and 52% respectively, the medical importance of the finding would be questionable, since the difference between the two treatments is so small. The question of what size of result can be considered important however is one for the clinician and practising doctor and not for the statistician to answer. If the results of a particular study are not deemed to be medically important, little more can be done. No amount of mathematical or statistical manipulation can make a silk purse out of a sow's ear. A study, for instance, that shows only a very small difference between two groups in the variable under examination is of little interest unless it is carried out to show the equivalence of the groups in the first place. Such is not usually the case.

   If the results of a particular study do seem medically important, then further analysis leading to a formal statistical hypothesis test must be performed. The purpose of such a test is to enable a judgement to be made on whether reliance can be placed on the (important) result obtained. The precise form of this hypothesis test will depend on, among other things: the sample size in the study, the number of groups being compared, how the groups were formed, the scale of measurement of the variable under analysis and the precise hypothesis being tested. Rather than examining at this stage the particular hypothesis tests which might be appropriate for the data in the above example, a more conceptual approach to the problem is now considered.

5.4   The null hypothesis

The medical hypothesis which the research group wish to test in the example is that in terms of five-year survival drug A is better than drug B. There is no doubt, of course, that in the patients studied drug A is indeed better, but the basic question is whether or not it is legitimate to extrapolate from the particular situation of these 50 patients to the general situation of all patients. The problem is one of statistical inference and requires a decision to be made concerning drug effectiveness on the basis of a small group of patients.

   The notion of making a decision on the basis of a sample, and thus on incomplete evidence, is not unique to statistics. The holding of an examination to decide if an individual should obtain a degree is but one example. Performance in a particular examination will not necessarily reflect true ability — the person may have an off-day; the questions asked may be in his/her one weak area — or, of course, the opposite could occur with a bit of luck (chance). The decision however is made on the basis of the examination taken. The decision may be fair or it may not and an element of doubt always remains. This element of doubt is the price paid for incomplete information, and is the only reason that statisticians have a part to play in medical, or any other, research.

   The first step in performing a statistical hypothesis test is to reformulate the medical hypothesis. In many situations, it is far easier to disprove a proposition than to prove it. For instance, to prove that (if it were true) all cows were black would require an examination of every cow in the world, while one brown cow disproves the statement immediately. In branches of mathematics, such as geometry, many proofs commence with the supposition that the required result is not true. When a consequent absurdity occurs the supposition is rejected and the result required is thus proved. In statistical analysis, a very similar approach is used. Rather than trying to 'prove' the medical hypothesis (drug A is better than drug B) an attempt is made to 'disprove' the hypothesis that drug A is the same as drug B. This reformulation to what is essentially a negative hypothesis is central to an understanding of most statistical analyses. In fact, the reformulated hypothesis is generally referred to as a *null hypothesis* and in most cases the researcher wants to disprove or reject it. In general, such hypotheses refer to no differences being present in groups being compared. Although in many situations the null hypothesis may not be explicitly stated, it is the cornerstone of every statistical or hypothesis test.

Having reformulated the original medical hypothesis in the form of a null hypothesis, the further premise that it can be 'proved' or 'disproved' in some way must be examined. Unfortunately real life is not like geometry, and when dealing with biological variability and the uncertainty introduced by not being able to study everybody, proof or disproof of a proposition can never be absolute. This is why rejection or acceptance of a null hypothesis is referred to, rather than the proof or disproof of it. In fact, for reasons discussed later, it is preferable to refer to the non-rejection of a null hypothesis rather than to its acceptance.

An interesting analogy may be drawn with the judicial process. An individual is assumed innocent until proved guilty. The assumption of innocence corresponds to the null hypothesis and 'proven guilty' (which corresponds to rejection of this hypothesis) does not refer to absolute truth but to the decision (possibly fallible) of a jury on the basis of the (possibly incomplete) evidence presented. Absolute truth is no more discernible in statistics than in a court of law.

The first step then in hypothesis testing requires that a hypothesis of medical interest must be reformulated into a null hypothesis which, on the basis of the results of a particular study, will or will not be rejected, with a margin of error in whatever conclusion is reached.

A null hypothesis always makes a statement about reality, or in more technical terms, about a population or populations. The results of a study are based on a subset of (or sample from) the population(s) of interest. In medical situations, however, it is sometimes very difficult to identify the precise population(s) referred to in a null hypothesis, as in many situations the study groups are not random samples from fully specifiable populations. In the example, the null hypothesis that drug A has the same effect on five-year survival as drug B refers, in a vague sense, to all patients similar to those included in the study. In some way, however, the results are important only insofar as they can be applied to patients in the future, while the study groups themselves are based on patients already diagnosed and treated in the past. As is discussed in Chapter 10, hypothesis testing in the context of a clinical trial such as this requires a slight alteration in the interpretation of the null hypothesis, but for clarity at this point it will be assumed that the two treated groups (drug A and drug B) are representative of two populations. The 25 persons on drug B are representative of the population of all patients with breast cancer if they had all been given the standard treatment, and the 25 persons on drug A are representative of the population of patients if they had all been treated with that particular drug. The fact that the populations do not exist in reality does not detract from the approach, and the conclusion of the study will relate to the question — 'What would happen if all patients were treated with either one of the preparations?'

The above discussion may seem somewhat convoluted, but it is important to realize that the results of any study are useful only insofar as they can be generalized and that for statistical analysis the existence of certain populations may have to be postulated for valid application of the techniques.

5.5   Testing the hypothesis

Fig. 5.1 illustrates the two states of reality referred to in the hypotheses. Reality, according to the null hypothesis, is that the two drugs are equivalent

Fig. 5.1. Reality and results in hypothesis testing.

(in terms of 5-year survival). Corresponding to any null hypothesis there is always an alternative hypothesis which includes all possible realities not included in the null hypothesis itself. In this example, reality according to the alternative hypothesis is that drugs A and B have different effects.

Of course, it can never be known what actually corresponds to reality, and the whole purpose of hypothesis testing is to enable a decision to be taken as to which of the two alternatives (a null hypothesis or the alternative hypothesis) should be decided upon. Important results, of course, immediately suggest that the alternative hypothesis is more tenable than the null hypothesis (which states there is no difference between the two groups). The main problem however is whether or not enough reliance can be placed on the results to actually reach such a conclusion. The question which should be asked is whether or not the results are spurious (due to chance and sampling variation) or whether they reflect a real difference between the effects of the two drugs. What is meant by spurious is best illustrated by examination of Table 5.2. This shows the number of heads and tails obtained by tossing a 50p coin and a 10p coin 25 times each. The figures are identical to those obtained in the clinical trial example (Table 5.1) with the coins replacing the two treatments and heads and tails replacing the outcomes of 'alive' and 'dead'.

Because the two coins were unbiased, a large number of tosses would in the long run have resulted in 50% tails (approximately). The results in Table 5.2 did, however, actually occur. Knowing how the results were obtained, it can be said with hindsight that the percentages of heads and tails do not indicate differences between the two coins and in that sense it may be said that the observed result is spurious or due to chance. Since the figures obtained in the clinical trial are, however, identical to those of the coin-tossing experiment it can only be concluded that they can throw no light on the efficacy of the drugs in question and that interpretation of the results is difficult. Drug A could be better than drug B, but it could also have an identical effect. In statistical terms, there is no firm evidence to reject the (null) hypothesis that the two drugs are the same.

As well as illustrating the two possible states of reality, Fig. 5.1 also shows the sample results and how they might be achieved. If the null hypothesis were true it would be expected that the results in the two groups would be fairly close, and if it were false the observed results would be expected to reflect the true actions of the drugs. It is, of course, necessary to work

Table 5.2   Results of tossing 2 coins 25 times each.

Coins	Heads	Tails	Total
10p	17(68·0%)	8(32·0%)	25(100·0%)
50p	12(48·0%)	13(52·0%)	25(100·0%)

backwards from the results to reality. If there is a large (important) difference between the groups then either the null hypothesis is false, or it is true, in which case sampling variation is the explanation for the observed spurious result. Hypothesis testing provides a method whereby it is possible to differentiate between these two alternatives.

The approach taken is to calculate (as described in the next chapter) the probability of obtaining the observed result or one even more at variance with the null hypothesis if, in fact, the null hypothesis were true. In the example, the probability of getting a mortality difference between drugs A and B of 20% or greater, in a study of two groups of 25 patients on two similar drugs, is calculated. If the size of this probability is large (often arbitrarily set at 5% or greater), it is accepted that the result could be spurious and due to chance and that, therefore, the null hypothesis cannot be rejected. In the example, it was seen that the results of the trial could have been obtained in practice by tossing two coins, and it might therefore be predicted that there is a fairly large probability of this result being spurious. (The actual probability is, in fact, greater than 10%.)

If, on the other hand, the magnitude of this probability is small, it may be decided that, since the result is unusual, there is evidence to reject the null hypothesis and to accept the alternative hypothesis. Of course, to reject the null hypothesis could be wrong, but the smaller the calculated probability, the less the chance of making a wrong decision. Going back to the analogy with the judicial process, the jury must decide whether the evidence (corresponding to the observed result) is consistent with the accused being innocent (the null hypothesis). If the evidence is such that it is difficult to explain its existence if the person is innocent, then the jury will probably declare a verdict of guilty (rejecting the null hypothesis).

It has already been pointed out that when the probability of a spurious result is large, it is not possible to distinguish between the realities postulated by the null and alternative hypotheses (between spurious and real results). Because of this ambiguity the statement 'do not reject the null hypothesis' is generally used instead of the clearer 'accept the null hypothesis'. This corresponds to the possible judicial verdict in Scottish law of 'not proven' rather than 'not guilty'. Rejection or non-rejection of a null hypothesis depends on the magnitude of the probability of getting the observed result, or one even more discordant, if the null hypothesis were true. If the probability is small, the null hypothesis is rejected and the alternative hypothesis accepted. The value for this probability is often called the p-value for the significance test. The purpose of every statistical hypothesis test is to enable calculation of a p value under a specified null hypothesis and, in a sense, it is far more important to understand the meaning of a p value than to know how to calculate it. This p should not be confused with the p used in the last chapter to denote a sample proportion.

The rule of thumb mentioned above, i.e. that a value of p less than 5% ($p < 0.05$) leads to a rejection of the null hypothesis, is fairly arbitrary but universally used. Cut-off points other than 5% can be taken and whichever is chosen is called the significance level of the test. Sometimes, a significance level of 1% is taken, in which case the p value (chance of a spurious result) must be less than 1% before the null hypothesis can be rejected. The smaller the p value, the more reliance can be placed on the sample results as reflecting reality, but when a p value very close to 5% is calculated it is obviously nonsense to reject a null hypothesis at, say, a p of 4.99% and to fail to reject it at a p value of 5.01%. The 5% level is purely a guideline.

In a statistical analysis, rejection of a null hypothesis is often referred to as a *significant result*. Thus, a significant result is a result which is not likely to have occurred by chance. Although the significance level should be stated explicitly, usage often takes a 'significant result' to imply the rejection of a null hypothesis at a 5% level and a 'highly significant result' to imply a 1% level of significance. A non-significant result means that the null hypothesis is not rejected (usually at a 5% level). Table 5.3 lists the various meanings or descriptions which could be put on a significant result.

For those persons unhappy about postulated populations to which the null hypothesis refers, an alternative interpretation of hypothesis tests can be suggested. As has been said, the reason for any statistical analysis in the first place is the problem of sampling variation or the uncertainty introduced into results due to the small number of subjects studied. If any given study was repeated on millions of subjects and showed the same results as obtained on the smaller, actual number studied, no statistical analysis would be necessary, since (apart from problems due to bad study design or implementation) the results would speak for themselves. In this light, a significant result can be interpreted to mean that if large numbers were, in fact, studied, similar results to those obtained in the smaller study actually carried out would be expected. A non-significant result, on the other hand, would mean that if a study were to be performed on a very large number of subjects, there could be no certainty that the actual sample results would be observed in the larger study.

Table 5.3 Equivalent descriptions of a statistically significant result.

Reject the null hypothesis
Accept the alternative hypothesis
There is strong evidence to doubt the null hypothesis
The chance of the result being spurious is small
$p < 5\%$ or $p < 0.05$
The observed result is not compatible with the null hypothesis
Sampling variation is not sufficient to explain the observed result
Result is unlikely to be due to chance

For instance, if the two coins were tossed millions of times, the percentage of tails in each coin would be very close to 50%, unlike the percentages obtained in the small number of tosses in the example.

At this point, the difference between a statistically significant result and a medically important result must be reiterated. Medical importance relates to the magnitude of the observed effect while significance refers to the statistical question of whether or not the result is spurious. What is ideal in any situation is an important result that is also significant. An important result that is non-significant (as in the example discussed above) may provide some grounds for optimism but no reliance may be placed on the results. Non-important results, statistically significant (as they can be) or not, usually give very little information to the researcher.

5.6   Summary

The general form of a hypothesis or significance test thus runs as follows: a null hypothesis is postulated, and it is usually hoped to be able to reject it; the results of the particular study are examined and, if medically important, are subjected to further mathematical manipulation which depends on the type of study, the measurements made and other relevant factors. This eventually leads to the calculation of a p value, which is the probability of the observed results (or results even more at variance with the null hypothesis) being spurious if the null hypothesis were true in the first place. If the p value is small (usually less than 5%), the null hypothesis is rejected and the result declared statistically significant. If the p value is large, it is concluded that the result is non-significant, and that no decision can be made about whether or not there is a real effect. Therefore, the null hypothesis cannot be rejected.

The following chapter considers hypothesis testing from a more mathematical viewpoint, examining one specific test in some detail. In particular, points not considered above, relating to the interpretation and further examination of non-significant results and different forms of the null hypothesis, are considered.

CHAPTER 6
Hypothesis Testing: General Principles Illustrated by One-Sample Tests

6.1 Introduction

In the previous chapter, some of the concepts underlying *hypothesis testing* or, as it is often called, significance testing were considered. The null hypothesis was introduced in the context of a specific example and the important distinction between medical importance (based on the magnitude of an observed result) and statistical significance (based on a p value) was made. In this chapter it is described how the p value is calculated in a particular situation, and some of the concepts underlying this approach to statistical analysis are considered in more detail. The problems of negative results and appropriate sample sizes are also raised.

The examples considered are based on hypotheses concerning population parameters in studies consisting of one sample only, although most practical applications of hypothesis testing in medical statistics involve two samples. However, at this stage, the theory is best illustrated in the one-sample situation.

Prerequisites for this chapter, apart from the previous chapter, include knowledge of the properties of the normal and t distributions and of the sampling distributions of means and proportions.

6.2 The null and alternative hypotheses

The example which is taken has already been considered in Chapter 4 in the context of statistical estimation using confidence intervals. A sample of 100 lung cancer patients on a new drug are observed to have a mean survival of 27·5 months with a standard deviation of 25·0 months. Suppose now, that from previous studies it is known that the mean survival of such patients (before the new drug was introduced) is 22·2 months. The investigators want to know if, on the basis of these data (the adequacy of which will be discussed in Chapter 10), they can conclude that the new drug prolongs survival.

The investigators' first step is to form a null hypothesis — in this case, stating that the new drug has no effect on survival. This is equivalent to saying that the population mean survival with the new drug is 22·2 months, the same as observed in a large series of patients who did not have this particular treatment. Another way of looking at the null hypothesis is that it states that the 100 patients are a random sample from the population of all lung cancer patients who, because the drug has no effect, have a mean survival of 22·2 months. Notationally, this may be written

$$H_0 : \mu_D = 22\cdot2 \text{ months}$$

where H_0 means 'the null hypothesis is', and μ_D represents the mean survival in the population of patients treated with the new drug.

Having stated the null hypothesis the investigators must then specify what the alternative hypothesis is. Without prior knowledge, they cannot be sure that the new drug does not actually reduce survival, so their alternative hypothesis is that the survival of patients with this drug is different from that of patients not so treated, and

$$H_A : \mu_D \neq 22\cdot2 \text{ months}$$

where H_A refers to the alternative hypothesis and $\neq$ means 'not equal to'. In most situations in medicine, the alternative hypothesis is stated in this simple way unless prior knowledge outside of the study data suggests otherwise (see below). As with the null hypothesis, the alternative hypothesis may be interpreted as implying that the 100 patients were a random sample from a population of treated lung cancer patients whose mean survival was not 22·2 months. Since these 100 patients may have been the only group ever treated on the drug, a slight modification of the theory is required in that they should be considered to be a sample from a hypothetical population of lung cancer patients treated with this drug. The fact that the population only exists in the mind of the investigators does not matter, since the sample was treated and, of course, the inference is being made to a population of potentially treatable patients.

6.3 The significance test

For a significance test, it was said in the last chapter that it is necessary to calculate the probability that a result, such as the one obtained, or one even more unlikely, could have arisen if the null hypothesis were true. If this probability is small, the hypothesis is rejected. The significance level, which defines the size of probability, should be stated before the test and it will be assumed here that it is set at the 5% level. The p value for this example can now be calculated.

From the results of Chapter 4, it is known that 95% of all possible samples, sized $n = 100$, from a population of mean $\mu_D = 22\cdot2$ (as specified by the null hypothesis) and standard deviation $\sigma = 25\cdot0$ will lie between

$$\mu_D \pm 1{\cdot}96\ \sigma/\sqrt{n}$$

where $\sigma/\sqrt{n}$ is the standard error of the mean, and is equal to $25/\sqrt{100}=2{\cdot}5$. (Note that it is assumed that σ is known exactly.) Thus, there is a 95% chance that a particular sample mean will lie between these limits, i.e.

$$22{\cdot}2 \pm 1{\cdot}96(2{\cdot}5)$$

or $22{\cdot}2 \pm 4{\cdot}9$

that is, between 17·3 and 27·1. Alternatively, it could be said that there is only a 5% chance that the mean of such a sample is greater than 27·1 or less than 17·3, or equivalently more than 4·9 months away from the hypothesized mean. (Note that the addition law of probability [see Chapter 3] was used in making this statement.)

Now, the sample mean happens to be 27·5 (5·3 months above the hypothesized mean of 22·2) and thus it may be said that if the null hypothesis were true the chances of getting a sample result more than 5·3 months above or below 22·2 are less than 5%. But by definition this is the p value, so that as a result of the calculation it can now be stated, for this example, that p is less than 5% or $p<0{\cdot}05$. Thus, statistical significance at a 5% level can be declared and the null hypothesis rejected, leading to the conclusion that sampling variation is an unlikely explanation of the observed sample result. In more medically meaningful terms it might be said that the new drug gave a statistically significant increased survival in lung cancer patients compared with that of previously available treatments.

If instead of a 5% level of significance the researchers had decided to declare a significant result only if the p value was less than 1%, they could not have rejected the null hypothesis. Again, using the properties of the normal distribution, it is known that if the null hypothesis were true only 1% of possible sample means would lie outside

$$\mu_D \pm 2{\cdot}576\ \sigma/\sqrt{n}$$

or $22{\cdot}2 \pm 2{\cdot}576(2{\cdot}5)$

and be less than 15·8 or greater than 28·6 months. The observed sample mean of 27·5 months does not lie outside these limits, and therefore by definition p must be greater than 1%. Thus, the null hypothesis cannot be rejected at a 1% level of significance and a non-significant result must be declared at that level. It can be seen from this that a result which is significant at one level may not be significant at a higher level. (A 1% significance level is usually referred to as a higher significance level than 5%.) To be more certain of the result, a more stringent criterion for rejecting the null hypothesis is necessary. On the other hand, a result which is significant at the 1% level is obviously also significant at the lower 5% level.

Values such as 17·3 and 27·1 as obtained in the example for the 5% significance level are referred to as the *critical values* (lower and upper respectively) for the test. Obviously, they depend on the actual study situation and the chosen significance level. If the test statistic, which for this formulation is the sample mean, falls between the two values, the null hypothesis is accepted at the defined significance level, and the interval from 17·3 to 27·1 is called the acceptance region for the test. The critical region for the test comprises all values below and including the lower critical value (17·3) and all values above and including the upper critical value (27·1). If the test statistic falls in the critical region, the null hypothesis can be rejected.

6.4   Relationship with confidence intervals

In the one-sample hypothesis test for a mean it was stated that a result significant at the 5% level would be obtained if the sample mean ($\bar{X} = 27·5$) lay outside the critical values given by

Hypothesized mean $\pm 1·96$ standard errors   (6.1)

which, in the example, were 17·3 and 27·1. When, in Chapter 4, the estimation of the population mean survival of all lung cancer patients that could have been treated with the new drug was considered, a 95% confidence interval was calculated as (see Eqn. 4.3)

Sample mean $\pm 1·96$ standard errors   (6.2)

which was from 22·6 to 32·4. This was interpreted to mean that it is 95% certain that the unknown mean survival lies between these values.

It is seen immediately that if the population mean specified by the null hypothesis is outside the 95% confidence interval the sample mean is outside the limits given by Eqn. 6.1 and, thus, an alternative approach to hypothesis testing is to declare a statistically significant result at the 5% level if the hypothesized mean is outside the 95% confidence interval. This is quite logical and in many cases provides an acceptable alternative method of testing hypotheses. Note, however, that the confidence interval approach and the significance test approach are not equivalent in all situations (comparing proportions for instance) and the preferred approach for significance testing is that outlined in Section 6.3. To reiterate the distinction, the hypothesis test is performed by seeing if the observed sample mean is further than $\pm 1·96$ SE away from the hypothesized mean (Eqn. 6.1). The confidence interval approach, on the other hand, is based on whether or not the hypothesized mean is more than $\pm 1·96$ SE away from the sample mean. The two approaches happen to give identical results for the one-sample test given here, but for reasons too complex for this text this is not true in general.

6.5   One-sided and two-sided tests

The example which has been considered so far of a sample of 100 lung cancer patients has been analysed with a null hypothesis of

$$H_0 : \mu_D = 22 \cdot 2 \text{ months}$$

and an alternative hypothesis of

$$H_A : \mu_D \neq 22 \cdot 2 \text{ months}$$

This alternative hypothesis does not distinguish between the situations where the new drug has a beneficial as opposed to a deleterious effect on survival. Consequently, the criterion for a significant result is whether or not the sample mean is further away from 22·2 months *in either direction* by 1·96 standard errors or 4·9 months. The $\pm 1 \cdot 96$ SE is based on the areas in both tails of the normal distribution, adding up to the chosen significance level of 5% (see Fig. 6.1). For this reason, the test as described above is referred to as a *two-tailed* or *two-sided* significance test.

The two-sided significance test as outlined is appropriate to most medical applications when the direction of the anticipated results (i.e. greater or less than the value specified by the null hypothesis) cannot be determined beforehand. In the example, for instance, it would be dangerous if the researchers assumed, prior to the study, that the drug could only have a beneficial effect on survival. They were, therefore, correct in using a two-sided test, allowing for either increased or decreased survival compared with the hypothesized population value of 22·2 months. One-sided tests (to be discussed below) may be legitimate, however, when either a result in one particular direction is of no interest to researchers, or they are sure that the true result will be in one direction only.

Suppose that in the general male population the mean cholesterol level is known to be 6·5 mmol/l with a standard deviation of 1·2 mmol/l. If researchers are interested in studying cholesterol levels in male agricultural

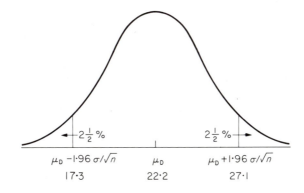

Fig. 6.1. Sampling distribution of the mean for samples sized $n = 100$ taken from a population of mean $\mu_D = 22 \cdot 2$ and standard deviation $\sigma = 25 \cdot 0$.

How do they know that?

labourers, and know that whatever the mean level may be it cannot be below 6·5, they might decide on a one-sided significance test for the study. In such a case, the alternative hypothesis would be expressed as

$$H_A : \mu_L > 6\cdot5$$

where μ_L refers to the population mean cholesterol level in agricultural labourers. If the null hypothesis is rejected, only the alternative of mean cholesterol levels being greater than 6·5 mmol/l can be accepted. To continue with this example, suppose that the researchers studied 25 agricultural labourers and discovered a mean cholesterol level of 6·9 mmol/l; what can they conclude? In such a situation, it has been asserted beforehand that observed mean results less than 6·5 are due to chance and, therefore, spurious. It is only of interest to decide if mean values greater than 6·5 could be spurious or if they reflect a real difference in cholesterol levels of agricultural labourers. Again, using the properties of the sampling distribution of the mean, it can be asserted that if the population mean cholesterol of agricultural labourers is 6·5 mmol/l only 5% of possible sample means will lie above

$$\mu_L + 1\cdot645\ \sigma/\sqrt{n}$$

or $6\cdot5 + 1\cdot645\ (1\cdot2/\sqrt{25}) = 6\cdot89$

(see Fig. 6.2 and Table B.2).

For a one-sided significance test, there is only one critical value. In this case, with the sample mean as the test statistic, it is the upper critical value of 6·89. The observed result obtained by the researchers was a sample mean of 6·9 mmol/l, which is just above the critical value, so that the null hypothesis may be rejected at a 5% one-sided level of significance. Agricultural labourers may be said to have statistically significant higher cholesterol levels than those observed in the general male population.

Note that if a two-sided test had been specified, the observed mean

FIG. 6.2. Sampling distribution of the mean for samples sized $n = 25$ taken from a population of mean $\mu_L = 6\cdot5$ and standard deviation $\sigma = 1\cdot2$.

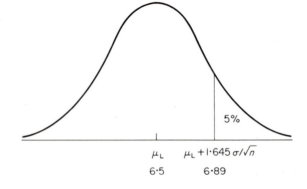

5%

μ_L $\mu_L + 1\cdot645\ \sigma/\sqrt{n}$

6·5   6·89

cholesterol level of agricultural labourers would have had to lie outside

$$\mu_L \pm 1\!\cdot\!96\,\sigma/\sqrt{n}$$

and be greater than or equal to 6·97 or less than or equal to 6·03. The observed sample value of 6·9 mmol/l is inside the acceptance region, so the result would be non-significant for a two-sided significance test. In general, two-sided tests are more conservative than one-sided tests and make it harder to reject the null hypothesis. If in doubt, however, two-sided tests should always be employed, since definite prior information is required before the one-sided test is legitimate. Note that if the null hypothesis for the one-sided test had specified a difference in the opposite direction to that discussed above, the plus sign should be replaced by a minus sign and the critical region would be below the point defined by $\mu_L - 1\!\cdot\!645\,\sigma/\sqrt{n}$.

6.6   General structure of a significance test

So far, two examples have been worked through in detail, showing how a particular null hypothesis could be accepted or rejected at a specified significance level. The examples taken dealt with the one-sample situation, and hypotheses concerning means. As has already been stated, the particular hypothesis test used in a specific situation will depend on many factors, but the underlying approach is the same. The one-sample test described in the previous sections will now be reformulated into a format that will be generally applicable in nearly all situations. This is achieved by changing the scale of measurement used in the example. It was seen in Chapter 3 that a normal variable with a given mean and standard deviation can be transformed so that the resulting variable has a mean of 0 and standard deviation of 1. This is achieved by using the equation

$$Z = \frac{\text{Value of variable} - \text{mean}}{\text{Standard deviation}} \tag{6.3}$$

where Z is the transformed or standardized variable (see Eqn. 3.5).

In the example of the lung cancer patients, the sampling distribution of the mean under the null hypothesis had a mean of $\mu_D = 22\!\cdot\!2$ and a standard deviation (called the standard error of the mean) of 2·5 calculated from $\sigma/\sqrt{n}$ with $\sigma = 25$ and $n = 100$. If instead of looking at the distribution of possible sample means ($\bar{X}$) the distribution of

$$Z = \frac{\bar{X} - \mu_D}{\sigma/\sqrt{n}} \tag{6.4}$$

is examined, it could be said that it follows a standard normal distribution of mean 0 and standard deviation 1. Thus, 95% of the time the value of Z should lie between -1.96 and $+1.96$. In 5% of samples, Z, calculated from Eqn. 6.4, would lie outside these limits. The Z value corresponding to the sample mean of 27.5 is

$$Z = \frac{27.5 - 22.2}{2.5} = 2.12$$

which is greater than 1.96. Thus, if the null hypothesis were true, a value of Z as extreme as 2.12 would occur less than 5% of the time, so that the p value for the test is less than 5%. This is, therefore, a significant result and the null hypothesis that a population of patients treated with this new drug would have the same survival as all previous patients can be rejected. This, of course, is the conclusion that was reached before, using a slightly different but equivalent mathematical approach. In general for a one-sample two-sided hypothesis test on a mean, the null hypothesis specifying the mean of a population to be μ_0 (a particular numerical value) may be rejected at a 5% level if

$$Z \geqslant 1.96 \text{ or } Z \leqslant -1.96$$

where

$$Z = \frac{\bar{X} - \mu_0}{SE(\bar{X})} \tag{6.4}$$

is the test statistic for this formulation of the test. Tests which employ the standard normal deviate (Z) as a test statistic are generally called Z tests. The critical and acceptance regions for this test are illustrated in Fig. 6.3. If $Z \geqslant 1.96$ it can be concluded that the true population mean is greater than that specified by the null hypothesis, while if $Z \leqslant -1.96$ it can be concluded that the population mean is, in fact, less than that specified by the null hypothesis.

Going back to the properties of the standard normal distribution, it is

FIG. 6.3. The standard normal curve showing the critical region for rejection of H_0 and the acceptance region for non-rejection of H_0 for the Z test at a two-sided significance level of 5%.

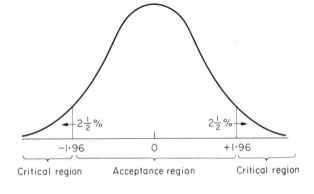

known that ± 1.96 cuts off 5% of the area in the two tails. If a significance test at a 1% level is required 1.96 would be replaced by 2.576 which corresponds to 1% of the area in both tails of a standard normal curve. Similarly, for a one-sided test, where the alternative hypothesis states that the population mean should be greater than that specified by the null hypothesis, a significant result at a 5% level would be obtained if $Z \geqslant 1.645$ where 1.645 corresponds to a 5% area in the upper tail of the standard normal distribution. Table B.2 in Appendix B gives the critical values for various significance levels of one- and two-sided Z tests. The table does not, however, allow for the calculation of an exact p value. In the example, for instance, with a Z of 2.12 it was calculated that p was less than 5%. Obviously, if the area in the tails of the distribution outside ± 2.12 could be calculated, the exact p value could be calculated. In fact, extensive tables of the standard normal distribution are available which would enable such an exact calculation, but the fact that p is less than 5% is sufficient for most practical purposes. Note that the higher the absolute value of the test statistic, Z, the smaller are the corresponding areas in the tails of the distribution and, thus, the greater the level of statistical significance achieved. Often, the results of a significance test may be expressed by giving a range within which the p value lies. Thus, using the table, if Z was 1.72, the two-sided p value would be given as greater than 0.05 but less than 0.10. This would be written: $0.05 < p < 0.10$ which, of course, is not a significant result at the 5% level. The highest significance level achieved should be given if p happens to be less than 5%; thus 'p less than 1%' would be quoted rather than 'p less than 5%'. On the other hand, most researchers just write down NS (for non-significant) for all values of p above 5%, although it might perhaps be better if a more exact range were given. The results of a significance test are often written as $Z = 2.12$; $p < 0.05$ or $Z = 1.72$; NS.

As shall be seen later, many test statistics are also formulated in a similar manner to the one-sample Z test as

$$\frac{\text{Sample estimate}}{\text{Standard error of the estimate}} \tag{6.5}$$

and the format of the one-sample Z test has general applicability to most statistical tests of significance (see Table 6.1). A null hypothesis is postulated, a significance level is set and a one- or two-tailed test chosen. A test statistic is calculated on the basis of the sample data and null hypothesis. The particular statistic will, of course, depend on the data, the type of study and many other factors, but whatever the statistic, it is known from theoretical considerations to have a specific distribution if the null hypothesis is true. Tables of this distribution are examined to see if the statistic lies in the acceptance region or inside the critical region for the particular test chosen. The critical region usually corresponds to areas in the tail or tails of the distribution in question.

Table 6.1   General structure of a significance test.

General test	Example of one-sample Z test
State the null hypothesis (H_0)	$\mu_D = 22 \cdot 2$
$\downarrow$	
Set the significance level	5%
$\downarrow$	
One- or two-sided test?	two-sided
$\downarrow$	
Calculate the test statistic	$Z = \dfrac{\bar{X} - \mu_D}{\sigma/\sqrt{n}} = 2 \cdot 12$
$\downarrow$	
Find the critical values of the distribution of the test statistic for the given (one- or two-sided) significance level	Critical values are $-1 \cdot 96$ and $+1 \cdot 96$
$\downarrow$	
If the test statistic lies within the acceptance region do not reject H_0. If the statistic lies in the critical region reject H_0 and claim a significant result	Acceptance region: $-1 \cdot 96 < Z < 1 \cdot 96$ Critical region: $Z \leqslant -1 \cdot 96$ or $Z \geqslant 1 \cdot 96$ So H_0 rejected with $Z = 2 \cdot 12$

If the test statistic lies within the critical region, a significant result may be claimed. In practice, what is often done is to calculate the highest level of significance for the given statistic without prior setting of the level required. By convention however, a significance level of 5% is usually assumed to be necessary for rejection of the null hypothesis.

6.7   Power considerations, sample size, type I and type II errors

Having looked in detail at the calculation of significance levels and their interpretation in the context of the one-sample Z test, the interpretation of non-significant results is now considered. This is sometimes referred to as 'the other side of significance testing'. This leads on to the important question of determining adequate sample sizes for specific studies.

The example of the 100 lung cancer patients and the one-sample Z test will again be used to illustrate the ideas. As was seen, the level of statistical significance attained depends on the magnitude of the test statistic

$$Z = \frac{\bar{X} - \mu_0}{\sigma / \sqrt{n}} \qquad (6.4)$$

where $\bar{X}$ is the observed sample mean, μ_0 is the hypothesized mean, σ is the standard deviation in the population, and n is the sample size. The larger the value of Z, the greater the level of statistical significance achieved, and the less likelihood that the observed result is spurious. What, then, are the factors which lead to statistically significant results? Firstly, the magnitude of $\bar{X} - \mu_0$ is important; all else being equal, sample means far away from the hypo- thesized population value will give significant results more readily than values close to it. This is an intuitively obvious result, in the sense that a sample with a mean very much larger (or smaller) than what was hypo- thesized tends to throw doubt on the hypothesis. So the degree of statistical significance depends on the true (unknown) population value when the null hypothesis is false. The second factor which will affect the likelihood of a significant result is the population standard deviation σ. Statistically signifi- cant results are more likely with small values of σ. Again this is reasonable, since if the spread or variation in the population is small it should be easier to detect samples not originating from that population. The third and perhaps most important factor which will determine whether or not significance may be achieved is the sample size, n. For a given observed difference, $\bar{X} - \mu_0$, and given σ, larger sample sizes will more easily give significant results. In fact, it is easily seen that any difference (no matter how small or unimportant) can be made statistically significant if the sample size is large enough. This highlights the distinction made in the last chapter between medically important and statistically significant results, and also justifies the claim that with an important result based on large enough numbers statistical analysis is almost entirely redundant.

From the opposite point of view, a non-significant result can be due to the true population mean lying very near the hypothesized value, too large a spread in the population, too small a sample size or any combination of these three factors. Although illustrated in the context of the one-sample Z test, the above points may be taken as being generally applicable to most statistical tests of significance.

Fig. 6.4 illustrates the main elements of the decision process involved in hypothesis testing, using the one-sample drug trial as a practical example. On the top of the figure two possible states of 'reality' are shown; either the null hypothesis is true, and the mean survival of patients treated with the drug is 22·2 months, or the null hypothesis is false. On the left side of the figure are noted the two possible decisions which can be made — rejection or acceptance of this null hypothesis. In the body of the figure are the

REALITY

		Null hypothesis true	Null hypothesis false (alternative hypothesis true)
		$H_0: \mu_0 = 22 \cdot 2$	$\mu_0 \neq 22 \cdot 2$
DECISION	Do not reject H_0 (non-significant result)	Correct decision	β or type II error
	Reject H_0 (significant result)	α or type I error	Correct decision

FIG. 6.4. Type I and type II errors in hypothesis testing.

implications of any particular decision for either of the two realities.

If the null hypothesis is true and a non-significant result is obtained everything is fine and the correct decision has been made. If, however, the null hypothesis is true and a significant result is obtained, the decision to reject the hypothesis is incorrect and an error has been made. This form of error is called an alpha (α — the Greek letter 'a') error or type I error. The probability of making a type I error, denoted by α, is by definition the probability of rejecting the null hypothesis when it is in fact true. This, of course, is nothing more than the significance level of the test. (Remember — a significant result obtains if, traditionally, p is less than 0·05 and, by definition, p can be less than this value for 5% of the possible samples when the null hypothesis is true.) The p value for any result can be alternatively interpreted as the chance of making a type I or alpha error (see Table 6.2). Returning to Fig. 6.4: if the null hypothesis is false a statistically significant result leads to a correct decision. If, however, in this situation a non-significant result is obtained, a decision error has again been made, and this is called the beta (β — the Greek letter 'b') or type II error. For non-significant results, it is, therefore, necessary to calculate the probability of making this error. It has already been mentioned that a non-significant result should be expressed as a non-rejection of the null hypothesis rather than an acceptance of it since, in this case, the two states of reality cannot be

Table 6.2 Definition of type I and type II errors.

α	β
Probability of making a type I error	Probability of making a type II error
Probability of rejecting H_0 when it is true	Probability of not rejecting H_0 when it is false
Significance level of the test	

distinguished. The problem is, of course, that the alternative hypothesis (in the example for instance) encompasses every possible mean survival not exactly equal to 22·2 months. If, in fact, the mean population survival of the drug-treated group was 22·3 months (3 days greater than in the group without the drug) it would be technically wrong to fail to reject the null hypothesis. Such an error, however, would not be very important, since an increase of mean survival of this magnitude would be irrelevant in cancer therapy. Obviously, if the true mean survival was as close to 22·2 months as above, it would be very difficult to obtain a significant result (the sample mean $\bar{X}$ would most likely be very close to the hypothesized mean of 22·2) and there would be a high chance of a beta or type II error. On the other hand, if the true survival was much greater or less than 22·2 the chances of a type II error should decrease. This illustrates one of the important facts concerning type II errors — the chances of their occurrence depend on the true value of the population mean. The actual size of the β probability depends on the overlap between the sampling distributions of the mean under (a) the null hypothesis and (b) a specific alternative hypothesis for which the type II error is to be calculated. Fig. 6·5 shows the sampling distribution of the means for the reality specified by the null hypothesis, and a reality specified by an alternative hypothesis, suggesting a mean drug group survival of 30 months. It has already been shown that the null hypothesis would not be rejected at the 5% level if the sample mean was less than 27·1 months, or did not lie in the shaded area of the upper distribution. If, however, the real population mean was 30·0 months (and thus the null hypothesis was false) a

FIG. 6.5. Sampling distributions of the mean for (a) the null hypothesis $\mu_D = 22·2$ and (b) a specific alternative hypothesis $\mu_D = 30·0$.

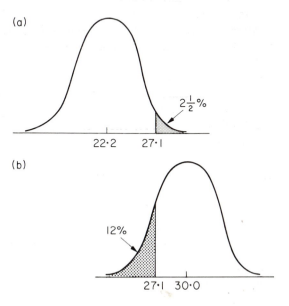

mean value of less than 27·1 could arise in a sample from this population. The probability (denoted β) that it would arise with a consequent type II error is given by the heavily shaded area in the second curve. This can be calculated to be about 0·12 or 12%. The calculations are not detailed in this text.

Fig. 6.6 shows a graph of calculated β values for various alternative survival times in the drug-treated population, with a sample size of 100 and a two-sided significance level of 5%. Such a graph is called the *operating characteristic curve* for a test. From this it can be seen that if, for example, the true mean survival is 24 months, then β equals 0·9 and thus there is a 90% chance of making a type II error. For a mean survival of 30 months however, the probability of a type II error reduces, as was said above, to about 12%. Sometimes, the value of $1-\beta$ is quoted rather than the value of β itself. $1-\beta$ is called the *power* of the test. For a true mean survival of 30 months, the power of the test is $1-0·12=0·88$ or 88%. The power of a test increases as the difference between the hypothesized value of the mean and the real value increases, and a high power means a low chance of a type II error, or alternatively, a large chance of detecting (significantly) a particular result.

How, then, can the probability of a type II error be reduced? Looking at Fig. 6.5, it can be seen that there are two main possibilities. Firstly, the significance level could be reduced to greater than 5%, thus increasing the shaded area in the upper curve. This, in turn, will decrease the dark area in the lower curve, corresponding to the β probability. This is a fairly general result: for a given sample size and a specified difference between the true population mean and the hypothesized mean, increases in α will decrease β and vice versa. What you lose on the roundabout, you gain on the swings. However, since the α value or p value of the test is specified beforehand, decreasing the type II error in this manner is not to be encouraged. The other

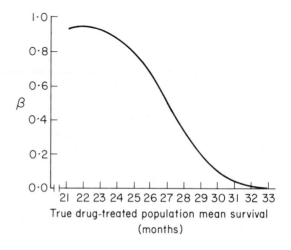

Fig. 6.6. Operating characteristic curve for a two-sided 5% test of significance of the null hypothesis that the mean survival in the treated group is 22·2 months for samples sized 100 and population standard deviation of 25·0 months.

β

True drug-treated population mean survival (months)

way of reducing β is by reducing the spread of the sampling distribution of the mean, thus reducing the overlap of the two curves. Now, remember that the spread of the sampling distribution of the mean is determined by the standard error of the mean or $\sigma/\sqrt{n}$. The population standard deviation, σ, cannot be controlled, but the sample size can be increased, thus reducing the standard error. This is a second important result: for a given significance level and specified difference between the hypothesized population mean and the true population value, the β error may be reduced by increasing the sample size.

The further analysis required for negative or non-significant results can now be explained. So far, the interdependence of four quantities has been seen — the significance level (α); the probability of a type II error (β); the sample size (n); and the difference between the hypothesized mean μ_0 and that actually obtaining in the population sampled. Given three of these factors, the fourth may be calculated, assuming that the population standard deviation is known.

If the study gives a significant result, then quoting the significance level is sufficient, since it gives the probability of the only error which could have been made — the type I error (see Fig. 6.4). If the study, however, gives a non-significant result at a specified level (usually 5%) the reader should be told what the chances of missing a real result were, i.e. the β probabilities should be presented for a range of possible values for the mean of the population from which the sample was taken. This may show that, in fact, the chances of missing a result where the true mean lay a fair distance from that given by the null hypothesis were quite high, and that from the beginning the study could have been judged inadequate to detect important medical findings. This is often expressed by saying that the power $(1 - \beta)$ of the study was too small. For negative results, confidence interval presentations can also show how inadequate a study sample size may be.

The usual reason for missing important results is that the sample size is too small, and investigations have shown that many medical studies with non-significant results were too small to detect anything but the most marked departures from the null hypothesis. When the sample size is too small, it is impossible to distinguish between real and spurious results. The solution, of course, is to estimate the required sample at the beginning of a study, in the planning stages. In certain situations this is relatively easy, and Appendix D gives some sample-size formulae which may be useful in certain simple situations. In general, however, professional statistical advice should be obtained at the planning stages to determine how large a study is required. Usually, the requirements needed to calculate a sample size are a specification of the significance level, the chance one is willing to take in making a type II error (β), the size of the effect one doesn't want to miss (i.e. the magnitude of what would be considered an important result in terms of departure from the null hypothesis) and an estimate of the population variability σ. (This last requirement is not necessary when estimating sample sizes for comparing proportions.) From these factors, a required sample size can usually be calculated. Unfortunately, sample sizes often turn out to be much larger than expected by the investigator, and the final size of the study is often a compromise between the numbers required from the statistical point of view and the practical situation relating to the resources available. In this situation at least, whatever sample size is chosen the investigator can know what the chances are of detecting an important result, and if these prove to be too low the study should probably not be undertaken in the first place.

6.8   The one-sample t test

So far in this chapter, it has been assumed that the population standard deviation σ is known, and this led to the derivation of the one-sample Z test. The other assumptions underlying this test were that a random sample in the population of interest had been taken and that this parent population was not very skewed (see Section 4.4 also). As discussed in Section 4.6 in the context of confidence intervals, the Student's t distribution should be used in place of the normal distribution (Z) when the sample standard deviation S is used instead of the population standard deviation σ for sample sizes of less than 60 or so. In this more realistic situation, the appropriate one-sample test statistic is, instead of Eqn. 6.4,

$$t_{n-1} = \frac{\bar{X} - \mu_0}{S/\sqrt{n}} \tag{6.6}$$

where $\bar{X}$ is the sample mean, μ_0 is the hypothesized population mean, n is the sample size and S is the sample standard deviation. The t_{n-1} indicates that it is necessary to look up a table of the t distribution on $n-1$ degrees of freedom, rather than the table of the normal distribution, for obtaining the critical values. The resulting significance test is called the t test.

   The one-sample t test will be illustrated using the example already discussed in Chapter 4. In that example, a researcher studied 9 children with a specific congenital heart disease, and found that they started to walk at a mean age of 12·8 months with a standard deviation of 2·4 months. Assume now that it is known that normal children start to walk at a mean age of 11·4 months. Can the researcher conclude that congenital heart disease delays the age at which children begin to walk? Since the sample size is much less than 60, and only a sample estimate of the standard deviation is available, a t test must be employed. The null hypothesis is that children with congenital heart disease start to walk at a mean age of $\mu_W = 11·4$ months, and a two-sided significance level of 5% is chosen. The test statistic is from Eqn. 6.6

$$t = \frac{12\cdot8 - 11\cdot4}{2\cdot4/\sqrt{9}} = 1\cdot75$$

on 8 degrees of freedom. Looking up Table B.3 for the Student's t distribution, it is seen that the critical values for a two-sided 5% level of significance are $\pm 2\cdot306$. The calculated t of $1\cdot75$ falls within the acceptance region for the test and thus the null hypothesis cannot be rejected. The effect of the congenital heart disease on mean age at starting to walk is non-significant ($t = 1\cdot75$; $d.f. = 8$; NS).

6.9　One-sample tests for a single proportion

The significance test for comparing an observed sample proportion with some hypothesized value is similar in form to the one-sample Z test for means. If the population proportion specified by the null hypothesis is called π_0 and the proportion observed in the sample is denoted by p, then an appropriate test statistic which has the standard normal distribution is

$$Z = \frac{p - \pi_0}{SE(p)} \qquad (6.7)$$

where $SE(p)$, the standard error of the sample proportion, is given by Eqn. 4.8. Thus,

$$Z = \frac{p - \pi_0}{\sqrt{\dfrac{\pi_0(1 - \pi_0)}{n}}} \qquad (6.8)$$

where n is the sample size. Note that, assuming the null hypothesis is true, an exact expression for the standard error of the sample proportion can be given, rather than the approximation with the confidence interval approach, where Eqn. 4.10 was used instead. Note that the restriction mentioned in Chapter 4 on the adequacy of the normal approximation to the binomial distribution applies here as well. Both $n\pi$ and $n(1 - \pi)$ must be greater than 5 for the valid use of the Z test on proportions.

Take as an example the study of 200 death certificates of which 32% or $0\cdot32$ recorded coronary heart disease as the cause of death. Are these data compatible with a null hypothesis stating that the proportion of deaths due to coronary heart disease is actually $0\cdot4$ in the population? The test statistic is, from Eqn. 6.8,

$$Z = \frac{0.32 - 0.4}{\sqrt{\dfrac{0.4(0.6)}{200}}} = -2.309$$

Since the two-sided 5% critical values for the Z test are ± 1.96, the hypothesis may be rejected at a 5% level of significance. Note that the hypothesis cannot be rejected at a 1% level since the critical values in this case are ± 2.576.

6.10   The one-sample χ^2 test for many proportions

Sometimes researchers may have sample values of a qualitative variable taking on more than two values which they wish to compare with a known population distribution. For instance, a survey of the smoking habits of 250 female nurses gave 108(43·2%) current smokers, 24(9·6%) ex-smokers and 118(47·2%) non-smokers. Are these percentages significantly different from those obtained in females in the general population — 36·4, 15·7 and 47·9% respectively? (Assume that these define the population distribution exactly. See Table 1.1.) Since this smoking variable has more than 2 categories, the test described in the last section for single proportions cannot be applied. A special test is available for this situation however. It is called the chi-square test and is denoted χ^2 (χ, chi — the Greek letter corresponding to 'ch'). The formulation of this test is quite different from anything encountered so far. The test is based on calculating expected numbers in the different categories of the variable if the null hypothesis were true, and comparing these with the numbers actually obtained (the observed frequencies).

In the example, the null hypothesis would specify that the percentages in the nursing population of current, ex- and non-smokers were 36·4, 15·7 and 47·9% respectively. Of the 250 nurses sampled, it would therefore be expected that 36·4% or 91·0 (250×0.364) would be current smokers, 15·7% or 39·25 (250×0.157) would be ex-smokers, and 47·9% or 119·75 (250×0.479) would be non-smokers. These are called the expected numbers. (In statistics, fractions of people are often allowed to end up in different categories, and this should not worry you!) Table 6.3 shows these expected numbers (E) and the numbers actually observed in the sample (O). The expected numbers will add up to the total sample size. The hypothesis test is now based on the discrepancy between the observed and expected values. If the observed and expected values are close, it would be reasonable to think that there would be little evidence to reject the null hypothesis. On the other hand, large discrepancies may make it possible to reject it. In fact, it is the relative differences which are perhaps more important, and the test statistic that compares these quantities and has a known theoretical distribution is χ^2. χ^2 is obtained by subtracting each expected quantity from each observed quantity, squaring the answer, dividing by the expected number and adding the result over the categories of the variable.

$$\chi^2 = \sum \frac{(O-E)^2}{E} \tag{6.9}$$

This calculation is illustrated in Table 6.3 where a χ^2 value of 9·127 is obtained. Note that the $O - E$ quantities themselves always sum to zero.

The critical values of the chi-square distribution must now be looked up in tables, just as for the Z and t tests in previous sections. Table B.4 gives such a table of critical values for χ^2 and the actual properties of this distribution are not of concern here. Note from the table that, like the t distribution, the chi-square distribution also has many different degrees of freedom. How are these degrees of freedom to be determined in the example? In the t test the degrees of freedom depended on the sample size; in the χ^2 test, however, the degrees of freedom depend on the number of categories in the variable being examined, and the appropriate degrees of freedom are given by one less than the number of categories. In this case, the degrees of freedom are related to the number of independent comparisons which can be made between the observed and the expected numbers. The more categories in the variable, the more comparisons can be made and the higher the value for chi-square. A chi-square distribution with high degrees of freedom has higher critical values than a chi-square with lower degrees of freedom. Thus, since smoking had 3 categories the χ^2 test with 2 degrees of freedom is appropriate for the example.

A further point to note about the chi-square distribution is that the critical values are all positive; this is because χ^2 must itself be positive due to the squared term in Eqn. 6.9. The critical values given must then be exceeded for a significant result. For this one-sample test, only two-sided significance levels are appropriate, as the specification of differences in one particular direction has no real meaning. For a 5% two-sided test on 2 degrees of freedom, the critical χ^2 value is 5·991 from the table. The calculated χ^2 value of 9·127 is

Table 6.3 Calculations for the one-sample χ^2 test.

Smoking category	Observed numbers (O)	Hypothesized proportions	Expected numbers (E)	$(O-E)$	$(O-E)^2/E$
Current smokers	108	0·364	91·00	17·00	3·176
Ex-smokers	24	0·157	39·25	−15·25	5·925
Non-smokers	118	0·479	119·75	−1·75	0·026
	250	1·0	250·00	0·00	9·127

$$\chi^2 = 9\cdot127; \, d.f. = 2; \, p < 0\cdot05$$

greater than this, so it can be concluded that there is a significant difference between the smoking habits of nurses and those of the general female population. ($\chi^2 = 9.127$; $d.f. = 2$; $p < 0.05$).

The one-sample χ^2 test as described above requires that theoretical population proportions are hypothesized without reference to the sample values. Such situations will often arise in genetical calculations for example. The one-sample χ^2 test can also be used in slightly different situations to test the goodness of fit of (grouped) data to a theoretical distribution like the normal. In these situations, the degrees of freedom are calculated differently however, and a more advanced text should be consulted.

The χ^2 test requires that the actual sample frequencies observed in the different categories of the variable be known — it is not sufficient to know only the percentages or proportions occurring in the sample. The test is limited in that it does not easily lead to confidence interval estimation, but with only two categories of a qualitative variable it is mathematically equivalent to the one-sample test for proportions discussed in the last section. (The chi-square distribution with one degree of freedom is the square of the standard normal distribution.) This test should only be used if not more than 20% of the expected frequencies are less than 5, and no single expected frequency is less than 1. If these assumptions are not met, combination of adjacent categories may increase the expected frequencies to the required levels.

6.11   Assumptions in significance testing

A fundamental requirement for tests of significance is that the sampling distribution of the test statistic of interest corresponds to a particular theoretical distribution. Many of the tests discussed in this chapter require that the sampling distribution is normal. Other sampling distributions such as the binomial distribution, Student's t distribution and the chi-square distribution have also been referred to. Certain assumptions must often be made before it can be accepted that a given test statistic will conform to a theoretical distribution, and if these assumptions are invalid then the related tests of significance and the conclusions drawn from them are also invalid.

This important point is often overlooked. Thus, it cannot be automatically taken that the sampling distribution of the mean will be normal, even for quite large samples. If the parent population is normally distributed, the sampling distribution of the mean will also be normal, even for quite small samples. If the parent population is moderately skewed, the sampling distribution of means will tend to a normal distribution as the sample size increases, and may be assumed to be normal for large samples ($n > 30$). However, if the population is highly skewed, it cannot be taken that the sampling distribution will be normal, even for large samples. An assumption of 'approximate normality' of a variable in the population is necessary for many significance tests. It is, therefore, very important to examine the characteristics of a distribution before using any particular type of test of significance. For this purpose, it is useful to draw a histogram or frequency polygon of the sample drawn from the population, since this gives an indication of how skewed the population might be.

While this subject is not pursued here, it may be noted that various techniques are available for reducing the degree of skewness in a distribution. For example, while a variable X may be markedly skewed, it may be that log X is normal or nearly so. If log X is normally distributed it is referred to as a *log-normal distribution* and tests of significance may be used which are based on the characteristics of a log-normal distribution. Again, if a variable X is markedly skewed, it may be found that the transformed variable $1/X$ (the reciprocal transform) is normally or near-normally distributed. The use of transformations of this kind is quite common in medical statistics; many important variables, such as blood pressure and lipid levels, are found in practice to be markedly skewed, and skewness can be reduced by transforming the original data.

If there are still doubts relating to the veracity of assumptions underlying the tests described, alternative *non-parametric* tests are sometimes available. Some of these are discussed in the next chapter.

6.12   Summary

In this chapter the development of the one-sample normal (Z) test was described in detail to illustrate the underlying structure of hypothesis tests.

Table 6.4   Summary of one-sample tests.

Hypothesis test on	Test statistic
One mean:	
σ known	$Z = \dfrac{\bar{X} - \mu_0}{\sigma/\sqrt{n}}$
σ unknown	$t_{n-1} = \dfrac{\bar{X} - \mu_0}{S/\sqrt{n}}$
One proportion	$Z = \dfrac{p - \pi_0}{\sqrt{\dfrac{\pi_0(1-\pi_0)}{n}}}$
Many proportions	$\chi^2 = \sum \dfrac{(O-E)^2}{E}$

The relationship of confidence intervals to hypothesis tests was discussed, as were the concepts of one- and two-sided tests and the principles of power and sample size calculations. Later sections in the chapter detailed calculations for the more widely applicable one-sample t test. The Z test for a single proportion and the χ^2 test for many proportions were also described. Table 6.4 summarizes the one-sample tests discussed in this chapter, and the computational steps are outlined in Appendix C.

The following chapter details tests for the comparison of two or more samples, which is a much more common situation in the medical area. The general principles discussed above however, in the context of the one-sample test, are applicable to all tests of hypotheses and are necessary for a full grasp of the remaining chapters.

CHAPTER 7
Hypothesis Testing: Comparison of Two or More Groups

... of means — Two-sample tests
... of % — chi²
... & ... rank tests

7.1 Introduction

The general concepts of statistical hypothesis testing, together with a fairly complete discussion of the one-sample situation, have now been presented. This chapter considers the much more widely used tests for comparing two or more groups. It is explained how the number of groups in the analysis, the measurement scale of the data being analysed, any assumptions concerning the distributions of these data and the method of collection all determine which statistical test to employ.

The commonly encountered two-sample tests for comparison of means, the chi-square test for comparison of proportions and some of the more common rank tests are described. Although the derivation of these tests is not given, their application is demonstrated on simple examples. It is hoped that this 'cookbook' chapter will be of practical use to medical researchers who wish to perform simple analyses on their data. Appendix C provides a step-by-step guide to all the tests discussed. It must be pointed out, however, that many studies in medicine result in data which cannot be analysed by these particular methods, and more advanced text books may have to be consulted to find an appropriate test.

Since all statistical tests are based on the same underlying philosophy, the tests themselves are described only briefly; therefore, a good grasp of the concepts of hypothesis testing as given in the last two chapters is necessary for the material which follows.

7.2 Independent and paired comparisons

One of the most common errors in statistical hypothesis testing is a failure to take cognizance of how the data were collected in the first place. Statistical analysis is not simply a tool applied to numbers, it is a methodology for examining real data which a researcher may have spent many months or years gathering together.

This chapter considers the comparison of two or more groups and is, therefore, in essence, concerned with the analysis of two or more samples taken from corresponding populations. Apart from issues relating to the accuracy of data collection, and whether or not the resulting numbers are truly a measure of what is being studied (see Sections 13.4 and 13.5), the way in which samples are chosen from the populations is of vital importance.

Suppose that a sample has been taken from a population and it is of interest to compare blood pressures in current, ex- and non cigarette-smokers. Each of these three groups can be considered to be a sample from one of the three populations defined by current, ex- and non-smoking. This is a common situation in medical research, where the comparison groups are defined by the value of some qualitative variable (such as smoking) in a single study group. Sometimes, however, the sampling from population groups is more explicit. Separate samples may, for instance, be taken of schoolchildren from rural and urban areas to compare IQs. The samples may be of equal size or may reflect the distribution of urban and rural children in the country as a whole.

Both of these examples have one important factor in common; the samples are *independent samples* from the populations being studied. By independent it is meant, in simple terms, that the actual selection of individuals for one sample group is not affected by the individuals already selected for one of the other groups. It is vital to understand this notion of independence if the correct statistical test is to be chosen, and before undertaking any statistical analysis a researcher must be sure whether or not the comparison groups are independent.

At the other extreme from the comparison of independent samples is the comparison of *paired samples* or, with more than two groups, *individually matched* samples. A paired sample arises in two-group comparisons when every individual in one of the groups has a unique match or pair in the other group. A researcher, for instance, might be interested in comparing the smoking habits of a group of lung cancer patients with a control or comparison group of persons who do not have this cancer. Such a study is referred to as a *case-control study*, and is discussed in some detail in Chapter 9. The researcher, however, knows that smoking habits are related to both a person's age and sex, and wants to avoid a biased analysis which might arise if the age and sex distributions were different in the two groups being studied. One solution to this problem would be to use paired samples. For every lung cancer case in the first group, the researcher would choose, from the general population, a control of the same age and sex who does not have lung cancer. In this way, each individual in one group is matched with an individual in the other group. This technique is sometimes called *artificial pairing*.

In animal experimentation, litter mates often provide the experimental material. Two treatments may be compared in a group of rats by assigning one animal to one treatment and one of its litter mates to the other treatment. Thus, every animal in one group would have a litter mate in the other group.

Such situations result in what is called *natural pairing*.

A third form of pairing is *self-pairing*, when the same individuals belong to both comparison groups. This can arise when, say, a new chemical is being tested for allergic reactions and compared with a non-allergic preparation. The chemical might be applied to a person's right arm, and the other preparation to his left arm. The arms of the people under study would be compared and for every right arm there is a left arm. A further example of a self-paired situation is when some variable is measured before and after a particular therapy. The measurements made before the therapy are matched with the measurements on the same individual after the therapy. The same situation arises when two different treatments are tested on the same individuals on two different occasions.

Although the examples of paired data above were for two-group comparisons, similar data may arise with more than two groups, although it is relatively uncommon in the medical literature. A point to note also is that in a paired situation the sample size in each of the groups must necessarily be the same, while this need not be so for independent comparisons. Situations can arise however when data in two groups are not independent, but do not consist of individually paired individuals either. Methods for dealing with such a situation are not considered in this text, but see the discussion of *frequency matching* in Chapter 9.

7.3 Parametric and non-parametric significance tests

Apart from how the data were collected, the measurement scale of the variable being studied can also determine the statistical hypothesis test to be used. In the discussion so far, it was sufficient to distinguish between quantitative and qualitative variables. In the medical literature, the vast majority of significance tests compare either proportions or means in two or more groups, thus operating on qualitative or quantitative data respectively.

It was noted in Chapter 1 that a qualitative variable can consist of ordered categories which will often take a numerical label or tag, although the concept of distance between these categories does not arise. Thus, it can be said that a systolic blood pressure of 200 mm Hg is twice as high as a systolic blood pressure of 100 mm Hg but it cannot be said that an individual in social group I is twice as privileged as an individual in social group II. On this basis, a hierarchy of variables can be created: qualitative variables with no intrinsic order; qualitative variables with order; and quantitative variables based on measurement. For convenience, these three types of variables will from here on be referred to as nominal, ordinal and quantitative variables respectively. It is important to note that a quantitative variable, such as age, can be expressed in ordinal form (e.g. by ranking from youngest to oldest) or in nominal form (e.g. by categorizing into young, middle-aged or old). This means essentially that a significance test suitable for a low level of measurement can be applied to any higher level, if the scale of measurement is adjusted appropriately. Thus, tests suitable for nominal data can be applied to ordinal or quantitative data, and tests for ordinal data can also be applied to quantitative data.

One of the rules of good statistical analysis, all else being equal, is to use the highest level of test available for the data; but usually all is not equal, and in particular, many tests suitable for quantitative data make large assumptions about the distribution of variables in the populations being compared. It was seen in the last chapter, for instance, that an underlying assumption of normally distributed data was required for a valid application of the one-sample t test, but that with a large sample size violations of this assumption could be tolerated. Significance tests which make distributional assumptions about the variable being analysed are called *parametric tests*.

In most situations, it is not possible to check whether such assumptions are true, particularly when the sample size tends to be small, and there is often doubt about whether or not a particular test is valid for a set of quantitative data. As has been said however, quantitative data can be analysed as ordinal data, and most of the statistical tests of ordinal data are assumption-free. Such tests are called *non-parametric*, *distribution-free* or *rank tests* and provide a useful fallback in many situations.

A further point about many of the rank tests is that they test a null hypothesis relating to median values rather than mean values. The median however is probably much more appropriate for skewed data (see Section 2.2) and is close to the mean if the data have a nearly symmetrical distribution in the first place. It must be pointed out, however, that in general parametric tests are somewhat more powerful (in the sense of Section 6.7) in detecting differences between populations when the underlying assumptions hold, and many of the more complex parametric tests do not have a non-parametric equivalent. In general too, the non-parametric tests are not useful for estimation purposes, and confidence intervals for estimates are usually difficult to calculate.

In the two-sample situation however, non-parametric tests can be exceptionally useful in the analysis of quantitative data. With small sample sizes, many of the underlying assumptions of parametric tests are invalid, and the non-parametric tests are probably the only valid ones to use. For this reason, such tests are sometimes called *small sample tests*, and, in fact, tables for the non-parametric tests in this text are only given for studies of up to moderate size. With fairly large sample sizes, on the other hand, many of the assumptions for the parametric tests may hold approximately, and they can be employed with a large degree of confidence. For large sample sizes too, the non-parametric tests are computationally more tedious.

The remainder of this chapter outlines the application of the more common parametric and non-parametric significance tests. Statistical tables are given in an appendix, and an appendix also summarizes the application of each test for easy reference.

7.4   Comparison of two independent means: the *t* tests

The parametric *t* test used for the comparison of means in two samples is one of the most commonly used tests in medical statistics. The test to be described in this section is for independent samples only and should not be used when the data are paired or matched (see Section 7.2). Failure to take note of this is an oft-repeated error and results in a loss of power in the comparison. In other words, an independent *t* test performed (incorrectly) on paired data will increase the chances of declaring a non-significant result when, in fact, the null hypothesis is false.

Suppose 20 regular users of oral contraceptives were studied to determine if cholesterol levels in such women are significantly different from those of women who do not use oral contraceptives. Because the cholesterol levels in the population were not known, a comparison or control group of 20 similarly aged women who were not on the 'pill' was also taken, without pairing or matching. The results of the study are shown in Table 7.1. The mean cholesterol levels in the contraceptive-users and controls were 5·20 and 4·81 mmol/l respectively with corresponding standard deviations of 0·53 and 0·48 mmol/l.

The null hypothesis is that the mean cholesterol levels in the populations of oral contraceptive-users and non-users are the same. The results of the samples suggest a difference of 0·39 mmol/l between the two groups. Could this be due to chance or does it reflect a real difference?

The statistical approach is similar to the situation with one sample only. If there really was no difference between the two groups, it would be expected that repeat samples, sized 20, from each group would generate a series of

Table 7.1   The independent *t* test comparing cholesterol levels in users and non-users of oral contraceptives.

	Contraceptive-users	Controls
Sample size	20	20
Sample means	5·20	4·81
Sample standard deviations	0·53	0·48
Difference between means	0·39 mmol/l	

$$t = 2 \cdot 439; \ d.f. = 38; \ p < 0 \cdot 05$$

mean differences distributed around the value of 0. As in the one-sample case, a test statistic is calculated based on the difference obtained (0·39 mmol/l), divided by a factor which is the standard error of this difference. This test statistic has a known distribution from theoretical considerations, and tables can be used to see if the calculated value lies in the tails of the distribution. Moreover, since no prior knowledge is available concerning the direction of the difference in cholesterol levels, a two-sided test must be employed.

The actual test statistic to employ is defined

$$Z = \frac{\bar{X}_1 - \bar{X}_2}{SE(\bar{X}_1 - \bar{X}_2)} \tag{7.1}$$

where $\bar{X}_1$ and $\bar{X}_2$ are the means in the groups being compared and $SE(\bar{X}_1 - \bar{X}_2)$ is the exact standard error of the difference between the means. In general,

$$SE(\bar{X}_1 - \bar{X}_2) = \sqrt{\frac{\sigma_1^2}{n_1} + \frac{\sigma_2^2}{n_2}} \tag{7.2}$$

where σ_1 and σ_2 are the population standard deviations and n_1 and n_2 are the two sample sizes.

When, as is usual, the population standard deviations are not known, the sample values S_1 and S_2 must be used instead. How these sample values are employed depends on the assumptions which can be made. If it can be assumed that the two population standard deviations are equal, then what is called a *pooled variance* is calculated as the weighted average of the two sample variances.*

$$S_p^2 = \frac{(n_1 - 1)S_1^2 + (n_2 - 1)S_2^2}{n_1 + n_2 - 2} \tag{7.3}$$

An appropriate test statistic for the comparison of two means is then obtained by substituting S_p^2 for each of the two population values in Eqn. 7.2.

$$t = \frac{\bar{X}_1 - \bar{X}_2}{\sqrt{\dfrac{S_p^2}{n_1} + \dfrac{S_p^2}{n_2}}} \tag{7.4}$$

on $n_1 + n_2 - 2$ degrees of freedom. When the sample sizes are equal ($n_1 = n_2$

---

* For technical reasons, a weighted average of the variances, rather than the standard deviations, is calculated.

$=n$) this reduces to the simpler expression

$$t = \frac{\bar{X}_1 - \bar{X}_2}{\sqrt{\dfrac{S_1^2 + S_2^2}{n}}} \tag{7.5}$$

on $2n - 2$ degrees of freedom.

In the example, the two sample standard deviations are fairly close in value, and since the sample sizes are equal, Eqn. 7.5 is an appropriate test statistic. Substituting in the sample values

$$t = \frac{5 \cdot 20 - 4 \cdot 81}{\sqrt{\dfrac{(0 \cdot 53)^2 + (0 \cdot 48)^2}{20}}} = 2 \cdot 439$$

This value must now be looked up in the tables of the t distribution for 38 degrees of freedom. Table B.3 does not give values for 38 degrees of freedom, but 40 is near enough for a valid approximation. The critical 5% (two-sided) level for t is $2 \cdot 021$ and the statistic exceeds this, so $p < 0 \cdot 05$. Note too, that the critical 1% value is $2 \cdot 704$, and that the result, although achieving a 5% level of significance, does not reach the 1% level. It can, therefore, be concluded that chance is not a likely explanation of the observed differences between the cholesterol levels of users and non-users of oral contraceptives.

A few words need to be said concerning the assumptions underlying this particular application of the t test. The first assumption is, of course, that the two samples are random and independent. The two-sample t test, like the one-sample test, also assumes that the populations from which the samples were taken are not too markedly skewed. The final assumption is that the standard deviations in the two populations are the same (the technical term for this is *homoscedasticity*). If there is reason to doubt this assumption, it is not valid to pool the two sample variances into a single estimate; instead it is necessary to calculate

$$t' = \frac{\bar{X}_1 - \bar{X}_2}{\sqrt{\dfrac{S_1^2}{n_1} + \dfrac{S_2^2}{n_2}}} \tag{7.6}$$

using the separate sample values for the variances. This statistic does not have a Student's t distribution, and although some approximate solutions involving the t distribution with a complex formula for the appropriate degrees of freedom are available, they are not given here. If the sample sizes are large enough, it is suggested a normal approximation setting $t' = Z$ is used, or with smaller sample sizes, the non-parametric test outlined in the next section.

The confidence interval for the mean difference between two population values is given by

$$(\bar{X}_1 - \bar{X}_2) \pm t_c \, \text{SE}(\bar{X}_1 - \bar{X}_2) \tag{7.7}$$

where t_c is the appropriate critical value of the t distribution, and the standard error term is given by the denominator of the appropriate t test. In the cholesterol example, the standard error is given by the denominator of Eqn. 7.5 and is 0·160. The critical t value for 40 (close enough to 38) degrees of freedom and a 95% confidence interval is 2·021, so that the confidence interval for the mean cholesterol difference between the contraceptive-users and non-users is

0·39 ± 2·021 (0·160)

or

0·39 ± 0·32

Thus, it is 95% certain that the mean cholesterol level in contraceptive-users is at least 0·07 mmol/l higher than in controls and could be as much as 0·71 mmol/l higher. The independent t tests are summarized in Section C.5 of Appendix C.

7.5   Comparison of two independent medians: the Wilcoxon two-sample rank sum test

In many situations, especially with small sample sizes, the assumptions underlying the parametric independent t test described in the last section may not hold. In such cases it may be wiser to employ a non-parametric alternative. Also, if the measurement scale of the data is ordinal, and not quantitative, the mean values are uninterpretable and the t tests cannot be employed.

Suppose that systolic blood pressure has been measured on 9 young adults with diabetes mellitus and on 8 control patients of similar age (not matched) without this condition. The diabetes mellitus patients had systolic blood pressures of 114, 120, 120, 128, 130, 135, 138, 140 and 141 mm Hg. The control patients had blood pressures of 110, 112, 112, 118, 120, 122, 125 and 130 mm Hg. The purpose of the study is to see if there is a relationship between blood pressure and diabetes mellitus, and there is no prior conception about what the direction of this relationship may be. Also, since the sample size is small and the distribution of blood pressures may be quite skewed, it is decided that the two-sample t test is likely to be invalid. The most commonly used test in this situation is the *Wilcoxon two-sample rank sum test* or the entirely equivalent *Mann–Whitney U test* or *Kendall's S test*. The formulation which will be considered is that of Wilcoxon.

This test, like most non-parametric tests, is based on ranking or ordering the data. The data from the two groups are combined and ordered from lowest to highest, giving a rank of 1 to the lowest value and, in the example, 17 (the sum of the two sample sizes) to the highest observed value. The groups from which the different observations are taken must also be noted. If there are ties in the data (i.e. more than one individual has the same value for a measurement) the average of the ranks that would have been given to the observations are assigned instead.

In the example, the data would be laid out as in Table 7.2, underlining the observations from (say) the control group, and calling it group 1. The easiest way to assign the ranks correctly is to number the observations from lowest to highest. If there are no ties, these numbers are the ranks. If there are ties as, for example, the two blood pressures of 112 mm Hg, these are assigned a rank calculated as the average of the observation numbers. In this case the two measurements are given numbers 2 and 3, and are therefore assigned the average rank of $2\frac{1}{2}$ $[(2+3)/2]$. The three observations of 120 mm Hg with numbers 6, 7 and 8 are all assigned rank 7 $[(6+7+8)/3=7]$.

The Wilcoxon test is based on examining the sum of the ranks in each

Table 7.2 The Wilcoxon rank sum test comparing systolic blood pressures in 9 diabetics (group 2) and 8 controls (group 1).

Systolic blood pressures (mm Hg)*	Ranks (observation numbers)	Ranks adjusted for ties*
<u>110</u>	<u>1</u>	<u>1</u>
112	2	$2\frac{1}{2}$
112	3	$2\frac{1}{2}$
114	4	4
<u>118</u>	<u>5</u>	<u>5</u>
<u>120</u>	<u>6</u>	<u>7</u>
120	7	7
120	8	7
<u>122</u>	<u>9</u>	<u>9</u>
<u>125</u>	<u>10</u>	<u>10</u>
128	11	11
<u>130</u>	<u>12</u>	$12\frac{1}{2}$
130	13	$12\frac{1}{2}$
135	14	14
138	15	15
140	16	16
141	17	17

*Control (group 1) values and ranks underlined.

T_1 = sum of ranks in group 1 = 49·5; T_2 = sum of ranks in group 2 = 103·5; $p_s < 0.05$

group. If the two populations have similar distributions, then it would be expected that the sums of the ranks in each group would be close to each other. If the distributions are different, it would be expected that the group with the lower median would have a lower sum of ranks. In the example, the sum of the ranks of the observations in group 1 (the control group) is denoted

$$T_1 = 1 + 2 \cdot 5 + \ldots + 12 \cdot 5 = 49 \cdot 5$$

and the sum of the ranks in group 2 is

$$T_2 = 4 + 7 + \ldots + 17 = 103 \cdot 5$$

This immediately suggests that the median value in group 1 might be less than that in group 2.

The test statistic for the Wilcoxon rank sum test is the sum of the ranks in one of the groups — say group 1. As with all significance tests, this statistic is referred to tables of a particular distribution. The critical values for the Wilcoxon statistic are to be found in Table B.5 (Appendix B). Unfortunately the table is rather cumbersome and spread out over 12 pages of the appendix. The table allows for sample sizes of n_1 up to 25 and n_2 up to 35. The groups can be relabelled if one has more than 25 observations. For sample sizes outside this range a more detailed text should be consulted (see Appendix B).

Table B.5 is in three parts for values of n_1 of (a) 1–9, (b) 10–17, (c) 18–25. Firstly choose the appropriate part of the table depending on the value of n_1. For each range of values of n_1 there are four pages of tables, one for each of the two-sided (one-sided) significance levels of $0 \cdot 10(0 \cdot 05)$, $0 \cdot 05(0 \cdot 025)$, $0 \cdot 02(0 \cdot 01)$ and $0 \cdot 01(0 \cdot 005)$. Having chosen the required significance level the lower (T_l) and the upper (T_u) critical values for the sample sizes in group 1 (n_1) and in group 2 (n_2) can be read from the table. If the test statistic T_1 is greater than or equal to T_u or less than or equal to T_l a significant result can be claimed.

In the example the controls were labelled as group 1 and $T_1 = 49 \cdot 5$. The lower and upper critical 5% two-sided values are, for $n_1 = 8$ and $n_2 = 9$, $T_l = 51$ and $T_u = 93$. The sum of ranks at $49 \cdot 5$ is less than T_l so there is a significant difference between the blood pressures of the two groups. Since T_1 is less than the lower critical value, it can be concluded that the blood pressure of controls is less than that of the diabetic patients.

Unfortunately however, as with many non-parametric tests, no direct measure of the magnitude of the difference between the groups is available, and it is necessary to rely on, perhaps, the examination of group means or medians to determine the importance of a given result. With the t test, on the other hand, the magnitude of the difference between the two groups, $\bar{X}_1 - \bar{X}_2$, entered directly into the calculation of the test statistic.

The main assumption for the Wilcoxon test is that there is an underlying continuous distribution of the variable of interest (even if the measurements are only on an ordinal scale). In essence, the test compares the two distributions in their entirety, so it is a valid test for the comparison of means or medians. It is nearly as powerful as the parametric t test, even when all the assumptions for that test are valid, and when the assumptions do not hold it is always to be preferred. There are some slight problems if there are many ties in the data, but the test as outlined should be adequate for most practical situations. The application of the test is summarized in Appendix C, Section C.6.

7.6 Comparison of means in paired samples: the paired t test

When data have been collected on pairs of individuals, and each member of one of the groups has a match or pair in the other group, the independent t test cannot be used. The statistical analysis must take account of how the data were collected. Suppose that a study on the effect of a particular drug on pulse rate is performed on 8 volunteers; their pulses are measured before and after the administration of the drug, giving the data shown in Table 7.3. The mean pulse rate prior to drug administration is 67·0 beats per minute and afterwards it has increased to 70·375 beats per minute. One point to note is that in any paired situation such as this the sample sizes in the two groups must necessarily be the same.

The approach to hypothesis testing in a paired situation is to take advantage of the fact that observations in the groups come in pairs. If, under the null hypothesis, the means of the two populations (pulse rates before and after administration of the drug) are the same, then the mean of the

Table 7.3 The paired t test. Pulse rates in 8 subjects before and after administration of a drug.

Subject (pair)	Pulse rate (beats/min)		
	Before drug	After drug	After minus before d
1	58	66	8
2	65	69	4
3	68	75	7
4	70	68	−2
5	66	73	7
6	75	75	0
7	62	68	6
8	72	69	−3
mean	67·0	70·375	3·375($\bar{d}$)

$t = 2\cdot167$; $d.f. = 7$; NS

differences calculated on a sample of pairs of individuals should be close to 0. Column 4 of Table 7.3 shows the differences in the pulse rates calculated by subtracting the 'before' reading from the 'after' reading. The mean of these differences denoted $\bar{d}$ is 3·375, which is the same as the difference between the means of the original two groups, 67·0 and 70·375 beats per minute. This is a general result, that the mean of the differences is the same as the difference of the means.

For the analysis of a paired experiment attention should be focused on the column of differences, essentially reducing the situation to a single sample of differences. The null hypothesis states that the population mean difference should be 0 and so, using an adaptation of the one-sample test (Eqn. 6.6), an appropriate test statistic for the paired situation is

$$t = \frac{\bar{d} - 0}{S_d / \sqrt{n}} \tag{7.8}$$

on $n-1$ degrees of freedom. $\bar{d}$ is the observed mean of the differences, and the 0 in the formula is the hypothesized value for the mean population difference. S_d is nothing more than the standard deviation of the differences calculated in the usual manner. Note though, that if any of the differences have a minus sign, this must be taken into account, and also that zero differences should be included. n is the number of pairs in the entire study, which, of course, is the number of calculated differences. There are $n-1$ degrees of freedom since, essentially, the paired data have been reduced to a one-sample situation, with n observations of differences.

The mean of the figures in column 4 of Table 7.3 is $\bar{d} = 3·375$ and the standard deviation can be calculated as $S_d = 4·406$. With n equal to 8

$$t = \frac{3·375}{4·406 / \sqrt{8}} = 2·167$$

There are seven degrees of freedom and it will be assumed that a two-sided test at a 5% level of significance is to be performed. The critical 5% value for a two-sided t test on 7 degrees of freedom is 2·365 (Table B.3) and since the calculated t of 2·167 does not exceed this value a statistically significant result cannot be claimed. Although the drug increased the mean pulse rate by over 3 beats per minute in the subjects studied, this could be a spurious result due to sampling variation.

A confidence interval for the mean difference between the pulse rates can be calculated using

$$\bar{d} \pm t_c S_d / \sqrt{n} \tag{7.9}$$

where $S_d / \sqrt{n}$ is the standard error of the mean difference. In the example the 95% confidence interval turns out to be

3·375 $\pm$ 2·365 (1·558)

This gives confidence limits of -0.31 and 7.06 beats per minute; thus the confidence interval includes 0 as might have been expected from the result of the significance test.

The approach to this analysis of paired quantitative data is to reduce the two sets of observations to one set of differences, and the assumption underlying the use of the paired t test is that the distribution of differences in the population is not markedly skewed. The assumption required for the independent t test of equal population standard deviations is not required, since there is now only one population of differences. Section C.7 (Appendix C) summarizes these calculations.

7.7 Comparison of medians in paired samples: the sign test

An alternative to the parametric paired t test is the non-parametric *sign test*. Essentially, this examines the null hypothesis that the medians in the two populations are the same, and it is an exceptionally easy test to perform. As with the Wilcoxon rank sum test, the data may be quantitative or ordinal, but an underlying continuous distribution is assumed.

Suppose that the reactions of 10 patients to two different analgesics (A and B) have been studied, with the patients rating the effectiveness of each preparation on a scale from 0 to 9. On the basis of these scores, it is necessary to determine which analgesic might be judged more effective. The results of this study are laid out in Table 7.4. It can be seen immediately that analgesic A is superior to B according to 8 of the persons studied. They are scored equally by one person, and another person judges B to be superior to

Table 7.4 The sign test (paired data). Scores assigned by 10 patients to two analgesics A and B.

Patient (pair)	Analgesic A	Analgesic B	Sign of $A - B$
1	2	2	0
2	4	3	+
3	7	4	+
4	3	0	+
5	0	1	−
6	3	2	+
7	6	4	+
8	4	2	+
9	5	4	+
10	8	6	+

$n_+ = $ number of '+' signs $= 8$; $n = $ number of untied pairs $= 9$;
$p < 0.05$

A. If the median effects of the two analgesics were the same, it would be expected that, on average, half the persons would prefer A and the other half would prefer B; the sign test is, in fact, based on the number of preferences for one drug over the other, the superior drug being likely to have more preferences.

A preference (or superiority of one drug over the other) can be detected by the sign of the difference between the measured scores, a plus sign, say, representing a preference for A, and a minus sign a preference for B. Tied results (e.g. subject number 1 who scored both drugs with a 2) must be ignored, and the number of preferences or 'pluses' denoted by n_+ should be recorded. In this case $n_+ = 8$, out of 9 untied pairs. This number of preferences can be referred to critical values for the sign test, which depend on the number of untied pairs (n) and, as usual, on the significance level for the chosen one- or two-sided test. Table B.6 in Appendix B gives the lower (S_l) and upper (S_u) critical values. For $n = 9$, the two-sided 5% critical values are 1 and 8, and in this example n_+ at 8 is equal to the upper critical value. Thus, it can be concluded that there are more preferences for analgesic A in this study than could reasonably have arisen by chance, and a significant result can be claimed at the 5% level.

Note that this test does not, by its nature, take any account of the magnitude of the differences between the groups. The example shows, however, that small differences in a consistent direction, even with a small sample size, can lead to significant results. Section C.8 of Appendix C summarizes the applications of the sign test.

7.8 Comparison of medians in paired samples: the Wilcoxon signed rank test

The non-parametric sign test for paired data described in the previous section took account only of the sign of the differences between the observations in the two groups, and took no cognizance of the magnitude of these differences. The test described below is more powerful than the sign test, in that the magnitude of the differences contributes to the test statistic.

The *Wilcoxon signed rank test* will be illustrated on the same data employed for the paired t test — the difference in pulse rates before and after administration of a drug (see Table 7.3). As with the paired t test (Section 7.6) the first step is to calculate the difference between the values for each pair ('after minus before' values). The next step is to rank these differences from smallest to largest, ignoring the sign of the difference. This is done in Table 7.5. As usual, tied ranks are given the average of the ranks that would have been given if the values were not tied. Note that the zero difference on subject 6 is not included for the purpose of ranking. (In the paired t test, this

Table 7.5 The Wilcoxon signed rank test (paired data).
Differences between pulse rates before and after
administration of a drug (see Table 7.3).

Subject (pair)	Difference* in pulse rates (after − before) beats/min d	Rank	Signed rank
6	0	—	—
4	−2	1	−1
8	−3	2	−2
2	4	3	3
7	6	4	4
3	7	5·5	5·5
5	7	5·5	5·5
1	8	7	7

*Ordered by magnitude.

T_+ = sum of positive ranks = 25; n = number of united pairs = 7;
NS

zero difference did contribute to the test statistic.) Thus, the observed
difference of −2 is given rank 1 and the difference of −3 is given rank 2. The
difference 4 is the next largest, and is given the rank of 3. The remainder of the
ranks are assigned similarly. Once the ranks have been calculated in this
manner, the sign of the difference is given back to each rank, to form the
signed ranks as shown in the last column of Table 7.5. The test statistic is then
taken as the sum of the positive ranks, which is denoted T_+ and is in this
example 25 $(3+4+5·5+5·5+7)$.

Again, this test statistic is intuitively reasonable. The null hypothesis states
that the distributions from which the two sets of observations are sampled are
identical and thus that the means, and/or medians, are the same. If this were
the case, the differences (d) should be symmetrical about 0; that is, there
should be as many negative differences as positive differences. Also, the sum
of the positive ranks (T_+) should be close in value to the sum of the negative
ranks, the sum of the ranks with the minus sign. If, however, the population
mean (or median) of the 'after' group was greater than that of the 'before'
group, there would be more positive differences, and thus T_+ would tend to
be larger than expected under the null hypothesis. Similarly, if the differences
were in the other direction T_+ would be smaller than expected. Table B.7 in
Appendix B gives the lower (T_l) and upper (T_u) critical values of T_+ for
different numbers of non-zero differences, since obviously these critical values
will depend on the total number of differences that were ranked. In the
example, there are 7 untied pairs, and T_+ is equal to 25. The critical values

for a 5% two-sided test are, from the table, 2 and 26; thus T_+ does not lie in the critical region, and, as with the paired t test, it must be concluded that the difference between the pulse rates before and after treatment with this particular drug is non-significant, and could be ascribed to chance.

Like many of the non-parametric tests considered so far, it is necessary to assume an underlying continuous distribution for the variable, and there should not be too many ties among the differences. Section C.9 in Appendix C summarizes the use of the sign test.

7.9 Comparison of two independent proportions: the Z test

In many medical investigations, the variable of interest is binary and takes on two values only. Thus, it might be required to compare the proportions or percentages alive or dead in two groups. In this and the following section, techniques for the comparison of proportions in two or more groups are described. This section deals with the comparison of proportions in two independent samples. As with the one-sample situation, the analysis here is in terms of proportions, and if working with percentages is preferred, translation back to this measure at the end of the analysis is suggested.

As an example, take the clinical trial discussed in Chapter 5, where the 5-year survival, expressed as a proportion, of the two treated groups, each of 25 subjects, was found to be 0·68 in those on drug A and 0·48 in those on drug B. Table 7.6 presents these data in a 2×2 table, often called a 2×2 *contingency table*. The test to be described for use in this type of situation is approximate, insofar as the normal distribution is being used to approximate the binomial distribution (see Section 6.9). For this reason, the applicability of the test is in doubt with small sample sizes. The test, however, is non-parametric in that it makes no assumptions in relation to the distribution of the variables being examined.

Table 7.6 Results of a clinical trial comparing survival in two drug-treated groups. (Proportions given in parentheses.)

	5-year outcome		Total
	Alive	Dead	
Drug A	17 (0·68)	8 (0·32)	25 (1·0)
Drug B	12 (0·48)	13 (0·52)	25 (1·0)
	29 (0·58)	21 (0·42)	50 (1·0)

$Z = 1·433$; NS

As with the two-sample test for means, the test statistic for the comparison of the two proportions is in the form

$$\frac{\text{Difference between the proportions}}{\text{SE (Difference)}} \tag{7.10}$$

The standard error of the difference between the two proportions depends on the value for the proportions specified by the null hypothesis. The null hypothesis specifies that the proportions in the two populations from which the samples were taken are the same. If, in the example quoted, survival is being analysed then letting π_1 and π_2 represent the population proportion of survivors in the drug A- and drug B-treated groups respectively,

$$H_0 : \pi_1 - \pi_2 = 0$$

or $\quad H_0 : \pi_1 = \pi_2$

If this common value for the proportion of survivors as specified by the null hypothesis is denoted π then it can be shown that

$$\text{SE}(p_1 - p_2) = \sqrt{\pi(1 - \pi)\left(\frac{1}{n_1} + \frac{1}{n_2}\right)} \tag{7.11}$$

where p_1 and p_2 are the observed proportions of survivors in samples size n_1 and n_2 taken from the two populations of interest, and $\text{SE}(p_1 - p_2)$ is the standard error of the difference between these two proportions. In practice, of course, this common value of π in the populations is not known and the best estimate of the quantity is the proportion of survivors observed in the two treated groups combined. In the example, there were 29 survivors in the two groups out of a total of 50 patients studied (see Table 7.6), so that the overall proportion of survivors is 29/50 or 0·58. Denoting this pooled value by p

$$\text{SE}(p_1 - p_2) = \sqrt{pq\left(\frac{1}{n_1} + \frac{1}{n_2}\right)} \tag{7.12}$$

where q is defined as $1 - p$.

Combining these results, the following test statistic is appropriate for testing the difference between proportions in independent samples

$$Z = \frac{p_1 - p_2}{\sqrt{pq\left(\frac{1}{n_1} + \frac{1}{n_2}\right)}} \tag{7.13}$$

This should be referred to tables of the standard normal distribution (Table B.2).

Substituting in the results in the clinical trial example, this equation becomes

$$Z = \frac{0.68 - 0.48}{\sqrt{0.58(0.42)\left(\dfrac{1}{25} + \dfrac{1}{25}\right)}} = 1.433$$

For a two-sided test at a 5% level of significance, the critical Z value is 1·96 and, since the calculated value of 1·433 is not greater than this, it must be concluded that the difference between the drug effects is not statistically significant. In fact, examining the table of the standard normal distribution, it can be seen that the p value is just greater than 10%.

In some texts, the estimate of the standard error of the difference between two proportions may be given as

$$SE(p_1 - p_2) = \sqrt{\frac{p_1 q_1}{n_1} + \frac{p_2 q_2}{n_2}} \tag{7.14}$$

This is an acceptable approximation so long as n_1 and n_2 are nearly equal and p_1 and p_2 do not differ substantially. This formula for the standard error results in a figure of 0·137 for the example, as opposed to a value of 0·140 obtained with the more exact expression given by Eqn. 7.12. The standard error formula given by Eqn. 7.14 should, however, be used for estimating confidence intervals for the difference between two proportions, and 95% or 99% confidence intervals are given by

$$(p_1 - p_2) \pm Z_c \sqrt{\frac{p_1 q_1}{n_1} + \frac{p_2 q_2}{n_2}} \tag{7.15}$$

where Z_c is the 5% or 1% critical value for the normal distribution. For example, the 95% confidence interval for the difference between the proportions alive on drug A and drug B is

$$0.2 \pm 1.96(0.137)$$

or from -0.069 to 0.469.

The conditions under which the normal distribution can be used as an approximation to the binomial are that the total sample size be greater than 20, and that $n_1 p$, $n_2 p$, $n_1 q$ and $n_2 q$ are all greater than 5 for sample sizes between 20 and 40. The approximation should be quite valid for a total sample size, that is in the two groups above 40. These criteria are satisfied in the example. If the criteria do not hold, then an exact test for the comparison of proportions based on the binomial distribution is available (see Section 7.11). The Z test for independent proportions is summarized in Section C.10 of Appendix C.

7.10 Comparison of two independent proportions: the χ^2 test

A more common alternative to the Z test discussed in the last section is to employ a χ^2 test to compare differences between two independent proportions. This test is easier to apply, but the computational approach, though mathematically equivalent, is quite different.

The data are laid out in a 2×2 table, and the test statistic is based on the observed and expected (under the null hypothesis) frequencies in each of the four cells of the table. It is essential, however, that the actual numbers in the cells are used rather than the percentages or proportions. Table 7.7 shows the results obtained when cigarette smoking in a group of 150 patients with an upper respiratory tract infection (URTI) is compared with that of a control group of 140 patients without URTI. The aim is to determine if

Table 7.7 The χ^2 test. Smoking status in 150 patients with upper respiratory tract infection (URTI) compared to 140 controls.

Observed numbers

	URTI	Controls	Total
Smokers	95 (63·3%)	70 (50·0%)	165 (56·9%)
Non-smokers	55 (36·7%)	70 (50·0%)	125 (43·1%)
	150 (100·0%)	140 (100·0%)	290 (100·0%)

Expected numbers

	URTI	Controls	Total
Smokers	85·345	79·655	165
Non-smokers	64·655	60·345	125
	150	140	290

Observed O	Expected E	$O-E$	$(O-E)^2$	$(O-E)^2/E$
95	83·345	9·655	93·219	1·092
55	64·655	−9·655	93·219	1·442
70	79·655	9·655	93·219	1·170
70	60·345	−9·655	93·219	1·545
				5·249

$$\chi^2 = 5\cdot249; \quad d.f. = 1; \quad p < 0\cdot05$$

smoking is associated with URTI or, equivalently, if there is a difference in the proportion of smokers amongst the population of URTI patients and the comparison population. As in previous examples, it will be assumed that the comparison is valid, and that the design of the study has been adequate. It is important, however, that the two samples should have been independently chosen. The null hypothesis then states that the proportion of smokers in each group is the same.

The first step in applying the test which is being considered is to calculate the numbers of people expected to be observed in the four cells of the table if, in fact, the null hypothesis were true. If there really is no difference between the groups, it would be expected that the proportion of smokers observed in the total sample, $165/290 = 0.5690$, would be seen in each of the groups; thus out of 150 cases of URTI it would be expected that $0.5690 \times 150 = 85.345$ individuals would be smokers. Similarly, for the controls, $0.5690 \times 140 = 79.655$ persons would be expected to be smokers. Now, the overall proportion of non-smokers in the two groups combined is $125/290 = 0.4310$, so that in 150 cases of URTI $0.4310 \times 150 = 64.655$ non-smokers are expected and a similar calculation leads to 60.345 expected non-smokers in the comparison group.

The middle of Table 7.7 shows these expected numbers filled into the corresponding cells of a 2×2 table. Note that when these expected numbers are added up across the rows and columns, the same total numbers of cases and controls and smokers and non-smokers as were in the original table are obtained. This is an important property of the expected numbers, and it can be seen that, in fact, for such a table only one of the expected numbers need be calculated and that all the others may be obtained by subtracting from the totals at the edge of the table (the marginal totals).* In practice, it is advisable to calculate all the expected values, and to check the calculation by ensuring that they do add up to the original totals. It is usually sufficient to keep to three decimal places in the calculation.

Once the expected numbers have been calculated in this way, the significance test is fairly straightforward. Obviously, the greater the difference between the observed and the expected figures, the more evidence there is to reject the null hypothesis. The test statistic is based on this observation, and also includes a factor to allow for the relative magnitude of these differences (e.g. a difference of 10 is much more striking if it arises from values of 30 and 20 than from values of 310 and 300). The test statistic used is

$$\chi^2 = \sum \frac{(O-E)^2}{E} \qquad (7.16)$$

---

* This is another example of degrees of freedom. Once one expected value is calculated in a 2×2 table, the other three are predetermined, and such a table is said to have one degree of freedom.

where the Os are the four observed numbers in the body of the table and the Es are the four expected numbers. Summation is over the four cells of the table. The bottom of Table 7.7 illustrates the calculation of this sum which turns out to be 5·249. Note that the magnitude of the $O - E$ quantities is the same for each cell of the table in the 2×2 case but this is not so for larger tables. (The sum of the $O - E$ quantities is always 0 however.)

5·249 is then referred to tables of the χ^2 distribution on one degree of freedom (Table B.4). Note that the chi-square test statistic as calculated must always have a positive sign, and unlike the other tests considered so far, it does not indicate which of the groups has the larger proportion. The critical values given in the χ^2 table must be *exceeded* for a significant result.* The two-sided critical value for χ^2 with one degree of freedom is 3·841 for a 5% level of significance, and since the calculated value of 5·249 is greater than this, it can be concluded that there is a significant difference in the proportion of smokers among the URTI cases and controls. The exact same result would have been obtained if the methods of the last section, using the Z test, had been employed. Which test to use is quite arbitrary, though the χ^2 test is by far the most popular. Although it does not enable confidence intervals to be calculated, it has the great advantage, as is seen in Section 7.12, that the method extends to tables larger than 2×2.

The applicability of the χ^2 test for 2×2 tables depends on the same criteria as used in the Z test, which can be restated in terms of the expected values. For total sample sizes less than 20, it is advisable that a more exact test should be used (see next section). For sample sizes between 20 and 40, the test is quite valid as long as none of the expected frequencies falls below 5. For sample sizes greater than 40, there should be no problem with the use of the χ^2 test. The application of this test is summarized in Appendix C, Section C.11.

7.11 Comparison of two independent proportions: Fisher's exact test

As has been pointed out, the χ^2 test is not valid whenever the expected frequency in any of the cells in a 2×2 table falls below 5. In this case, an exact test is available called *Fisher's exact test*. Unlike all the other significance tests so far described, this test involves the calculation of the p value directly, without the use of a particular test statistic. Of all the tests encountered, Fisher's exact test is, without any doubt, the most difficult to calculate but,

---

* The χ^2 table gives both one- and two-sided critical values for various significance levels. The one-sided critical values, however, do not refer to areas in one tail of the χ^2 distribution, but the interpretation of a one-sided test is as described before. The one-sided test is really only valid for the 2×2 tables being considered in this section.

nonetheless, is useful in many situations, and the computational method is outlined below.

The χ^2 test for a 2×2 table has been described as a test for the comparison of proportions in two independent samples. In such a situation, the numbers of individuals in each sample are determined by the investigator, and thus, depending on the layout of the table, the column totals are fixed while the row totals are free to vary according to the results of the study.

The χ^2 test, however, may also be used where one sample is classified by two binary variables; thus, the numbers of smokers and non-smokers in males and females in a single sample from a population might be examined. In this case, both the row totals and the column totals are free to vary; they are determined by the sex and smoking distributions in the sample, and are not fixed in advance of the study. The only quantity fixed is the total sample size. The χ^2 test is also appropriate for 2×2 tables arising in this manner. It is also possible that in a 2×2 table both the row and column totals are fixed beforehand by the investigator. This type of situation rarely arises in medical applications, but again the χ^2 test is appropriate.

Now Fisher's exact test is in fact based on fixed row and column totals, and so, theoretically, is not applicable to 2×2 tables arising from either the two-sample or one-sample situations described above. However, the test is often used in these cases also, with the proviso that it is conditional on (i.e. assumes) fixed row and column totals (fixed marginals), and, in practice, will not give misleading results where the χ^2 test is inapplicable due to small sample sizes.

Underlying the approach to all hypothesis tests is the distribution of a specific test statistic, and the calculation of the area (areas) — corresponding to probabilities — in the tail(s) of the distribution cut off by the test statistic actually calculated on the basis of the observed results. In Fisher's exact test, the distribution of all possible 2×2 tables with the same fixed column and row totals as the one observed in the study are examined. The probability of obtaining each of these tables, if there is no relationship between the two factors being studied, can be calculated. For a general 2×2 table laid out as shown in Table 7.8, this probability is

$$P = \frac{r_1! \, r_2! \, s_1! \, s_2!}{n! \, a! \, b! \, c! \, d!} \tag{7.17}$$

The letters r and s with the subscripts refer to the row and column totals, and a, b, c and d are the numbers in each of the cells; n is the total sample size. The exclamation mark denotes 'factorial' and means successive multiplication of the integers in descending order, thus $5! = 5 \times 4 \times 3 \times 2 \times 1 = 120$. $0!$ is defined as equal to 1.

Now, to calculate a p value for Fisher's exact test, it is necessary to add up the probabilities of the observed table, and any even more unlikely ones, in

Table 7.8 Fisher's exact test: general layout for a 2×2 table and its exact probability (p).

| a | b | r_1 |
c	d	r_2
s_1	s_2	n

$$p = \frac{r_1!\, r_2!\, s_1!\, s_2!}{n!\, a!\, b!\, c!\, d!}$$

the tail of the distribution of all possible tables. This will give a one-sided test if only tables showing a more extreme result than that actually obtained are included, which at the same time also suggest the same direction of difference in the result. A two-sided test is obtained by doubling the one-sided p value.

Suppose that 16 elderly insulin-dependent patients with diabetes mellitus were studied and that 6 of these were classified as having had poor diabetic control during their illness. The patients were also examined to determine if they suffered any of the long-term complications of diabetes, such as deteriorating eyesight or circulatory problems. Table 7.9a displays these results in a 2×2 table. The aim is to determine if good control of diabetes is associated with a lower rate of complications. Among the 7 patients with complications, 4 or 57.1% had poor control, while among the 9 patients without complications, only 2 or 22.2% could be so classified. Thus, on the basis of the sample results, there seems to be an association between the two factors, but is it statistically significant? The χ^2 test cannot be used here, since the sample size is less than 20 and 3 of the 4 expected frequencies are less than 5; Fisher's exact test should be employed instead.

The easiest way to apply Fisher's exact test is firstly to rearrange the observed 2×2 table so that the number in the top left cell is the smallest of the observed cell frequencies. In this example the smallest cell frequency is 2, and the rearranged table is shown in Table 7.9b. Labelling the table by the number in the top left cell, this is called set 2. The tables with more extreme results are then obtained by successively reducing the top left figure by 1 with the remainder of the table determined by the fact that the row and column totals are fixed. This process is repeated until a table with a top left cell having a 0 entry is obtained. In the example, set 1, with a 1 in the top left cell, has 5, 8 and 2 in the other three cells determined by the fixed rows and columns (Table 7.9c). This table has more extreme results in the same direction as the original, in that only 1/9 (11.1%) of those with no complications had poor diabetic control compared to 22.2% in the original table. The final set in the example, set 0 with a zero in the top left, has again even more extreme results.

Table 7.9   Fisher's exact test: diabetic control and complications in 16 patients.

(a) Original table

Diabetic control	Diabetic complications		Total
	Present	Absent	
Good	3 (42·9%)	7 (77·8%)	10 (62·5%)
Poor	4 (57·1%)	2 (22·2%)	6 (37·5%)
	7 (100·0%)	9 (100·0%)	16 (100·0%)

(b) Rearranged table (set 2)

Diabetic control	Diabetic complications		Total
	Absent	Present	
Poor	2	4	6
Good	7	3	10
	9	7	16

(c) Set 1

1	5	6	
8	2	10	
9	7	16	

(d) Set 0

0	6	6	
9	1	10	
9	7	16	

The one-sided p value for the test is now obtained by summing the probabilities of these three sets or tables. In general, the number of such tables will be one more than the smallest frequency observed in any cell of the original. The probability of set 0 is calculated first. Using Eqn. 7.17,

$$P = \frac{6!\ 10!\ 9!\ 7!}{16!\ 0!\ 6!\ 9!\ 1!}$$

and cancelling this reduces to (using the subscript 0 to denote the set)

$$P_0 = \frac{10!\ 7!}{16!\ 1!}$$

This probability can be computed directly by cancelling a little more, noting that $10!/16! = 1/(16 \times 15 \times 14 \times 13 \times 12 \times 11)$. Calculated in this manner, $P_0 = 0\cdot0008741$.* If some of the numbers are fairly large, tables of log

---

* Many small calculators now have a factorial key, which can make this calculation even easier.

factorials may be employed. Table B.8 gives the logarithms of all the factorials from 0 to 99. From this table, $\log P_0 = \log 10! + \log 7! - \log 16!$ $- \log 1! = 6.55976 + 3.70243 - 13.32062 - 0.0 = -3.05843$. The decimal part of this log value must be positive to get the antilog from a table, so that $\log P_0 = \bar{4}.94157 \, (-4.0 + 0.94157)$. The 0.94157 must now be looked up in an antilog table* (Table B.9) where its antilog is found to be 8.742. Thus, the antilog of $\bar{4}.94157$ is 0.0008742 which is almost identical to the value previously obtained for P_0.

Once P_0 (the probability of set 0) is calculated, the probabilities for the remaining sets (if any) are easily obtained. If the four entries in the body of set i, where i is any number, are denoted as a_i, b_i, c_i and d_i then

$$P_{i+1} = P_i \times \frac{b_1 \times c_i}{a_{i+1} \times d_{i+1}} \tag{7.18}$$

That is, to obtain the probability of a set it is necessary to multiply the probability of the previous set by b and c from that set and divide by a and d from the new set. Thus

$$P_1 = P_0 \times \frac{6 \times 9}{1 \times 2} = 0.0236007$$

$$P_2 = P_1 \times \frac{8 \times 5}{2 \times 3} = 0.157338$$

In this case, $P_0 + P_1 + P_2 = 0.1818$. Under the assumption of fixed rows and columns, and independence of the two factors being studied, this is the probability that the result, or one even more extreme, is spurious. This, of course, defines the one-sided p value and the two-sided value is obtained by doubling this figure (0.3636). Thus, in this example, diabetic complications are not significantly associated with poor control (Fisher's exact test; two-sided; $p = 0.36$).

As can be seen, this test is quite complex to perform, but a little practice does help. Section C.12 in Appendix C summarizes the steps involved.

7.12 Comparison of many proportions in two or more samples: the χ^2 test

In Section 7.10 the use of the χ^2 test for analysing independent data laid out in a 2×2 table was described. In many cases, however, data will be laid out in a larger table than a 2×2. Either a qualitative variable with perhaps more than 2 categories is to be compared in two or more independent samples, or the relationship between two qualitative variables is being examined in one sample. (The discussion in the previous section on Fisher's exact test drew

*Looking up 0.9416.

attention to such situations in a 2×2 context.) The χ^2 test is the appropriate test to employ for such tables larger than 2×2 also.

The use of the χ^2 test for a 3×2 table with three rows and two columns will be illustrated. Chapter 1, Table 1.1, gave the smoking status of males and females in a study of 2724 persons, and is reproduced in Table 7.10. The null hypothesis in this case would be that the distribution of smoking category is the same in males and females. The figures in the table suggest a definite difference, and with such a large sample size it could be presumed that the observed result actually does reflect a population difference between males and females. For illustrative purposes however, a χ^2 test will be performed on these data. The approach is identical to that used in the 2×2 table. Firstly, the expected numbers (E) under the null hypothesis are calculated. For instance, since there were *in toto* 1168 current smokers from a total of 2724 persons ($42 \cdot 9\%$) this percentage of males would be expected to be current smokers; $42 \cdot 9\%$ of 1353 males is $580 \cdot 14$ which is the expected number of male smokers. All the other expected numbers may be calculated in a similar manner, and are also given in Table 7.10. In general, to calculate the expected number in any cell, multiply the corresponding row total by the corresponding column total and divide by the total sample size. Thus, the expected number of male smokers can be obtained from $1168 \times 1353/2724 = 580 \cdot 14$. Note that in this example, once two of the expected numbers in a particular column are calculated, the remainder follow by subtraction from the row and column totals which remain fixed as usual.* It is suggested however that each expected number be calculated directly as above, and that a check on the calculations be made by confirming that they do add up to the correct row and column totals.

Once the expected numbers are calculated, the quantities $(O - E)^2/E$ are determined as before for each cell of the table, where O represents the observed numbers in the cells. (Note again that the $O - E$ quantities should sum to zero, apart from rounding errors.) The test statistic is then

$$\chi^2 = \sum \frac{(O - E)^2}{E} \tag{7.16}$$

as in the 2×2 table, but with two degrees of freedom in this example. In general, for a table with I rows and J columns there are $(I - 1)(J - 1)$ degrees of freedom which, with $I = 3$ and $J = 2$, is 2 degrees of freedom here, and of course 1 degree of freedom for a 2×2 table. In the smoking example, an extremely large value for χ^2 of $137 \cdot 579$ is obtained which, when referred to Table B.4 on two degrees of freedom, is seen to be highly significant. Unless the sample size is very large, χ^2 values of this magnitude are most unusual.

---

* In the light of the discussion of the 2×2 table in Section 7.10 it can be said that a 2×3 table has two degrees of freedom.

Table 7.10 The χ^2 test. Smoking status by sex in 2724 persons (see Table 1.1). O'Connor & Daly (1983) with permission.

(a) Observed numbers

	Male	Female	Total
Current smokers	669 (49·5%)	499 (36·4%)	1168 (42·9%)
Ex-smokers	328 (24·2%)	215 (15·7%)	543 (19·9%)
Non-smokers	356 (26·3%)	657 (47·9%)	1013 (37·2%)
	1353 (100·0%)	1371 (100·0%)	2724 (100·0%)

(b) Expected numbers

	Male	Female	Total
Current smokers	580·14	587·86	1168
Ex-smokers	269·71	273·29	543
Non-smokers	503·15	509·85	1013
	1353	1371	2724

(c) Calculation

Observed O	Expected E	$O - E$	$(O - E)^2$	$(O - E)^2/E$
669	580·14	88·86	7896·100	13·611
328	269·71	58·29	3397·724	12·598
356	503·15	− 147·15	21653·123	43·035
499	587·86	− 88·86	7896·100	13·432
215	273·29	− 58·29	3397·724	12·433
657	509·85	147·15	21653·123	42·470
				137·579

$$\chi^2 = 137 \cdot 579; \ d.f. = 2; \ p < 0 \cdot 001$$

Note that for tables larger than the 2×2 a one-sided χ^2 test is not applicable, since it is impossible to specify beforehand, or indeed interpret, a one-sided alternative hypothesis.

The χ^2 test can be employed so long as not more that 20% of the expected numbers in the cells are less than 5, with no cell having an expected frequency of less than 1. In the 2×2 situation, of course, this requires that all the expected numbers are greater than 5, which was the condition given already for this case.

Often, a quantitative variable, such as age, is categorized into, say, 'young', 'middle-aged' and 'old' and a χ^2 test rather than a parametric t test employed.

Obviously, a fair amount of the information obtained in a set of data is lost with a categorization such as this, but a χ^2 test is easier to perform than a t test, and avoids its parametric assumptions. However, the cut-off points for such categorizations must be selected carefully and they should be chosen before the data are analysed. The χ^2 test, however, is perhaps the most widely employed test in medical research, and the fact that it extends easily, as discussed here, to the comparison of more than two groups makes it one of the most useful tests to know. Its application is summarized in Section C.11 of Appendix C.

7.13 Comparison of paired proportions: the McNemar test

The tests for proportions in the previous sections assume that the groups being compared are independent. In this section, a simple test for use with paired samples, where the variable under examination is binary, is described. The test is sometimes called a test for correlated proportions.

Suppose that 18 patients on two different antihypertensive drugs were studied. Each patient was given either drug A or drug B for a one-month period, and a drop in systolic blood pressure of more than 15 mm Hg was considered a success, and a lesser drop or rise, a treatment failure. After a washout period the treatments were switched around so that those previously on drug A were now given drug B and *vice versa*. The same criteria were again used to assess the effectiveness of the treatment. Essentially then, there exists a paired sample with each of the 18 patients on each of the two treatments, with the effectiveness of the drugs determined on a qualitative binary scale as either a success or failure.

Paired data like this are often incorrectly analysed. The tendency is to create a 2×2 table for the results as shown in Table 7.11a and perform the usual chi-square test on it. Unfortunately however, this is incorrect; the two groups (drug A and drug B) are not independent and the analysis must take this into account. The table, although suitable for the presentation of results, cannot be used for significance testing since the 18 persons on each treatment are the same. The analysis must be performed in terms of the 18 pairs of observations — the result on drug A and the result on drug B for each individual. This requires more information than is contained in Table 7.11a and a table must be formed for analysis purposes as shown in Table 7.11b. The entry in the top left cell of 1 means that 1 person (one of the pairs) had a success with both treatments. The entry of 3 means that 3 persons were treated successfully with drug B but unsuccessfully with drug A. Nine persons, on the other hand, had a successful outcome on drug A and not on drug B. In 5 persons, neither drug worked. When analysing correlated or paired proportions, the data must be laid out in this way. Table 7.12 shows

Table 7.11 The McNemar test. Outcome of a paired experiment on 18 patients.

(a) Summary of results

	Drug A	Drug B	Total
Success	10 (55·6%)	4 (22·2%)	14
Failure	8 (44·4%)	14 (77·8%)	22
	18 (100·0%)	18 (100·0%)	36

(b) Layout for test

		Drug A		Total
		Success	Failure	
Drug B	Success	1	3	4
	Failure	9	5	14
		10	8	18

$$\text{McNemar's } \chi^2 \text{ on 1 } d.f. = \frac{(9-3)^2}{9+3} = 3 \cdot 0; \text{ NS}$$

this general layout. The plus and minus signs can refer to whatever the binary outcome is in the particular data being analysed. McNemar's test for this type of data is truly one of the few tests that can be done in one's head. A χ^2 on one degree of freedom is calculated as

$$\chi^2 = \frac{(b-c)^2}{b+c} \tag{7.19}$$

In the example, $\chi^2 = 6^2/12 = 3 \cdot 0$. For a two-sided, 5% significance level, the critical χ^2 value is 3·841 (Table B.4) so that no significant difference can be claimed between the effects of the drugs.

Table 7.12 The McNemar test: general lay-out.

		Variable 1	
		+	−
Variable 2	+	a	b
	−	c	d

$$\text{McNemar's } \chi^2 \text{ on 1 } d.f.; \frac{(b-c)^2}{b+c}$$

Note that only the untied observations contribute to this test statistic. The persons (pairs) on whom the effects of the two drugs were the same (two successes or two failures) do not enter into the calculation. These are called tied pairs; only the untied pairs are used. An alternative analytical procedure for such data (*sequential analysis*) is discussed in Chapter 10.

For small sample sizes, a different test statistic can be used. The number of pairs with a preference for one drug rather than the other one can be referred to the table for the sign test (Table B.6) entered at *n* equal to the total number of untied pairs. Thus, in the example, the test statistic could be 9 (the number of pairs denoting a preference for drug A). For a 5% two-sided significance test for 12 untied pairs, the lower and upper critical values are 2 and 10. The test statistic falls within the acceptance region, and therefore the results are non-significant. The use of this exact test is advisable when the sample sizes in the statistical table are adequate, even although the χ^2 approach is much easier to perform. Section C.13 in Appendix C summarizes the steps for this test, and includes more details on the interpretation of one-sided tests.

7.14   More complex statistical techniques

So far, this chapter has concentrated on the comparison of two groups only, outlining the statistical tests for quantitative and qualitative (ordinal and nominal) data. The χ^2 test for independent proportions was the only test that could be extended to the analysis of three or more groups. The techniques discussed were also limited in that they were applicable only to independent or individually matched data. Mention has already been made in Section 7.2 of data that are not independent but not individually matched either. Techniques for the analysis of such data are beyond the scope of this text but *standardization methods*, similar to those used in vital statistics (see Chapter 11), can be employed. See also Chapter 9 on the analysis of case-control studies.

Comparisons of quantitative variables between more than two groups should not be carried out using the two-group *t* tests applied to each pair of groups. For this purpose a very powerful set of techniques, *analysis of variance*, often referred to as ANOVA, is available. Essentially, these techniques, despite their name, allow for the comparison of means in more than two groups or in groups defined by more than one qualitative variable. Analysis of variance is based on an *F* test (a variance ratio test) to compare the variances by examining their ratio. Neither tables of the *F* distribution (which has two different degrees of freedom) nor computational details are given in this text, and only a brief introduction is presented below.

Suppose two samples are taken, and their variances S_1^2 and S_2^2 are calculated, with $S_1^2 > S_2^2$. If $F = S_1^2/S_2^2$ (a variance ratio) is close to 1, it can be concluded that the two population variances are likely to be equal. In general, the greater the value of *F*, the greater the likelihood that the two population variances are not the same, and the value of F can be referred to tables of the F distribution, to determine if a statistically significant result has been obtained under the null hypothesis that the population variances were equal. The F test is, strictly, applicable only to samples drawn from normal populations but can be used if there are no marked departures from this assumption.

Having explained the F distribution and variance ratio test, the much more general analysis of variance can now be discussed. As has been said, despite its name and the use of the variance ratio test, analysis of variance is primarily concerned with comparing sample means. Suppose a random sample of 100 observations is selected from a population and the sample mean and variance calculated. The sample mean and variance are unbiased estimates of the population mean and variance. Now, suppose this sample is divided into four subsamples, and the mean and variance calculated for each subsample. If the observations are randomly allocated amongst the subsamples, each subsample may be regarded as a random sample from the same parent population; the means and variances of the four subsamples should be similar to one another and to the population mean and variance.

Now, suppose that the sample observations were not randomly allocated between the four subsamples but were allocated to particular subsamples or classes according to some criterion. For example, if the original sample of 100 referred to weights of males, 21 years of age and over, these 100 weights might be classified into groups using a criterion of occupation. It may now be asked, 'Does weight vary with occupation?' If there is no connection between weight and occupation, then each subsample may be regarded, as before, as a random sample from the same population. The properties of the subsamples should be consistent with one another. If, however, they are shown to be significantly different, it may be concluded that the subsamples were not random samples drawn from a homogeneous parent population, but, in fact, were drawn from different populations. In other words, there is a connection between weight and occupation.

To answer this sort of problem it is necessary to set up the null hypothesis that *the variation in sample values is independent of the method of classification*. The null hypothesis is then tested by analysing the variation in values *within* each subsample and the variation in values *between* subsamples. As a first step, the total variation in all the sample values is calculated. This is done by calculating the deviation of each sample value from the total sample mean, squaring the deviations and adding them together. This gives a measure of the total variation in all the sample values. This total variation can then be split into two components: the variation within subsamples or classes, and the variation between classes. The methods by which this is done need not be explained here, but the general method of approach is illustrated in Table 7.13.

Table 7.13 A random sample of 16 examination papers with results classified by examiner.

	Examiner 1	Examiner 2	Examiner 3
	74	74	76
	72	77	78
	71	73	79
	74	75	78
	74	76	76
			75
Mean	73	75	77

Is there evidence of a difference between the three examiners with respect to marking? To answer this the hypothesis is formulated that variations in marks are independent of the examiner concerned, and then this hypothesis is tested by an analysis of variance.

It will first be noted that there are variations in the marks obtained within groups, which is to be expected. It may also be noted that there are variations in marks obtained between groups, as indicated by the fact that the average marks obtained in each group are different. The means of the three groups are 73, 75 and 77 marks respectively. The total variation in marks may be considered to consist of two components, the variation within groups and the variation between groups. The total variation may then be broken down to show (1) the *within-sample variance* and (2) the *between-sample variance*.

The reasoning is now as follows: if the null hypothesis were true, then each group could be regarded as a random sample from the same parent population — that is, the population of marks obtained by all candidates. Consequently, the variation in marks between samples should not be significantly different from the variation in marks within samples. If the null hypothesis is true, the within-sample variance and the between-sample variance are both independent estimates of the same population variance. If it can be shown that the within-sample variance and the between-sample variance are significantly different, by means of the variance ratio test, then doubt is cast on the hypothesis that the three samples were drawn from the same parent population. It would be concluded that marks obtained are not independent of the examiner.

In this particular example, the between-sample variance is 21·9, while the within-sample variance is 2·3. It seems unlikely that these two variances can be estimates of the same population variance. $F = 21\cdot9/2\cdot3 = 9\cdot5$, and this can be shown to be significant at the 1% level. The hypothesis that the three samples have been drawn from the same population is rejected. The between-sample variance is too large in relation to the within-sample variance. The variation in marks is not independent of the examiner. Often, what is called an analysis of variance table is presented for such an analysis. In fact, however, this provides little insight into the actual results except to a professional statistician or to a reader very familiar with the technique.

In the simple example quoted above, the sample data are classified according to one criterion of classification — in this case, by examiner. The analysis is called a *one-way analysis of variance*. The technique, however, is easily extended to more than one criterion of classification, and it is possible to have two-way and three-way analyses of variance. For example, the two-way analysis of variance can be used to analyse individually matched data in more than two groups and to control for the effect of confounding variables (see below).

As a simple example of a single classification analysis of variance, a study of 153 medical students will be taken, relating the score obtained in their university entrance examination to the results in their premedical (1st year) examination. Table 7.14 shows these results. The value of the F statistic (note the degrees of freedom are 4 and 148) is given below the table, and it can be concluded that premedical results are significantly related to the score in the university entrance examination.

An important assumption underlying analysis of variance is that the variances in the groups being compared are the same (homoscedasticity), and that there is a normal or near-normal distribution in the groups being analysed. If these assumptions do not hold, either a transformation of the data or a non-parametric test must be used. For independent groups, the non-parametric *Kruskall–Wallis test* is appropriate, and for individually

Table 7.14　Analysis of variance: university entrance examination score related to the results of the premedical examination in 153 medical students. Abbreviated from Horgan, Daly, Bourke & Wilson-Davis (1978) with permission.

Premedical category	Average entrance examination score
Failed each time	14·1
Failed twice only	14·9
Failed once only	12·6
Passed 1st time	17·4
Honours 1st time	22·1

$F = 19.58$; *d.f.* = 4, 148; $p < 0.001$

matched data the *Friedman test* can be employed. More advanced texts will
have to be consulted for these techniques.

7.15 Confounding in group comparisons

Thus far, the emphasis has been on the comparison of a single variable in two
or more groups. The first rule of any comparison is that like must be
compared with like — apart from the factor that distinguishes the groups in
the first place. Often, however, the distribution of variables other than the one
of interest will be different in the groups being compared and it may be
necessary to correct for this. To take a simple example: suppose that in a
study the blood pressure of males is seen to be much higher than that of
females. Suppose also that the males are much older than the females. Can it
be concluded that there is really a male/female difference in blood pressure or
could the observed difference be due to the fact that the males were older and
that blood pressure increases with age? Age may be a *confounder* of the
association between blood pressure and sex and, ideally, an analysis that can
'adjust', 'correct' or 'control' for age should be used, rather than the usual *t*
test, which cannot do this.

Statistical techniques are available to control for the effect of confounding
variables in group comparisons and in any such comparisons the possible
biasing effects of confounders should be examined. Some of the techniques
employed are indicated here. To be a confounder, a variable must have
different distributions in the groups being compared and must, at the same
time, be related to the primary variable of interest. Age is likely to be a
confounder in the example since it has a different distribution in males and
females and is also related to blood pressure.

One way to control for the confounding effect of age in the example would
be to examine the relationship between blood pressure and sex in, say, three
different age groups. If, in each of the three age groups, the males did have a
higher blood pressure than females then the original result would hold up. If,
on the other hand, males and females had more or less equal blood pressures
in each age group, the original result would be considered as a consequence of
the confounding effect of age. An adjusted comparison between blood
pressures in males and females would be obtained by some sort of averaging
of the differences observed in each of the three age groups. When, as in this
example, the primary variable of interest is quantitative and the confounder is
qualitative or has been grouped, then a two-way analysis of variance can be
performed which would compare the blood pressure between males and
females, adjusted for the effect of the grouped variable age. More than one
qualitative counfounding variable can be adjusted for in this way.

If it is desired to adjust for a quantitative confounder without categorizing it, then what is called an *analysis of covariance* can be carried out. The analysis of covariance will also facilitate the comparison of quantitative variables between groups while adjusting for the effects of any number of both qualitative and quantitative variables. This is, thus, a generalization of the analysis of variance.

If a qualitative variable is being compared between two or more groups, the χ^2 test would be used in the absence of confounders. If a potential confounder is present, it is usually grouped (if not grouped already), comparisons are made within each category of the confounder and an adjusted comparison obtained by averaging the differences obtained in each category. This is basically a standardization technique borrowed from vital statistics and the appropriate adjusted significance tests are based on techniques to combine χ^2 tests across the categories defined by the confounder.

Other techniques to control for confounding in group comparisons are available but are not discussed here. Regression techniques can be employed (see Chapter 8) and it is also seen in later chapters that confounding can be controlled in the design of an investigation, rather than in the analysis stage.

7.16 Summary

In this chapter an overview was given of the more common statistical tests employed in the comparison of two or more groups. The distinction between independent and individually matched data was made, and it was explained how this affects the significance test to be applied. The computational details for the more common two-sample tests were given, with appropriate examples, and details of non-parametric alternatives were also presented. A final section discussed the control of confounding in group comparisons. Table 7.15 illustrates the different tests discussed. Computational details of tests marked with an asterisk are not given in the text, and the χ^2 test is the only one detailed which is suitable for the comparison of more than two groups. It should be remembered that tests on quantitative data imply a comparison of means, tests on ordinal data imply a comparison of medians, and tests on nominal data, a comparison of percentages or proportions. It should also be stressed that statistical tests form a hierarchy, in that tests for nominal data can be applied to ordinal or quantitative data and that tests for ordinal data can be applied to quantitative data also. If quantitative data are ranked or ordered, then tests for ordinal data may be employed, and if ordinal or quantitative data are categorized into two or perhaps three groups, tests for nominal data, such as the chi-square, are appropriate.

A point that must be made is that it is not legitimate to apply all the possible valid tests to a given set of data and then to choose, for presentation

Table 7.15 Summary of statistical tests discussed in Chapter 7.

Type of data	Comparison of 2 groups		Comparison of > 2 groups	
	Independent	Matched	Independent	Matched
Quantitative	t test	Paired t test	One-way analysis of variance*	Two-way analysis of variance*
Qualitative (ordinal or ranked)	Wilcoxon rank sum test	Sign test Wilcoxon signed rank test	Kruskal–Wallis test*	Friedman's test*
Qualitative (nominal; 2 categories)	Z test χ^2 test Fisher's exact test	McNemar's test	χ^2 test	—
Qualitative (nominal; > 2 categories)	χ^2 test	—	χ^2 test	—

*Computational details not given in this text.

purposes, the one that gives a significant result. The most appropriate test must be chosen beforehand, and its results accepted.

It is hoped that this chapter will prove useful to researchers who wish to analyse their own data. Appendix C outlines, in step-by-step form, the computational details for all the tests described, and Appendix B provides a useful set of statistical tables. Beware however that different texts may give the statistical tables in a different format, and that the actual test statistic for a given test, particularly one of the non-parametric ones, may differ slightly from book to book. For this reason, it is advisable to become familiar with one particular set of tables, and the appropriate test statistic.

CHAPTER 8
Regression and Correlation

8.1 Introduction

The previous chapter of this book showed how one could statistically analyse differences between groups as regards quantitative variables (comparing mean values) and qualitative variables (comparing percentages or proportions). Such a comparison of two or more groups can be viewed as an examination of the association or relationship between two variables, one of which is qualitative and defined by group membership. If, for instance, the proportions of smokers in groups of individuals with and without lung cancer are being compared, essentially the relationship between two qualitative variables is being examined. These are the variable 'lung cancer' (present or absent) and the variable 'smoking category'. If blood pressure is being compared in males and females the relationship between a quantitative variable (blood pressure) and a qualitative variable (sex) is being examined.

The third possible combination of two variables is that both are quantitative and this chapter examines associations between two such variables. For instance, for a group of children, an association would be expected between height and weight. *On average*, taller children would weigh more. Similarly, an association might be expected between coronary heart disease mortality and increasing age. This chapter also considers, briefly, some allied but more complex techniques. Although details of some of the simpler calculations are included, these can be omitted at first reading.

8.2 Regression lines and regression equations

In Chapter 2 it was indicated that a scattergram could be used to display the relationship between two quantitative variables. Fig. 8.1 shows, for instance, the relationship between systolic blood pressure (SBP) in mm Hg and weight (W) in kg in 40 ten-year-old schoolchildren.* The points on the scattergram

---

* Adapted from Pollock, Wines & Hall (1981) with permission. Although the regression equation and correlation coefficient (to be discussed later) are taken from this article which is actually based on a study of 675 children, the scattergram presented here is not based on the actual data and is used for illustrative purposes only.

131

show a trend upwards and to the right; this indicates a direct or positive relationship between the two sets of readings. High (low) values of one variable, blood pressure, are associated with high (low) values of the other (weight).

Having identified an apparent relationship between two quantitative variables, it might be asked — 'Is it possible to describe or summarize the relationship in some compact way?' For instance, is it possible to obtain an equation that would express the relationship or association in numerical terms? Equations are often used to describe relationships; for instance, $Y = 2.54X$ describes the exact relationship between inches and centimetres, where Y represents centimetres, and X represents inches. Such a relationship could also be represented graphically by a straight line, with centimetres on the Y-axis and inches on the X-axis, as in Fig. 8.2. A 'straight line' relationship such as this is called *linear*. In a linear relationship, the change in one variable associated with a given change in the other variable is not dependent on the absolute magnitude of the values concerned. Thus, in the example, an increase in length from 10 inches to 12 inches means an increase of 5.08 centimetres, from 25.40 to 30.48 centimetres. An increase from 25 inches to 27 inches is, of course, also associated with a length increase of 5.08 centimetres.

More generally, the equation of a straight line can be expressed as $Y = a + bX$, where 'a' is the intercept of the line on the Y-axis and 'b' is the slope of the line. In the special case in which the line passes through the origin (0) of the two axes, as in Fig. 8.2, $a = 0$, and the equation of the line reduces to $Y = bX$. The coefficient b may take any value. In the equation $Y = 2.54X$

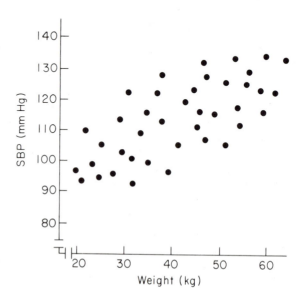

FIG. 8.1. A scattergram of systolic blood pressure (SBP) and weight in 40 ten-year-olds.

FIG. 8.2. A direct linear
relationship.

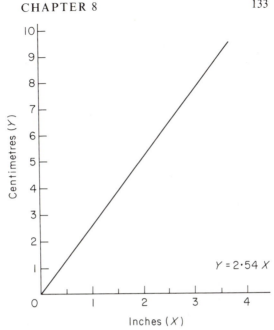

Inches (X)

for example, $b = 2\cdot54$. An equation always implies an exact relationship, which in the case of two variables X and Y means that given a value for X a value for Y can be precisely determined. A linear relationship is said to be *direct* if the two variables involved increase together, in which case the coefficient b has a positive sign. Linear relationships can also be *indirect* or *inverse*, as illustrated in Fig. 8.3. In this case, the coefficient b will be negative ($Y = a - bX$) and as one variable increases the other will decrease. In Fig. 8.4, a curvilinear (non-linear) exact relationship is shown, but the equation for such a relationship is more complex than for a linear one. $Y = bX^2$ is an example of such an equation.

Now return to the example of the relationship between weight and blood pressure for which the scattergram was given in Fig. 8.1. It is obvious that there is some form of relationship between the two variables but, obviously, this relationship cannot be described exactly by means of an equation. No line (straight or smoothly curved) could pass through all the points on the scattergram. However, some sort of 'average' equation could summarize the relationship, and might be obtained by drawing a smooth line through the middle of the data points. In Fig. 8.1 a straight line would seem to be the best choice, and although such a line could be fitted by using a ruler there would be a subjective element about this and different people would fit different lines. There is, however, a mathematical technique for fitting such a line to a set of data points, and the line so fitted to the data is called a

FIG. 8.3. An indirect or
inverse linear relationship.

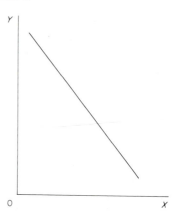

FIG. 8.4. An exact
curvilinear relationship.

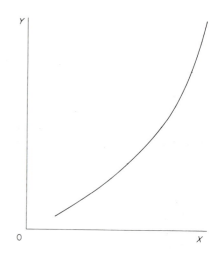

regression line, and its corresponding equation is called a *regression equation*. This text deals, for the most part, with linear regression, which means the relationship as seen in the scattergram should at least appear to be linear in the first place. For the moment also, only relationships between two variables, or what is technically referred to as *bivariate regression*, will be considered. The regression equation then, in some sense, measures the average relationship between two variables. It could be expressed in the form

$$\hat{Y} = a + bX \qquad\qquad (8.1)$$

where $\hat{Y}$ is the 'computed' or 'expected' value of Y given any value of X. 'a' and 'b' are constants, to be determined on the basis of the data, as described later, by the *method of least squares*. In many situations, the '^' above the Y variable will be omitted although it should always be remembered that in a regression equation it is an expected value which is being calculated. In the blood pressure study, the actual regression equation calculated turns out to be

$$SBP = 79.7 + 0.8W \qquad (8.2)$$

where SBP represents systolic blood pressure in mm Hg, W represents weight in kg, and the coefficients 79.7 and 0.8 are calculated from the data. This regression line is drawn in on the scattergram in Fig. 8.5. The line passes through the middle of the scatter points, and the regression line might reasonably be claimed to represent, approximately, the relationship between the two variables. On the basis of the regression line, it would be expected that a child weighing 40 kg, for instance, would have a systolic blood pressure of

$$SBP = 79.7 + 0.8(40) = 111.7 \text{ mm Hg}$$

This result could also have been read off Fig. 8.5 using the regression line. Note, however, that there may not have been anyone in the study who actually weighed 40 kg, and even if there was, he or she need not necessarily have had a blood pressure of 111.7. The figure of 111.7 mm Hg is interpreted

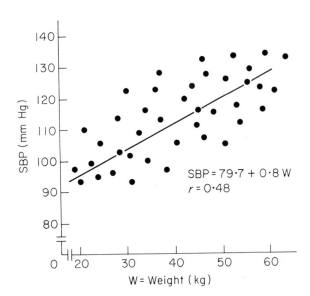

FIG. 8.5. Scattergram of systolic blood pressure (SBP) and weight with the regression line drawn in.

as the average blood pressure which would be expected among a large number of children, all of whom weighed 40 kg, or in other words, the average blood pressure associated with this weight.

The regression equation also implies that systolic blood pressure will increase by 0·8 mm Hg with every 1 kg increase in weight. The coefficient 0·8 in the equation is called the *regression coefficient* and, in general, means the change in Y per unit change in X. It is, in fact, the slope of the regression line. One further point may be noted; if a value of zero is substituted for weight in Eqn. 8.2, an expected systolic blood pressure of 79·7 would be calculated. It is plainly nonsensical to estimate a blood pressure for a child weighing nothing. The regression equation is derived from the observed values of the two variables, and it is only valid within the ranges actually observed for the variables. Extrapolation beyond this range may be misleading, and often totally invalid.

Another example of a regression analysis relates to indicators of prognosis after a myocardial infarction (heart attack). The left ventricular ejection fraction (LVEF) is one such indicator, but, unfortunately, is difficult to measure, and also expensive. On the other hand, the taking of an electro-cardiograph (ECG) is much faster and cheaper, and a particular index called the QRS score is easily derived from an ECG tracing. Twenty-eight patients had their LVEF measured three weeks after their heart attack. This was then compared with the patients' QRS score to evaluate the usefulness of this score in determining LVEF. Fig. 8.6 shows the scattergram and regression line for the relationship between these two variables. From inspection of the plot points on the diagram, it is clear that the relationship is linear but inverse. The regression equation can be calculated as

$$\text{LVEF} = 62 \cdot 01 - 3 \cdot 44 \text{QRS} \tag{8.3}$$

where the LVEF is measured as a percentage. In this case, the regression coefficient is $-3 \cdot 44$, which means that for every increase of 1 unit in the QRS score the value of the LVEF decreases by 3·44 (percent). An inverse relationship will always give rise to a negative regression coefficient.

In both of these examples, it was meaningful to consider how one variable depended on the other. In the first case, the aim was to determine how blood pressure depended on weight, and in the second case, how the LVEF could be determined by the QRS score. Blood pressure and the LVEF are both called *dependent* variables, while weight and the QRS score are considered the *independent* variables. (Note that this use of the word independent is different from that in Chapter 3, where the question of independent events was considered.) The question of which variable in a regression analysis is independent and which is dependent is decided on the basis of logic (a child's weight is hardly dependent on blood pressure) or on the precise question

FIG. 8.6. Scattergram
showing relationship
between the left ventricular
ejection fraction (LVEF)
and the QRS score in 28
patients after a myocardial
infarction. Palmeri,
Harrison, Cobb, Morris,
Harrell, Ideker, Selvester &
Wagner (1982) with
permission.

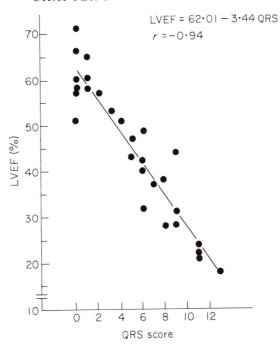

the researcher is trying to answer. (In the heart attack example, the purpose
was to predict a patient's LVEF on the basis of the QRS score.) It is important
to note however that a regression equation expresses a numerical association
between two variables, but it does not establish a causal link between the two,
or prove that one variable is causally dependent on the other.

In a regression equation, the dependent variable is written on the left-hand
side of the equation, and the independent variable is written on the right-hand
side; it is usual to talk about the regression of the dependent variable on the
independent one. Thus, the first example is of the regression of blood pressure
on weight. In the scattergram, the dependent variable is put on the Y-axis. It
is important in calculating regression equations that one is clear which
variable is to be considered independent. Without going into detail, the
regression of a variable Y on a variable X does not give the same mathematical
relationship as the regression of X on Y, although unless there is a large scatter
of points around the regression line the relationships are usually very close.

8.3　Correlation analysis

Consider the regression Eqn. 8.2. For a given value of W (body weight) a
corresponding value of SBP (systolic blood pressure) can be calculated. This

calculated value can be written $\hat{SBP}$. $\hat{SBP}$ can be interpreted as the expected or average value of systolic blood pressure associated with the given value of weight. Now, if all the points in the scattergram lay on the regression line, for any given value of W the expected and observed values of SBP would be identical. The regression equation would describe exactly the relationship between systolic blood pressure and weight. The variation in systolic blood pressure would be completely explained by, or be dependent upon, the variation in weight.

In practice, this is not the case. Systolic blood pressure can vary independently of variation in weight, so that two children of the same weight may have different blood pressures. Weight is not the only factor affecting systolic blood pressure. Given any particular value for weight, the expected blood pressure can be calculated. However, since blood pressures do vary independently of weight, the blood pressure associated with any particular weight cannot be predicted exactly. In this sense, the regression equation can be described as measuring the average relationship between the two variables. It does not measure the *strength* or *goodness of fit* of the relationship.

In the blood pressure and weight example (Fig. 8.5) there is a fairly large dispersion of the plot points around the regression line. This suggests a fairly weak relationship between the two variables. Given a weight of 40 kg a child's systolic blood pressure could be estimated as 111·7 mm Hg, but the child's actual blood pressure could vary quite appreciably around this. A considerable amount of the variation in the dependent variable is unexplained by the variation in the independent variable. Although, on average, systolic blood pressure increases with weight, there are obviously many other factors which influence this variable.

In Fig. 8.6, which shows the relationship between the LVEF and QRS score, the plot points lie close to the regression line, which suggests a strong relationship between the two variables. The observed values for LVEF do not differ markedly from the expected values represented by the regression line. This implies that most of the variation in LVEF can be 'explained' by the variation in the QRS score. Given a particular QRS score, the estimated left ventricular ejection fraction could be predicted, and it would be fairly certain that the actual value would be quite close to this predicted one.

A measure of the strength of the relationship between two variables is provided by the coefficient of correlation, denoted by 'r'. If the relationship between the two variables is of linear form, r is called *the coefficient of linear correlation*. r is also called *Pearson's product moment correlation*.

Values of r vary between $+1$ and -1, the sign of r depending on whether or not there is a direct relationship between the two variables, as in Fig. 8.5, or an inverse relationship, as in Fig. 8.6. If the relationship between the two variables is perfect or exact, that is if all the points on the scattergram lie on the regression line, r will be equal to $+1$ or -1. A positive sign indicates a direct relationship; a negative sign indicates an inverse one. If there is no relationship at all between the two variables, r will be 0. The greater the numerical value of r, the stronger the relationship between the two variables.

Methods for calculating the coefficient of correlation (or, as it is often called, the correlation coefficient) are given in the next section, but for the moment only the results for the two examples are given. The correlation coefficient for the relationship between blood pressure and weight in 10-year-old children is $r = 0.48$ which is not very high. On the other hand, $r = -0.94$ for the relationship between LVEF and the QRS score, which confirms the strength of that relationship as determined visually. (Note that r is negative for this inverse relationship.)

It has been said that r ranges from -1 to $+1$, but it is not immediately clear how to interpret different values of this coefficient. It happens however that the value of r^2 has a readily understandable interpretation in terms of the strength of a relationship. Take the example of blood pressure in 10-year-old children. Blood pressures will show a fair degree of variation from child to child due to the many factors, one of which is body weight, that affect blood pressure. This can be referred to as the total variation in the variable. Prediction of the systolic blood pressure of a 10-year-old without reference to these factors would be subject to quite a degree of uncertainty. If, however, only children of a particular weight were examined, the variation in their blood pressures would be considerably less. (See Fig. 8.5 where the scatter of blood pressures for a given weight is far less than the total scatter of blood pressure in all the children studied.) Some of the total variation in blood pressure measurements can be explained by the variation in children's weights (the 'explained' variation), while the remainder of the variation must be due to other factors which were not considered explicitly or are unknown (the 'unexplained' variation). The larger the first component is, relative to the second, the stronger is the relationship between the two variables.

It can be shown that r^2 (the square of the correlation coefficient — sometimes called the *coefficient of determination*) is equal to the proportion of the total variation in the dependent variable (SBP) that is explained by the regression line. If the relationship between the two variables is perfect, all the variation in the dependent variable is explained by the regression line, and thus r^2 equals 1 so that r equals ± 1. r is written plus or minus, according to whether the relationship is direct or inverse. The more closely the points in the scattergram are dispersed around the regression line, the higher will be the proportion of variation explained by the regression line, and hence the greater the value of r^2 and r. In the blood pressure example, it was said that r equals 0.48, so that r^2 equals 0.2304. Thus, the variation in the weights of the children explains just over 23% of the total variation in blood pressure. The other 77% of the variation is unexplained and must be due to many other factors not considered in this analysis. In the left ventricular ejection fraction example, $r^2 = (0.94)^2 = 0.8836$, which means that over 88% of the variation in LVEF is explained by the variation in the QRS score.

In most cases involving the use of regression analysis, it is advisable to include the value of the correlation coefficient or its square. There are situations, however, where determination of the exact form of a linear relationship is not relevant, or where identification of which of the variables being examined is dependent and which independent is not obvious. In these cases a correlation analysis examining only the strength of a relationship may be all that is required, and the actual regression equation(s) may be irrelevant. A regression analysis is not symmetrical, in that one variable must be taken as dependent and the other as independent. Correlation, however, results in a measure of association that does not imply any dependence of one variable on the other.

Fig. 8.7 is a case in point. This shows a scattergram for the relationship between the age at which 38 females with frequent urinary tract infections (UTI) developed their first kidney stone, and the age at which they first developed UTI. Rather than one age determining the other age, it is much more likely that another factor or factors determined the timing of each event. A regression analysis would not seem to be appropriate, but a correlation analysis examining the strength of the relationship would be. For this example, r turns out to be equal to 0.86 ($r^2 = 0.74$), showing a reasonably strong association between the age at first infection and the age at first stone. The interpretation of this association in terms of a causal hypothesis is much more difficult, however.

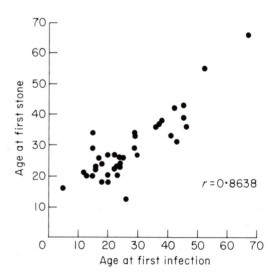

FIG. 8.7 Relation between age at first stone and age at first infection in 38 females with two or more stone-associated urinary tract infections (see Fig. 1.12). Parks, Coe & Strauss (1982) with permission.

8.4   Calculation of regression and correlation coefficients

In Section 8.2 it was pointed out that a regression line could be fitted by hand by drawing a line through the middle of the points on the scattergram. Obviously, as was said, this is rather a haphazard way of fitting the line, and a more systematic procedure is required. A number of different methods may be used, the best-known of which is the *method of least squares*. Assume that the scatter of points is such that a straight line would be appropriate to describe the relationship. From the infinite number of straight lines which could be drawn it is desirable to select that line to which the points on the scattergram are, in some sense, closest. That is, the line should be drawn in such a way as to minimize the distance between the scatter points and the line. In Fig. 8.8 a line has been fitted to minimize the sum of vertical distances between the four plot points and the line. Actually, since some of these distances will be positive (points above the line) and some will be negative (points below the line) the line is fitted to minimize the sum of squares of the vertical distance between the plot points and the line.* This is why it is called the method of least squares.

When the line is fitted in this way, the overall difference between the plot points and the line is minimized. This is the line of 'best fit'. The mathematical derivation of the regression coefficients a and b in the regression line

$$\hat{Y} = a + bX \tag{8.1}$$

are not given here, but they can be calculated from the following formulae

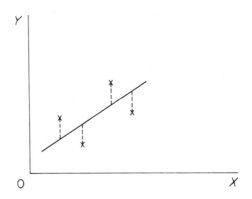

Fig. 8.8. Illustration of the 'method of least squares'.

---

* Since positive and negative distances would tend to cancel out, a regression line which was a 'poor fit' could still minimize the algebraic sum of the vertical distances between the plot points and the line. This is avoided by minimizing the *squares* of the distances, since all the values are then positive.

$$b = \frac{\Sigma(X - \bar{X})(Y - \bar{Y})}{\Sigma(X - \bar{X})^2} \tag{8.4}$$

$$= \frac{\Sigma(X - \bar{X})(Y - \bar{Y})}{(n-1)S_x{}^2} \tag{8.5}$$

$$a = \bar{Y} - b\bar{X} \tag{8.6}$$

These are the slope and intercept of the regression line as determined by the method of least squares. The numerator in the expression for b, $\Sigma(X - \bar{X})$ $(Y - \bar{Y})$, looks formidable, and as it stands requires subtraction of the mean of the X variable from each X value, the mean of the Y variable from each corresponding Y value, multiplication of the two results together, and summing over all the pairs of XY values. Appendix A, however, outlines an easier computational approach. The denominator of the expression for b is identical to $(n-1)S_x{}^2$ where $S_x{}^2$ is the variance (square of the standard deviation) of the X values (see Eqn. 2.3). The equation for a requires only the means of both X and Y, together with the calculated value of b.

Once the regression equation has been estimated, it can easily be drawn in on the scattergram. Choose two representative values for X; calculate the predicted or expected $\hat{Y}$ values; plot in these points and connect with a straight line.

The formula for the correlation coefficient r is also fairly cumbersome.

$$r = \frac{\Sigma(X - \bar{X})(Y - \bar{Y})}{\sqrt{\Sigma(X - \bar{X})^2 \Sigma(Y - \bar{Y})^2}} \tag{8.7}$$

$$= \frac{\Sigma(X - \bar{X})(Y - \bar{Y})}{(n-1)S_X S_Y} \tag{8.8}$$

where S_X and S_Y are the standard deviations of the X and Y variables respectively. Appendix A outlines in detail the calculation of these quantities for the left ventricular ejection fraction data of Fig. 8.6.

8.5 Statistical inference in regression and correlation

In the examples used so far, and in general, analysis is based on a sample of the pairs of variables of interest. Thus the data in Fig. 8.1 are based on a sample of 10-year-old children. Now, in the same way that the mean and standard deviation of a random sample are estimates of the mean and standard deviation of the population from which it is drawn, so the regression coefficient and correlation coefficient of a sample of pairs of two variables are estimates of the regression coefficient and correlation coefficient for the population of pairs of these values. Let the regression coefficient for the sample be denoted by b and the correlation coefficient by r; similarly, denote the regression coefficient for the whole population by β (beta) and the correlation coefficient by ρ (rho — the Greek letter 'r'). Then, the sample statistics b and r are estimates of the unknown population parameters β and ρ. The regression equation in the population may thus be written

$$Y = \alpha + \beta X \qquad\qquad (8.9)$$

where α and β are the regression coefficients in the population. ('a' and α are also called regression coefficients although the term is more usually employed for b and β.)

An interesting possibility now arises: suppose, for the whole population of pairs of values, that $\beta = 0$ and $\rho = 0$. This would occur in cases where there was no relationship between the two variables.* The two variables are said to be independent of one another. An example would be pairs of values which arise in throwing two dice simultaneously. There is no relationship (or should not be!) between the number which turns up on one die and the number turning up on the other. A regression analysis between pairs of values should yield $\beta = 0$ and $\rho = 0$.

However, if a sample of pairs of values is analysed, it is quite possible that, just by chance, non-zero values will be obtained for b and r. In the same way that the mean ($\bar{X}$) of a single sample is unlikely to be exactly equal to a population mean (μ), the values of a regression coefficient b and a correlation coefficient r derived from a sample are unlikely to be exactly equal to the population values β and ρ. Hence, it is likely that even if β and ρ equal 0, b and r will be non-zero. This means that the results of a regression analysis may suggest a relationship between two variables which is quite spurious. To guard against this possibility, some method is needed to make inferences about the population values of b and r (β and ρ respectively) on the basis of the sample results. In Chapters 4 and 6 it was explained how confidence intervals for, and significance tests on, unknown population parameters could be based on the sample statistics and their standard errors. Similarly, confidence intervals and significance tests are available for the regression and correlation coefficients (β and ρ) based on the standard errors of their sample values. Tests for the value of α (the Y-intercept) are also available, although less commonly employed.

As before however, some assumptions concerning the underlying distribution of the data must be made for valid use of these inferential approaches. For inferences relating to a regression analysis, it must be assumed that the

---

* β is a measure of the average change in one variable (Y) per unit change in the other (X). If there is no relationship between X and Y, an increase of 1 unit in X is equally likely to be associated with a decrease or increase in Y. Hence the average change in Y per unit change in X will be 0. Similarly, if no relationship can be postulated between X and Y, $\rho = 0$.

distribution of Y for each fixed value of X is normal (or nearly so), that the standard deviation of this normal distribution of Y is the same for each X, and that the mean values of the Y distribution are linearly related to X. These assumptions are examined below in the specific example of the regression of blood pressure on weight in 10-year-old children, considered earlier. The assumptions state that for children of a given weight (40 kg say) the distribution of systolic blood pressure is normal, with a standard deviation (σ), and that no matter which weight is chosen children of that weight will have a normally distributed blood pressure with this standard deviation. This assumption, which is often stated in terms of variances rather than standard deviations, is called the assumption of homoscedasticity. The final assumption is that the population mean systolic blood pressure for each different weight is a linear function of weight. Given these assumptions it can be shown that the standard error of b is

$$SE(b) = \frac{\sigma}{\sqrt{\Sigma(X - \bar{X})^2}} \qquad (8.10)$$

$$= \frac{\sigma}{\sqrt{(n-1)}\, S_X} \qquad (8.11)$$

where σ is the (unknown) standard deviation of the Y variable at each X value. The assumption of homoscedasticity is important, and more advanced techniques may have to be used if the assumption is not tenable, or perhaps a transformation of the data (see Section 6.11) may suffice. Note, of course, that σ is unknown, and must be estimated from the data. Again, without deriving the result, it can be shown that an estimate of σ is given by

$$S_{Y.X} = \sqrt{\frac{\Sigma(Y - \hat{Y})^2}{n-2}} \qquad (8.12)$$

where Y represents the observed Y values obtained, and $\hat{Y}$ is the predicted or expected Y calculated from the regression equation on the corresponding X (Eqn. 8.1). The similarity of this formula to that of the usual standard deviation should be noted. The quantity is some sort of average of the deviations of each point from its predicted value but, as for the standard deviation, it is the squared deviations that are averaged. It can be seen however, that $S_{Y.X}$ is a reasonable estimator for σ. (An easier computational form is given in Appendix A. The divisor of $n-2$ must be accepted on faith.) $S_{Y.X}$ is variously referred to as *the standard deviation from regression* or *the standard error of the estimate* or when squared as *the residual mean square*. $n-2$ is sometimes called the residual degrees of freedom. The subscript $Y.X$

on S means that we are talking about the regression of Y on X.

The standard error of b is estimated as (see Eqn. 8.11)

$$SE(b) = \frac{S_{Y.X}}{\sqrt{(n-1)}\,S_X} \tag{8.13}$$

This standard error of b has $n-2$ degrees of freedom so that

$$b \pm t_c\,SE(b)$$

gives a confidence interval for b where t_c is the critical value of the t distribution on $n-2$ degrees of freedom for the required confidence level. In the LVEF example, it can be shown that (see Appendix A) $S_{Y.X}$ equals 5·102 on 26 degrees of freedom, and S_X equals 4·118. It has already been seen that b equals $-3·438$ (to three decimal places) so that a 95% confidence interval for β is given by

$$-3·438 \pm 2·056(0·238)$$

where $SE(b) = 0·238$ from Eqn. 8.13, and $t_c = 2·056$ is the critical t value on 26 degrees of freedom, corresponding to 5% of the area in both tails. The lower and upper confidence limits are thus $-3·927$ and $-2·949$.

To recap — usually, a calculated regression equation is determined on a sample of values so that, in particular, the regression coefficient b is a sample estimate of the regression coefficient (β) in the population. As with sample means and proportions, it is possible (given certain assumptions) to calculate the standard error of the regression coefficient and thus give a confidence interval estimate for the unknown value of β. A hypothesis test for β is also easily derived. If the null hypothesis specifies a particular value β_0 for the regression coefficient in the population, the test statistic is

$$t = \frac{b - \beta_0}{SE(b)} \tag{8.14}$$

where b is the sample value of the regression coefficient, β_0 is the hypothesized value and $SE(b)$ is given by Eqn. 8.13. This provides a t test on $n-2$ degrees of freedom. The usual null hypothesis specifies a value of $\beta = 0$ so that the test is of the existence of any relationship in the first place, and Eqn. 8.14 becomes, when Eqn. 8.13 is used for $SE(b)$,

$$t = \frac{b S_X \sqrt{n-1}}{S_{Y.X}} \tag{8.15}$$

If t is greater than the appropriate (usually two-sided) critical value then the existence of a real relationship in the population can be accepted. For the LVEF data, $t = -14\cdot42$, $d.f. = 26$, $p < 0\cdot01$. Thus, the value of b is significantly different from zero. This, of course, is consistent with the confidence interval for β calculated above which did not include zero as a possible value.

Although formulae are not given in this text, it is also possible to derive standard errors for a predicted $\hat{Y}$ value, given a particular value for X, or for the population mean Y value for that X. Confidence intervals can then be obtained.

The null hypothesis of zero population correlation ($\rho = 0$) uses the test statistic

$$t = r\sqrt{\frac{n-2}{1-r^2}} \tag{8.16}$$

on $n-2$ degrees of freedom. For the LVEF data, $t = -14\cdot42$ on 26 degrees of freedom. This is numerically the same as that obtained using the t test of zero regression coefficient mentioned above (Eqn. 8.15). This is not an accident; it can be shown that the two tests are mathematically equivalent. Confidence intervals for ρ and tests of hypotheses for population values other than $\rho = 0$ are more complex and require additional assumptions relating to the distribution of the variables in the population. They are not considered here.

It is important to distinguish between the strength of a relationship as measured by the correlation coefficient, or its square, and its statistical significance for a null hypothesis of zero population correlation. A significant correlation does not mean a strong relationship, thus an r of $0\cdot12$ explaining only $1\cdot4\%$ $[(0\cdot12)^2 = 0\cdot0144]$ of the variation in the dependent variable could be highly significant from the statistical point of view, but would probably be of little consequence. On the other hand, a high value for r may be non-significant if based on a very small sample size. Correlation coefficients can only be interpreted if both their magnitude and significance are reported.

Section C.14 of Appendix C summarizes the statistical calculations of this section.

8.6 Non-linear regression

So far, all the examples have related to linear regression between two variables, where the scattergram suggested a linear form. What can be done if a plot of the data points indicates some kind of curve in the relationship? Transformation of the data may provide a solution to the problem. In some cases, taking the logarithm of the variables may lead to a linear relationship. For example, the curvilinear relationship $Y = bX^2$ can be linearized by transforming it to log $Y = \log b + 2 \log X$. See also Fig. 1.11 in Chapter 1, where a curved relationship was made linear in this way. A linear regression analysis would then be performed on the transformed data.* Another approach to curvilinear regression is to run a *polynomial regression* where, without transformations, a dependent variable Y might be related to an independent variable X with a polynomial of the following form

$$Y = a + bX + cX^2 \qquad\qquad (8.17)$$

with terms in X^3 and X^4 etc. if necessary. With such analyses, more than one regression coefficient must be estimated (e.g. b and c above). Many curvilinear relationships can be expressed in such polynomial form, and the analysis is very similar to that for *multiple regression* to be discussed in a later section.

8.7   Regression to the mean

The term 'regression' for the type of analysis which has been considered seems a bit strange and was first used by Sir Francis Galton in describing his 'law of universal regression' in 1889. 'Each peculiarity in a man is shared by his kinsman, but *on the average* in a less degree'. Thus, intelligent fathers will tend to have intelligent sons, but the sons will, on average, be less intelligent than their fathers. There is a regression, or 'going back', of the sons' intelligence towards the average intelligence of all men. Sons of intelligent fathers will, of course, be more intelligent than the average in the population. Galton's 'law' can be shown graphically, as in Fig. 8.9. For any parental IQ, the son's IQ is closer to the mean IQ (about 100) than his father's was. The word 'regression' is now applied to the analysis of any such relationship, as has been discussed in this chapter.

Regression to the mean, as this phenomenon is called, is not confined to genetic situations, and its existence can cause confusion in the interpretation of certain results. Take a simple example. Suppose the mid-year examination results of 100 first-year medical students in statistics have been obtained and the group of 25 who obtained the highest marks have been identified. The average mark for these 25 is 62% and, of all the students, is 50%. It can be predicted that when these 100 students sit their end-year examination the average mark of the 25 identified on the basis of the first examination will be less than 62%. This will occur even if the average mark for the whole group remains at 50%, with an overall similar spread of marks. Why this happens is not very hard to see. Some of the 25 students will have got very high marks in

---

* Transformations of variables can linearize relationships as well as reducing the degree of skewness in one variable (see Section 6.11).

FIG. 8.9. Regression to the mean of sons' IQ

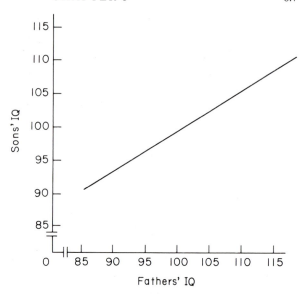

the mid-year examination that they are most unlikely to improve on. On the other hand, some of the 25 could drop their marks appreciably in the second examination; this could be due to luck on the first examination or a bad day on the second. As a consequence, the *average* mark of the group is likely to fall, or regress downward, to the mean of the full group. If instead the 25 worst students on the first examination had been taken, their average mark would have been likely to increase or regress upward to the mean.

Regression to the mean occurs when a variable is measured on two separate occasions, when that variable can change its value in the individual on whom it is measured and when a subgroup of a larger study group is defined on the basis of high (or low) values of the variable at the first measurement. Any subgroup so defined will have an average value for the variable that is lower (or higher) the second time it is measured. If, for instance, a group of patients was selected on the basis of systolic blood pressure being above 180 mm Hg at a particular examination, the average blood pressure of this group would be lower on a repeat examination. Such a decrease could be mistakenly interpreted as the effect of a particular treatment, whereas it would occur without any intervention whatsoever.

Regression to the mean relates to the experience of the whole group, and not to any defined individuals. Allowing for regression to the mean mathematically is not usually an easy procedure. The problem is probably best solved by ignoring the first measurement on the basis of which the individuals were categorized and to take, as a baseline, measurements taken at a subsequent examination when spuriously high (or low) levels have 'settled down'.

8.8 Multiple regression

The discussion and examples in the previous sections have been concerned with regression and correlation between just two variables. Often, analysis is concerned with the relationship between a number of quantitative variables. Analysis which involves more than two variables may be approached in two ways. Using the first approach, the relationship between pairs of variables may be examined independently of the other variables, in the manner already explained. Thus, if there are three variables, say X_1, X_2 and X_3, the relationship between the pairs can be examined: X_1 and X_2, X_1 and X_3, and X_2 and X_3, in each case ignoring the third variable. An example of this kind of analysis is shown in Table 8.1. There are four variables in this example: cigarette and dairy product consumption in 1973, and male and female coronary heart disease mortality in 1974, determined in 14 countries. The figures in the table are the values of the correlation coefficient between any pair of variables. Thus, in the first line, the correlation between cigarette consumption in 1973 and dairy products consumption in 1973 is negative, with a value of $r = -0.36$. The correlation between cigarette consumption in 1973 and male coronary heart disease mortality in 1974 is 0·17 and so on. In the second line, the correlation between dairy products consumption and cigarette consumption in 1973 is omitted, since it already appears in the first line. The correlation between any variable and itself is necessarily unity, as shown in the diagonal of the table.

Each correlation coefficient is calculated between two variables quite independently of the other two variables. The table therefore consists of a number of separate bivariate correlation coefficients calculated by the methods described in Section 8.3 and interpreted in the same way. Each correlation coefficient has been tested for significance, and those coefficients which are significantly different from zero at the 5% level are marked with an

Table 8.1 Zero order correlation coefficients between cigarette consumption (1973), dairy product consumption (1973) and male and female coronary heart disease (CHD) mortality (1974) in 14 countries. Adapted and abbreviated from Salonen & Vohlonen (1982) with permission.

	Cigarettes in 1973	Dairy products in 1973	Male CHD in 1974	Female CHD in 1974
Cigarettes in 1973	1·0	−0·36	0·17	0·33
Dairy products in 1973		1·0	0·78*	0·70*
Male CHD in 1974			1·0	0·96*
Female CHD in 1974				1·0

$*p < 0.05$.

asterisk. A table of this kind, sometimes referred to as a matrix of bivariate correlation coefficients, is a useful method of summarizing the independent relationships between a number of variables, and of showing which relationships are significant. In Table 8.1 there are three significant relationships; the remaining correlations can be ignored. This example shows some of the problems in the interpretation of bivariate correlation coefficients. The relationships between dairy product consumption and male and female CHD deaths could possibly be attributed to a causal connection between the factors, while the association between male and female deaths is of little relevance in developing a causal hypothesis. This latter relationship is likely to be due, almost totally, to the influence of dairy consumption (and other factors) on the CHD deaths in both sexes.

The second approach for analysing relationships between more than two quantitative variables is quite different, involving the simultaneous analysis of the variables. This is called *multiple regression analysis*, as distinct from simple bivariate analysis, which deals with only two variables. As an example, return to the study of blood pressure in 10-year-old children discussed in a previous section. In this study, many variables, other than weight, were examined for their influence on blood pressure. The authors present a multiple regression equation for systolic blood pressure as a dependent variable, with, in addition to weight as an independent variable, two further factors — diastolic blood pressure and the time of day at which the measurement was taken. They obtained the following multiple regression equation

$$SBP = 39 \cdot 6 + 0 \cdot 45W + 0 \cdot 69DBP + 0 \cdot 45T$$

where SBP and DBP are systolic and diastolic blood pressures in mm Hg, W is weight in kg and T is the time of day measured in number of completed hours. In this multiple regression equation SBP is the dependent variable and DBP, W and T are independent or explanatory variables. The coefficients 0·45, 0·69 and 0·45 are called *partial regression coefficients*. 0·69 is the average change in systolic blood pressure per 1 mm Hg change in diastolic blood pressure when weight and the time of day are held constant. This shows how systolic blood pressure is related to diastolic blood pressure independently of the other two factors. 0·45 is the partial regression coefficient for weight, which shows the relationship of systolic blood pressure and weight when diastolic blood pressure and time of day are held constant. The coefficient for T is also 0·45 and measures the relationship between systolic blood pressure and time of day when the other two factors are held constant. Note that the partial regression coefficient for weight (0·45) is much less than the simple regression coefficient of 0·8 obtained when weight was the only independent variable included in the analysis (see Eqn. 8.2). Thus, the relationship of systolic blood pressure with weight is not as marked when diastolic blood pressure is taken into account. For a fixed time of day and fixed diastolic blood pressure, systolic blood pressure will increase by 0·45 mm Hg for every 1 kg increase of weight, compared to 0·8 mm Hg when the other variables are not taken into account. Multiple regression can thus control for the confounding effects of other variables on any bivariate relationship.

The strength of the relationship between the dependent variable and the explanatory variables may also be estimated by calculating the *coefficient of multiple correlation* (r). This is analogous to the simple correlation coefficient and, as before, its square measures the proportion of the total variation in the dependent variable which can be 'explained' by variations in the explanatory variables. The 'unexplained' variation may be due, of course, to other variables which have not been included in the regression equation. If these variables can be identified, then a new multiple regression equation can be calculated with these additional variables included. The value of r^2 will be increased, since the proportion of 'explained' variation in the dependent variable will be higher. The value of r^2 for the multiple regression equation above is 0·53 compared to the value of 0·23 in the simple regression equation with weight only included. More of the variation in systolic blood pressure is explained by inclusion of the extra independent variables. Moreover, by calculating what are called *partial correlation coefficients*, the strength of the relationship between the dependent variable and any *one* of the independent variables may be calculated, assuming the other independent variables are held constant. These partial correlation coefficients differ from the simple bivariate (or zero order) correlation coefficients described earlier. In the former, the simultaneous influence of other independent variables is taken into account; in the latter, the correlation between two variables is calculated without any explicit attempt to remove the possible influence of other variables.

A multiple regression equation can be fitted to observed data by methods similar to those used for simple bivariate regression. If a three-dimensional scatter diagram is envisaged, the regression plane is fitted to the data, as before, as the plane of 'best fit'. The partial regression coefficients are calculated, as well as the constant term, and the resulting equation describes the average relationship between the dependent variable and the independent variables. In principle, there is no limit to the number of independent variables which may be included, but in practice of course it is necessary to keep the number of variables to a manageable level. Various methods are employed to choose the 'best' (in some sense) set of independent variables for inclusion in a multiple regression equation. *Forward (stepwise) inclusion* methods search through all the possible independent variables not already in the equation and add into the equation, at each step, the variables that increase the coefficient of multiple correlation to the greatest extent. (Other statistical criteria may also be used before a variable is entered into the equation.) The process is then continued until enough variables have been entered or the inclusion criteria cannot be satisfied. Other techniques such as *backward elimination*, where one starts with all the variables in the equation deleting them one by one, or even more complex methods, may also be used to obtain the 'best' set of independent variables. Due to their computational complexity multiple regressions are usually performed on a computer.

It must be stressed, however, that multiple regression techniques cannot be used blindly, including all possible variables in an analysis. In essence, a multiple regression analysis requires some model to be postulated that would determine beforehand which variables could be appropriately included on theoretical grounds. Thus an independent variable which is *known* to have no relationship with the dependent variable under examination should not be added into a multiple regression equation just to 'see what happens'. Multiple regression as described also assumes an additive effect of the different independent variables. Often in a multiple regression analysis, variables that do not have a significant relationship with the independent variable are deliberately not excluded from the final equation because, theoretically, their influence is important.

When two independent variables are highly correlated* the effect of one on the dependent variable will often totally mask the effect of the other. This can result in one of these variables having a small and non-significant partial regression coefficient. How to deal with such *multicollinearity* is a problem. Usually, only one of a set of such variables will be included in the final equation, since one variable may act as a proxy for all the others. Variables excluded for such reasons however may have important effects on the dependent variable.

8.9   Analysis of covariance and multiple logistic regression

So far, the regression techniques discussed have examined the relationship between a quantitative dependent variable, and one or more quantitative independent variables. When a qualitative independent variable is also to be included in such an analysis, the multiple regression approach can be modified to deal with the situation. The resulting analysis of covariance, as it is called (see Section 7.15), is beyond the scope of this text but has close connections with both analysis of variance and multiple regression.

A more common requirement, especially in epidemiological work, is the analysis of the relationship of a dependent qualitative variable to many

---

* This is not a contradiction in terms. The variables are called independent to distinguish them from the dependent variable in the analysis.

independent quantitative variables. With only one independent quantitative variable, the best approach would be via a t test, or a non-parametric equivalent. Suppose, for example, it is necessary to relate the independent variables blood glucose level (G), age (A), systolic blood pressure (SBP), relative weight (W), cholesterol (C) and number of cigarettes per day (NC) to a qualitative dependent variable, measuring the presence or absence of major abnormalities on electrocardiographs. It is possible to imagine a multiple regression analysis with the presence or absence of an ECG abnormality as a dependent variable, obtaining an equation such as

$$P = a + b_1 G + b_2 A + b_3 SBP + \ldots$$

where b_1, b_2 etc. are the partial regression coefficients for the corresponding variables, and P has a value of 1 for the presence of the abnormality and 0 otherwise. The problem about this approach is that the predicted values for P from the equation, for given values of the independent variables, could quite easily be less than 0 or greater than 1 and would thus be totally uninterpretable. If P could be constrained to lie between 0 and 1, it could be interpreted as the probability of an ECG abnormality given the set of values for the independent variables. *Logistic regression* is a technique which achieves this. Basically, one works with a transformed dependent variable, running a multiple regression on the transformed variable

$$Y = \ln \frac{P}{1 - P} \tag{8.19}$$

obtaining a regression equation like

$$\ln \frac{P}{1 - P} = a + b_1 G + b_2 A + b_3 SBP \ldots \tag{8.20}$$

where P is interpreted as the probability of an ECG abnormality. Given the form of this equation, P is constrained to lie between 0 and 1, and so has the required properties of a probability. The 'ln' denotes a logarithm based on the constant $e = 2.71828$. (If $10^2 = 100$, then $\log 100 = 2$ to the base 10; also $\log 24 = 1.38$ because $10^{1.38} = 24$. Now $e^2 = 7.38$, so that ln of $7.38 = 2$, also $\ln 24 = 3.18$, because $e^{3.18} = 24$.) This function has many desirable mathematical properties, and is preferred to the usual log to the base 10. Eqn. 8.20 can also be rewritten with P as a direct function of the independent variables

$$P = \frac{e^{\hat{Y}}}{1 + e^{\hat{Y}}} \tag{8.21}$$

where

$$\hat{Y} = a + b_1 G + b_2 A + b_3 SBP \ldots \tag{8.22}$$

is the predicted value of Y for a given set of values for the independent

Table 8.2 Multiple logistic regression coefficients for the relationship between six variables and ECG abnormalities in 3357 men aged 40–54. Abbreviated from Hickey, Mulcahy, Daly, Bourke & Moriarty (1979) with permission.

Variable	Logistic regression coefficients (b)
Glucose	0·0009
Age	0·1339*
SBP	0·0178*
Relative weight	−0·0079
Cholesterol	0·0034
No. of cigarettes	0·0075
Constant	−12·1041

*$p < 0.05$.

variables. Table 8.2 shows the multiple logistic regression coefficients obtained for a study on ECG abnormalities using the variables already discussed. Coefficients significantly different from 0 are marked with an asterisk; relative weight was defined as the percentage of desirable weight based on standard weight tables. To show how the results of such an analysis might be employed, the equation will be used to predict the probability of an ECG abnormality for a male aged 50 years, with a blood glucose level of 98·2 mg/dl, a systolic blood pressure of 140 mm Hg, a relative weight of 115%, a cholesterol level of 230 mg/dl and who smokes 25 cigarettes per day. The predicted $\hat{Y}$ value for this individual using the values of the coefficients in Table 8.2, is

$$\hat{Y} = -12{\cdot}1041 + 0{\cdot}0009\,(98{\cdot}2) + 0{\cdot}1339\,(50) + 0{\cdot}0178\,(140)$$

$$-0{\cdot}0079\,(115) + 0{\cdot}0034\,(230) + 0{\cdot}0075\,(25)$$

$$= -2{\cdot}768$$

When this value is substituted into Eqn. 8.21, the value for P is found to be 0·059 (This P is not to be confused with p denoting significance level.) Thus, on the basis of this study, an individual with the listed characteristics would have a 5·9% chance of having an ECG abnormality. The magnitude of the logistic regression coefficients gives some idea of the relative importance of various factors in producing the probability of an abnormality. Often, as in this case, variables having a non-significant influence on the dependent variable are still included in the regression equation because there are theoretical reasons for retaining them. Logistic regression can also be adapted to include qualitative independent variables.

8.10   Multivariate techniques

In multiple and logistic regression analyses, interest lies in the variation in one variable called the dependent variable. *Multivariate analysis,* on the other hand, is designed to handle cases of simultaneous variation in two or more dependent variables. Multivariate problems are common in medical research and in recent years there has been a substantial development in statistical techniques and applications of multivariate analysis. Only a brief excursion through these techniques is attempted here, and the reader should be warned that the techniques are difficult to use and can easily be misapplied. An example of a multivariate technique is *discriminant analysis.* Suppose two populations are defined by a set of characteristics such as height, weight, serum cholesterol level etc., and that for each characteristic the two distributions overlap so that, for example, the distribution of heights in population A overlaps with the distribution of heights in population B. Thus, although the mean height of individuals in population A may be less than the mean height of individuals in population B, one individual picked at random from population A may be taller than an individual picked at random from population B. Consequently, if an individual was encountered and it was not known which population that individual belonged to, he could not be definitely assigned to a particular population unless, for any one of the variables concerned, the distributions were known not to overlap.

The purpose of discriminant analysis is to enable individual units to be assigned to one or other of the populations with, in some defined sense, the greatest probability of being correct (or smallest risk of error). The techniques of analysis, which are not explained here, involve the specification of a discriminant function, in which the relevant variables are assigned a weight or coefficient. If the discriminant function is linear in form, it will 'look like' a multiple regression equation. For a particular individual or case, values of the variables (height, weight etc.) are substituted in the discriminant equation and a value for the function calculated. On the basis of this value the individual is assigned to a particular population. As an indication of the possible application of discriminant analysis, suppose it is desired to allocate individuals to a 'high risk' or 'low risk' category for a particular disease, the allocation being made on the basis of certain diagnostic variables e.g. blood pressure, age. Coefficients of the discriminant function are estimated using sample observations of those who have and have not contracted the disease in some past period. Individuals can then be assigned to one or other category using the discriminant function as the method of allocation. Discriminant analysis has very close theoretical connections with logistic regression, but can easily be extended to the case of more than two groups.

Other multivariate techniques do not require specification of group membership prior to analysis, and can classify individuals or allocate them to groups which are distinct in some sense. These groups are defined by the data structure, and may or may not be logical or natural in themselves. *Principal components analysis, factor analysis* and *cluster analysis* (numerical taxonomy) are different techniques used in this area. However, not many applications in the general medical literature are seen, although the techniques have for example been used to classify psychiatric diagnosis on the basis of patient symptoms.

8.11   Rank correlation

Rank correlation is a non-parametric procedure for calculating a correlation coefficient. As such, it does not require the assumptions made for the usual approach when Pearson's product moment correlation coefficient is employed. There are two common rank procedures which will be encountered in the medical literature. The first is called *Kendall's rank correlation coefficient* or *Kendall's tau* (tau is the Greek letter 't'). The calculations can be complex and are not given in this text. An alternative rank correlation method due to Spearman is given instead, which results in the calculation of *Spearman's rank correlation coefficient*. When in doubt about the underlying assumptions required for an ordinary correlation analysis, or when perhaps only a ranking of the data is available, recourse to this method should be made. The first step is to rank the observations on each variable. Suppose 10 children are subjected to a form of an intelligence test by two independent assessors. The ranks assigned to the children by each investigator are shown in Table 8.3.

The ranking order given by the two assessors, although similar, is different. It will be of interest to assess the degree of correlation between the ranking order of the two investigators. If the ranking orders were exactly the same, a coefficient of correlation of $+1$ would be expected. On the other hand, if the

Table 8.3   Spearman's rank correlation coefficient. Rank assigned to 10 children by two assessors.

Child	1	2	3	4	5	6	7	8	9	10
Assessor A	7	6	1	2	3	$8\frac{1}{2}$	$8\frac{1}{2}$	10	4	5
Assessor B	6	7	3	2	1	4	9	8	10	5
d	1	-1	-2	0	2	$4\frac{1}{2}$	$-\frac{1}{2}$	2	-6	0
d^2	1	1	4	0	4	20·25	0·25	4	36	0

$$\Sigma d^2 = 70\cdot5; \; r_s = 1 - \frac{6(70\cdot5)}{10(99)} = 0\cdot5727; \; \text{NS}$$

ranking order of assessor B were exactly the *reverse* of assessor A, the coefficient of correlation would be expected to be -1. If there is no relationship at all between the two rankings, the coefficient of correlation would be expected to be almost 0.

For each student, it is now necessary to calculate the differences between the ranks given by the two assessors: $d =$ 'the rank for assessor A' minus 'the rank for assessor B'. These differences are shown in Table 8.3. They are squared and summed up to

$$\Sigma d^2 = 70.5 \tag{8.23}$$

Spearman's rank correlation coefficient is then simply calculated as

$$r_s = 1 - \frac{6\Sigma d^2}{n(n^2 - 1)} \tag{8.24}$$

where n is the number of pairs (10 in this case). r_s in the example turns out to be 0.5727. This correlation coefficient can be interpreted in a similar manner to the parametric correlation coefficient discussed earlier. The formula given is not quite exact if there are a lot of tied ranks in the data.

A significance test can also be performed on Spearman's rank correlation coefficient. The test statistic is actually r_s itself, and Table B.10 gives the critical values for a given number of pairs. If the calculated correlation coefficient is equal to or outside the limits defined by $\pm r$ given in the table, a significant result can be declared. For 10 pairs and a two-sided significance level of 5%, r_s would have to lie outside ± 0.6485. The calculated r_s in the example is not outside these limits, and so it can be concluded that there is no significant difference between the ranks assigned by these two assessors. Section C.15 of Appendix C summarizes the steps required to do these calculations.

8.12 Summary

In this chapter, it has been explained how the relationship between a number of variables may be described by means of regression equations, and how the strength of the relationship between the variables may be measured. It has been shown, also, how the significance of statistics such as the regression coefficient and the correlation coefficient may be tested. A brief description of more complex techniques was also presented. It is appropriate to complete this chapter with a word of caution concerning the interpretation of measures of regression and correlation, and indeed any statistical analysis. The establishment of a functional relationship in the form of a regression equation between one variable and another, or others, does not establish a *causal* link between the variables concerned. It is possible to establish a positive relationship between the growth of private vehicle registrations and the average number of telephone calls in Ireland. Both may reflect a more affluent society, but it is not suggested that there is a causal link between the two. Both may depend on a third factor, such as income, but be independent of one another. Many variables move in the same direction, or in opposite directions, over time without being in any way causally related. In practice, measures of regression and correlation are used to support hypotheses of causality, but cannot of themselves provide *proof* of causal relationships.

CHAPTER 9
Medical Studies and Epidemiological Statistics

9.1 Introduction

So far in this book, the emphasis has been on the statistical analysis of medical data. One point which has been particularly stressed is that data are not only numerical values but also information collected in a particular way for a particular purpose. The method of data collection and the design of a medical study are intimately related to the purposes for which the data are collected, and if the study design is inappropriate to, or inadequate for, the purposes of the study, no amount of statistical manipulation or analysis can rescue it.

The sampling techniques which can be used in population surveys were discussed in Chapter 3, and it was pointed out that in many situations random sampling is not employed as a basis for studies in medicine. This chapter examines some standard designs employed in observational studies, and looks at some of the epidemiological measures used in the presentation of results.

9.2 Observational and experimental studies

Studies in medicine may be divided into two distinct categories: *experimental studies* in which the investigator manipulates the allocation of individuals to different groups (discussed in the next chapter), and *observational studies* or *medical surveys* where the investigator merely makes observations on individuals, without experimental manipulation. In an observational study, different groups are compared without group membership being determined by the investigator, or alternatively relationships between different factors are examined in a single study group. Observational studies are often concerned with identifying factors which could be regarded as causal in the development of a disease or condition (risk factors), or with determining predictors of outcome or prognosis (without experimental manipulation) in patients who already have a specific condition. Observational studies may be classified into three broad groups: the *cross-sectional study*, the *prospective (cohort follow-up or longitudinal) study* and the *retrospective (case-control)*

159

study. This terminology is by no means ideal, but is fairly commonly employed. These three study designs are discussed individually below. In essence, the cross-sectional study takes no account of time; the prospective study goes forward in time from a risk factor to the disease; the case-control study goes backward in time from the disease to the risk factor.

Although case reports and clinical observations do not fall into the framework of statistical studies in medicine, they of course form the basis and foundation-stone for most medical research. Clinical observations and 'hunches' often provide the initial ideas which may eventually lead to a formal study, and to new knowledge being scientifically tested. Perhaps one of the best-known examples of this process started with the observation of Gregg (1941), an ophthalmologist, who noted an unusual number of congenital cataracts appearing in Australia. He suggested that this might be related to the exposure of the pregnant mother to German measles, of which there had been a severe epidemic in the previous year. This clinical observation led eventually to the implication of rubella virus in congenital malformations. Clues provided by studies in vital statistics may also lead to new and important findings, and such studies are discussed in Chapter 11.

As has been said, most studies in medicine eventually involve the comparison of two or more groups, and the determination of differences between the groups as regards a single factor of interest. Statistical analysis of a study is performed on the results as obtained, with the assumptions that the groups were randomly sampled from defined populations, and that measurements taken on the sample were true reflections on what one was actually trying to measure. In practice, of course, there are many biases in both the selection of study subjects and the measurements actually taken. Such biases may distort or completely invalidate the conclusions drawn from any study. Statistical analysis however cannot correct for such biases, and they must be avoided by careful study design and implementation. In the sections that follow, the design and analysis of observational studies and a few of the biases that can occur and may be preventable are discussed. Chapter 13 of this book considers the subject of bias in medical research in more detail, and to some extent the rest of this chapter assumes that such problems have been overcome, and do not affect the validity of presented results and analyses. In Chapter 7 the problems caused by confounding variables in group comparisons were alluded to, and some statistical techniques were briefly described which would control or adjust for the effect of confounding variables. The alternative to the control of confounding at the analysis stage of a study is to use an appropriate study design to eliminate the effects of confounding variables. In discussing different study designs in this chapter it is also indicated how confounding effects can be eliminated in group comparisons.

9.3 Association and causality

It has been indicated at various stages in the book that a statistical association or relationship between two factors does not imply a causal connection. The identification of causal factors requires investigations which go far beyond mere statistical calculation. Criteria for evaluating the causal significance of an association between some factor and the occurrence of a disease have been suggested (*Smoking and Health*, 1964) and these are outlined below in the context of the causal link between cigarette smoking and lung cancer. These criteria include the *consistency, strength, specificity, temporality* and *coherence* of the association. An association between a risk factor and a disease which satisfies these criteria can be taken as a strong, if not absolute, indication of causality.

1. The consistency of an association requires that different methods of study design, and studies in different populations all lead to similar conclusions. With few exceptions, all the studies of the association of cigarette smoking and lung cancer show a positive result.

2. The strength of an association means that the effect of the risk factor is large, and it is seen below how this might be quantified in studies of disease aetiology.

3. In simple terms, the specificity of the association between cigarette smoking and lung cancer demands that most persons with lung cancer are, in fact, cigarette smokers. Of course, lung cancer can arise in non-smokers, due to the multifactorial causation of the disease, but the specificity of this association is fairly clear. Note, however, that this does not mean that most cigarette smokers get lung cancer.

4. Before a risk factor for a particular disease can be judged causal, it must be certain that in fact the risk factor was present before the disease occurred. Although fairly easy to show for cigarette smoking and lung cancer, this temporality requirement can cause difficulties for other diseases and other risk factors.

5. For an association to be coherent, the association should not be at odds with known facts concerning the natural history and biology of a disease, and there should be a reasonable explanation for the association in this light. The dose–response relationship in the development of lung cancer and the numbers of cigarettes smoked, and the known carcinogenic effects of tobacco smoke, all contribute to the coherence of the association.

These five criteria are fairly stringent, and it must be admitted that many statistical associations between risk factors and disease do not meet them all. The criteria do however provide a reference by which to judge the likely causal significance of an association, and act as a reminder that statistical association on its own does not necessarily imply causality. With this caveat

in mind, different study designs to detect associations in medicine are
examined.

9.4   The cross-sectional study

Essentially, a cross-sectional study takes no account of the temporal
relationship between the factors studied, and usually involves the examination of a cross-section of a particular population at one point in time. It gives
a 'snapshot' view. Cross-sectional studies may be based on a random sample
from a defined population, or on a presenting sample of patients with a
particular condition. The sampling techniques discussed in Section 3.6 are
relevant in this context. If a study is hospital-based, one must be careful not to
over-generalize results, and be wary of the selection biases which lead to
hospital admission (see discussion in Chapter 11 also).

Cross-sectional studies may be employed to study associations between
different diseases, but they cannot often determine which disease might have
occurred first. In terms of explaining disease aetiology (cause of disease),
they provide only limited information. The *prevalence* of a disease can be
broadly defined as the proportion of persons in a population who have the
disease in question at a particular point in time (point prevalence), or over a
short time period (period prevalence). Cross-sectional studies are ideally
suited to study prevalence. Such studies also have a use in estimating health
needs or health attitudes and behaviour in a community, and the results of
such studies may be a help in planning services or appropriate health
education programmes. Screening programmes also fit into this category.
(These programmes, however, are not designed for research purposes, but are
set up to identify persons in the community who may have early evidence of a
particular disease. The object of these studies is to commence early treatment
of such persons.)

Although cross-sectional surveys are not as common in medical research as
prospective or retrospective studies they are widely used in many areas of
social research including government surveys of household budgets and
unemployment. The opinion poll itself is also of course a cross-sectional
survey.

9.5   The prospective study

The *prospective* or, as it is often called, the *cohort, longitudinal or follow-up
study* requires that individuals be followed up over a, sometimes quite long,
period of time. This follow-up may require periodic examination of the
individuals studied, or may just be based on the notification of the date of

death for each individual as he or she dies. Prospective studies have two main areas of application.

In studies of disease aetiology, a group of individuals without the disease in question may be followed forward in time until the particular disease develops, or until they die. The purpose of such studies is to identify which factors are related to the particular end-point being studied and typically will start with a cross-sectional survey. In studies of prognosis, patients with a specific disease are followed up to determine which factors relate to further morbidity (illness) and/or mortality. Studies of prognosis are usually based on a presenting sample of patients with a disease, and thus patients do not enter into observation at the same point in calendar time, but often over an extended period. Prognosis studies should, however, start at some fixed point in the natural history of the disease, usually at its first manifestation. As with all prospective studies, complete follow-up of all patients is essential, and this will often necessitate much work on the part of the investigator. When the end-point of the study is not death a regular follow-up is also required to ensure that, say, in a study of cancer recurrence no events are missed.

Two famous and long-running prospective studies to determine risk factors for specific diseases deserve mention. The Doll and Hill smoking study, as it is generally called, surveyed in 1951 all the 59 600 doctors on the medical register who were resident in the United Kingdom. Postal questionnaires were used, and nearly 41 000 usable replies were received. The questionnaire elicited very simple information regarding the respondents' cigarette smoking habits; each person was asked to classify himself/herself as a current smoker, a person who had smoked but had given up, or a person who had never smoked at all. Current and ex-smokers were asked the age at which they started to smoke, and how much they smoked. Ex-smokers were asked the age at which they ceased, and all respondents were requested to give their age at the time of the survey. Subsequent to the recipt of these questionnaires, all deaths among the doctors were notified to the study team through medical associations and the Registrar General (who is in charge of death certification). The study still continues, and the 20-year report was published in 1979 (Doll and Peto). This study has shown, very conclusively, that the death rates (number of deaths per 1000 in a defined population over a specified period) from lung cancer, and indeed all causes, among the smokers were very much higher than among the non-smokers, with the ex-smokers in an intermediate position. Death rates also increased with increasing use of tobacco.

A large sample size was required for this study, since the death rate from lung cancer was low, and a sufficient number of deaths had to be obtained. In England and Wales in 1951, eight out of every 10 000 males aged over 25 would have been expected to die from lung cancer. Note, however, that the study was not based on a random population sample and the generalization of the results requires that the relationship between lung cancer and smoking be judged the same in the general population as in doctors. The very long duration of this study is also noteworthy, although initial results were available a few years after the study commenced. As has been said, the important point about any prospective study is that the end-point (death or development of disease) be determined in all subjects. The Doll and Hill study employed routinely available records, in that the basic source of information was the death certificate. Stringent confirmation of cause of death was sought, however, and error checks on the time of death were also made.

A second famous prospective study is the Framingham Heart Study (Dawber, 1980). This study also commenced in the early 1950s, with a random sample of nearly 5000 male and female residents, aged 30–59 years, in the town of Framingham, Massachusetts (U.S.A.). The purpose of this study was to determine the many risk factors for coronary heart disease (CHD). Subjects underwent an initial comprehensive medical examination, which concentrated on the suspected risk factors for CHD. Subjects were then, and still are, examined every two years to determine the change of risk factors with time, and also the occurrence of the many manifestations of CHD. This study has provided much of what is now known about the aetiology of this condition.

9.6   Measures of risk

At this stage, it is necessary to consider the analysis and presentation of the results of a prospective study. Central to this is the notion of *risk*. There are three terms in epidemiology, which are, for most practical purposes, synonymous. For a disease, it is usual to talk about its *incidence rate* — the number of *new* cases of the disease over a particular period of time (usually a year) per 1000 (usually) of the population. (Compare this with the definition of the point prevalence rate which is the number of cases per 1000 of the population *existing* at a point in time.) A mortality rate is similarly defined as the incidence rate for the end-point of death. The *risk* of a disease or of death is the number of events occurring in a specific period of time divided by the total number of persons alive at the start of the period. Thus, a risk and a probability are measuring exactly the same thing. In this text, the subtle distinctions between rates and risks* are not of concern and only risks, as defined above, are considered, with the denominator as the total number of persons at the start of an investigation. Thus, if out of 200 individuals 15 developed CHD in one year, the risk of CHD among similar persons is

---

* The distinction between a rate and a risk is that the denominator of the former is usually the average population over the study period, while for a risk it is the number of persons at the start of the study period. The terms rate and risk are often used interchangeably, however.

15/200 or 7·5%. Note that the estimation of an incidence rate or risk requires a prospective study design, and that the definitions only allow for one event per person to occur — usually the first occurrence of an illness; death can of course occur only once.

There are many descriptive measures that can compare two risks, and they will be illustrated on the results of a study of survivors of a first heart attack (Daly *et al.*, 1983). 368 male cigarette smokers aged less than 60 years, who survived their first heart attack by at least two years*, were categorized by whether or not they had ceased cigarette smoking at this time. The patients were then followed up to determine if cessation of cigarette smoking was related to subsequent mortality. The data presented in Table 9.1 relate to the mortality experience of these patients in the two years following their categorization into continued and stopped smokers (i.e. four years after the initial heart attack). The data are laid out in a 2 × 2 table and, as was seen previously, an appropriate significance test for the mortality difference would be the χ^2 test. These two-year mortality results are non-significant at a 5% two-sided level ($\chi^2 = 3·03$; $d.f. = 1$), although over a longer period of follow-up (see Section 9.7) a significant difference was obtained.

To distinguish it from other measures the risk of an event is often termed the *absolute risk*. The absolute risk of a continued smoker dying within the 2 years of the study period is given by the number of deaths in this group

Table 9.1   Risk comparisons in a prospective study. Subsequent two-year mortality related to cessation of cigarette smoking in 368 survivors of a first heart attack.

	Survival at 2 years		Total
	Dead	Alive	
Continued smokers	19 (12·3%)	135 (87·7%)	154 (100·0%)
Stopped smokers	15 (7·0%)	199 (93·0%)	214 (100·0%)
	34 (9·2%)	334 (90·8%)	368 (100·0%)

$$\chi^2 = 3·03; \; d.f. = 1; \; NS$$

Absolute risks of death:
  continued smokers: 19/154 = 12·3%
  stopped smokers: 15/214 = 7·0%
  total: 34/368 = 9·2%

Comparing continued and stopped smokers:
  relative risk: 12·3%/7·0% = 1·76
  attributable risk: 12·3% − 7·0% = 5·3%
  attributable risk per cent: 5·3%/12·3% = 43·1%

* Six patients who were not followed for this 2-year period are excluded from this illustrative analysis. See Section 9.7 where the complete results on 374 patients are presented.

divided by the total number in the group: $19/154 = 12\cdot3\%$. The absolute risk for a stopped smoker is, similarly, $7\cdot0\%$, and for the group as a whole it is $9\cdot2\%$ (see Table 9.1). The risks of $12\cdot3$ and $7\cdot0\%$ in continued and stopped smokers may be compared in two basic ways. Their ratio can be taken and the *relative risk* of death for continued smokers relative to stopped smokers can be derived as $12\cdot3\%/7\cdot0\% = 1\cdot76$. This means that a continued smoker has $1\cdot76$ times the risk of death of a stopped smoker. This relative risk measure is the most commonly employed comparative measure of risk.

The relative risk, however, does not take account of the magnitude of its two component risks. For instance, a relative risk of $2\cdot0$ could be obtained from the two absolute risks of 90% and 45%, or from the two absolute risks of 2% and 1%. For this reason, an alternative comparative measure between two risks is also used. This is the *attributable* or *excess risk*. It is calculated by subtracting the two risks in question; thus, continued smokers have an excess risk of death of $12\cdot3\% - 7\cdot0\% = 5\cdot3\%$ relative to stopped smokers. The term attributable risk is used because, all else being equal, continued smokers, had they not continued, would have experienced a risk of $7\cdot0\%$ so that (assuming a significant result) the $5\cdot3\%$ excess can be attributed to their smoking. Both these comparative measures of risk display different aspects of the data.

Another comparative measure which is sometimes used is the attributable risk per cent. This is the attributable risk as a percentage of the absolute risk in the group exposed to the risk factor (in this case exposed to continued smoking). The attributable risk per cent is then $5\cdot3\%/12\cdot3\% = 0\cdot431 = 43\cdot1\%$. This can be interpreted to mean that, again all else being equal, $43\cdot1\%$ of the total risk of death in a continued smoker is attributable to smoking. Which of these or any of the many other comparative risk measures to employ depends on the purpose of a particular analysis. The relative risk is generally accepted as the best measure of the strength of an association between a risk factor and disease, because it is less likely to be influenced by unmeasured confounding or nuisance variables. The attributable risk on the other hand, or the attributable risk per cent, is a more useful indicator of the impact of prevention. For instance, on the basis of the above study, just over 40% of the risk of death in two years among the continued smokers could be eradicated if they had been persuaded to stop smoking; or in other words, 40% of the deaths among continued smokers were, in theory, preventable.

Although many comparative risk measures are available, the appropriate test of significance remains the same — the χ^2 test. Confidence intervals can, of course, be placed on the different risk measures but are beyond the scope of this text.

In a prospective study, one might often be interested in the joint effect of two or more risk factors on the end-point being considered. Table 9.2 shows the (hypothetical) risk of developing a disease X in groups defined by

Table 9.2 Risks (per 100 000) of developing a disease X in groups defined by drinking and smoking habits.

	Non-drinkers	Drinkers
Non-smokers	24	36
Smokers	32	50

drinking and smoking habits. An important question in relation to such data is whether or not the combined effect of both factors is greater than that expected on the basis of their individual effects in isolation. A *synergistic* effect is said to be present if the observed effect is greater than expected, and an *antagonistic* effect obtains if the effect is less than expected.

In the example, the observed effect of drinking and smoking is given by an absolute risk per 100 000 of 50, and the main question is how to calculate the expected effect. There are at least two methods of doing this, and they are best illustrated on a more concrete example. Table 9.3 shows the same numerical data, but this time relating the price of a cup of tea or coffee to whether it is drunk on the premises, or bought to take away. The price of a cup of coffee to drink at a table is not given, however. What would it be expected to be, on the basis of the prices displayed? It could be argued that since it costs 8p extra (32p–24p) to drink tea at a table it should also cost 8p extra to drink coffee at a table; thus, the cost of this should be $36p + 8p = 44p$. The same result could be obtained by noting that coffee costs 12p more than tea (to take away), so that coffee at a table should be 12p dearer than tea at a table, i.e. 44p. For obvious reasons this is considered an *additive* model for the expected price of coffee at a table.

An alternative method of calculating the expected price of drinking coffee at a table is to note that drinking tea at a table costs one-third extra, so that the expected price of drinking coffee at a table would also be one-third extra or $36p \times 1\frac{1}{3} = 48p$. This is the expected price under a *multiplicative* model. Going back to the same data as representing risks, the expected risk of disease X in smoking drinkers can be calculated at 44 per 100 000 on an additive

Table 9.3 Costs in pence of buying tea and coffee either to take away or to drink at a table in the premises (1984 prices).

	Tea	Coffee
To take away	24	36
To drink at a table	32	?

Cost to drink coffee at a table. Additive model: $36 + 8 = 44$; multiplicative model: $36 \times 1\frac{1}{3} = 48$.

model, or 48 per 100 000 on a multiplicative model. It can be seen that the expected risk in the additive model is based on equality of attributable or excess risks, for one variable at each level of the other, and in the multiplicative model on equality of relative risks. There is no definite answer as to which of the two models is more appropriate, although many favour the additive one. In the example, the observed risk of 50/100 000 is greater than that expected on either model, so that a synergistic effect of tobacco and alcohol consumption can be claimed unambiguously. In other situations, model choice may affect the interpretation of results on the combined effect of two risk factors.

9.7   Description of the clinical life table

In situations where the subjects in a prospective study do not enter the study at a fixed point in calendar time but, rather, enter over an extended period of perhaps many years there are difficulties in estimating the rates or risks of a particular end-point. (This end-point can, of course, be an event other than death, but the situation will be discussed in terms of mortality or, equivalently, survival.) Suppose a clinical follow-up study of mortality started in 1970; the patients were entered over the succeeding 10 years, and an analysis was performed early in 1980. Due to the fact that analysis must necessarily take place at a fixed point in calendar time, patients will have experienced various lengths of follow-up. (A patient entered in 1970 would have 10 years of follow-up; a patient entered in 1979 would have been followed for less than a year.) Also, at the time of analysis many patients will not have experienced the end-point of interest, and some patients may have been lost to follow-up before the analysis date, due to emigration, missed visits or other reasons. Survival or mortality data collected in this way are often called *censored data* since patient follow-up is terminated early, or censored, due to the practical requirements of data analysis. Such patients, who are, consequently, known to be alive at the analysis stage of a study before experiencing the end-point of interest, are called withdrawals. They should be differentiated from actual losses to follow-up.

Many erroneous approaches have been used to analyse prospective data when the subjects have experienced variable follow-up. The approach described in the last section of calculating survival or mortality at a fixed point from study entry (e.g. 5 years) is only valid when each subject is known to be either alive or dead at this time-point. To use this approach in a variable follow-up study requires that the data collected on many patients must be discarded (see more detailed discussion in the next section). The calculation of a 'total study mortality', by dividing all the observed deaths by the total number studied, is not a mortality rate in any sense of the word, since it takes no account of the time over which the events occurred. With a follow-up of everyone to death, this figure would eventually reach 100%! Sometimes, a mean 'length of survival' is calculated by averaging the time of death of the decedents and the time to last follow-up of the live withdrawals. The resulting figure however measures the average length of follow-up rather than anything else, and is totally dependent on the study duration. It is not a suitable summary measure of survival.

There are two solutions to the analysis of mortality with a variable follow-up. The first, although often used, is not the best approach. It defines an overall mortality rate in the study as the number of deaths per person-year of observation. A person-year of observation means one person followed for one year. Thus, no distinction is made between 10 persons followed for 2 years and 2 persons followed for 10 years. The person-years of observation are calculated by noting the total time each person was under observation up to death, loss or withdrawal, and adding over all the subjects. The resulting rate however is not readily amenable to statistical analysis.

The second approach for the analysis of variable follow-up data uses what is often called the *clinical or actuarial life table method*. (See Chapter 11 for a discussion of the *population life table*.) Many variants of this are available, and the simplest is described below. Essentially, the entire study period is subdivided into small intervals of time; usually years or months are employed, but some techniques require that the intervals be defined by the actual times of each event (death, loss or withdrawal). In each interval the number of patients alive at the start, the number of deaths and the number withdrawn alive or lost to follow-up are used to estimate a 'within-interval' mortality. These interval mortalities can then be combined to give a mortality risk (rate) for any time since study commencement. This method is described in more detail in the next section. The clinical life table approach gives an unbiased estimate of mortality at yearly intervals (or whatever size intervals are chosen) from study commencement, and thus gives a far more complete picture of what is happening than the usual 2×2 table which compares mortality at a fixed time-point only. The clinical life table is either a table or graph showing the percentage mortality (or survival) at each time point from study commencement. These are sometimes called the cumulative mortality or survival rates. Fig. 9.1 shows the cumulative mortality over a 13-year follow-up of the continued and stopped smokers in the study of heart attack survivors discussed in the previous section. Although most of the patients were not followed for the full 13 years, the clinical life table method allowed calculation of the 13-year mortality, which was around 82% in the continued smokers and 37% in those who ceased. Mortality at all times from the start of the study can easily be read off the graph, and the visual presentation shows clearly how the two mortality curves diverge over time.

In addition to presenting a clear and unbiased picture of mortality over

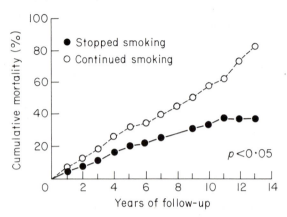

time, the clinical life table utilizes all the available data without discarding any of them. Losses to follow-up, as long as there are not too many, can also be accounted for by the method, given certain fairly reasonable assumptions. Statistical tests, the best-known of which is called the *logrank test*, are also available to compare the mortalities of two or more groups calculated by the life table method. In short, for the analysis of mortality or of any other end-point in a prospective study with variable follow-up, the clinical life table is the method of choice. In the next section the computations for constructing a clinical life table are outlined, and the logrank test is briefly described. The section can be omitted at a first reading.

9.8 Computation of the clinical life table

Fig. 9.2 shows, schematically, the follow-up of 14 patients entered into a prospective study between 1970 and 1979. The left-hand side of the figure shows the 'lifespan' of each of the patients (labelled from A to N) in calendar time. Patient A, for instance, entered into the study in 1970 and died near the end of 1973 (between 3 and 4 years from study entry). Patient C was lost track of during 1975, but was known to be alive just over 4 years after study entry (a loss to follow-up). Patient E entered the study in mid-1973, and was alive at the start of 1980 (more than 6 years after entry into the study). Similarly, patients H, J, K, L and N were all alive at the time the study was being analysed, and are considered as withdrawals. The right-hand side of Fig. 9.2 shows the patient histories plotted from study entry, rather than in calendar time. The light lines refer to the potential periods of follow-up had the patients not died or been lost to follow-up. Suppose now that it is wished to calculate a 4-year mortality rate or risk for these patients. Some of the incorrect methods already referred to in the last section will be illustrated

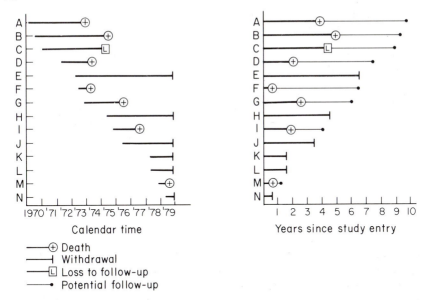

FIG. 9.2. Diagram showing follow-up of 14 patients entered into a prospective study.

first. Using the definition of number dead within 4 years divided by the total number of patients, the figure of 6 (patients A, D, F, G, I and M) divided by $14 = 42·9\%$ would be obtained. This, however, is unduly optimistic, because it assumes that patients J, K, L and N, the withdrawals, who were not actually followed for as long as 4 years, would in fact have remained alive until the end of the 4 years. This is an untenable assumption. Alternatively a 4-year survival rate might have been defined, putting the number alive at 4 years over the total number in the study. This gives 4 (patients B, C, E, and H) divided by 14, or 28·6%, which corresponds to a 4-year mortality of 71·4%. This is an unduly pessimistic figure, since its calculation assumes that the 4 withdrawals in the denominator would not have survived the full 4 years. In fact, the only unbiased estimator of a 4-year mortality rate is obtained by confining the analysis to only those patients actually followed for 4 years, or those who could have been followed if they had not died. This reduces the study cohort from the original 14 to 9 patients only (A to I) and gives a 4-year mortality of $6/9 = 66·7\%$. Because of the variable length of follow-up, the alternative to biased estimates of the mortality rate seem to require sacrificing much of the available information. It shall now be seen how the clinical life table approach avoids this problem, and provides an unbiased estimate of mortality.

As was said in the last section, this approach requires a division of the total follow-up period into intervals. Supposing the 10 years of the example study are now divided into 10 intervals of 1 year each; the data required for calculating a mortality rate using the clinical life table approach are then the total number alive at the start of the study and the numbers of deaths, withdrawals alive, and losses to follow-up observed in each interval.

The method is based on the law of combining conditional probabilities, discussed in Chapter 3 (Eqn. 3.3). To take a simple analogy, this law means that to get from London to New York via Shannon, for instance, it is necessary first to get to Shannon, and from Shannon it is necessary to travel to New York. Take an example of this principle in terms of survival rates or probabilities. Table 9.4 displays a simple mortality study. One hundred persons enter the study at time zero. Fifty-five die in the first year (leaving 45 alive) and 15 persons die in the second year, leaving 30 survivors at the end of 2 years. The 2-year survival is then $30/100 = 0.3$, expressed as the probability of surviving two years. Now the one-year survival probability is, obviously, given by $45/100 = 0.45$. Of these 45 persons who survived the first year, 15 die in the succeeding year, and 30 survive, so that the survival from the start to the end of year two, conditional on being alive at the start of year 2, is $30/45 = 0.6667$. Note, however, that $0.45 \times 0.6667 = 0.3$. This is an example of the application of Eqn. 3.3. To survive two intervals of time it is necessary to survive the first interval, and given that, to then survive the second interval. If the probability of surviving from time 0 (study commencement) to time i (the end of the ith interval or year) is denoted by P_i, and the conditional probability of surviving the ith interval (from time $i-1$ to i) by p_i, then the generalization of this is

$$P_i = p_i P_{i-1} \tag{9.1}$$

where P_0 is the probability of surviving to time 0 which must be 1.0. The P_i are called cumulative or unconditional survival probabilities.

The clinical life table utilizes this relationship by calculating the conditional probability of surviving each interval defined for the study, and then calculating the unconditional (cumulative) probabilities of survival from

Table 9.4 Simple example of conditional probabilities. P (event) means the probability of the event.

Time (years)	0		1		2
Interval no.		1		2	
No. alive	100		45		30
No. dying		55		15	

$P_1 = P(\text{survival } 0-1) = 45/100 = 0.45$
$P_2 = P(\text{survival } 0-2) = 30/100 = 0.3$
$p_2 = P(\text{survival } 1-2, \text{ given alive at } 1) = 30/45 = 0.6667$
$P_2 = p_2 P_1$.

study commencement to the end of each interval. The cumulative mortality probabilities are obtained by subtracting the survival probabilities from 1, and can then be converted to percentages. How then can the conditional probability of surviving each interval be calculated? First, some notation must be introduced. The intervals in the study are numbered from 1 to i, where 1 denotes the first interval, running from time 0 to time 1 (years or months). Table 9.5 displays the notation adopted. It has already been mentioned that the life table calculation requires that n_1, the number entering the study (and therefore the first interval), and the d_i and w_i, the deaths and withdrawals/ losses in each defined interval, are known. No distinction is made between withdrawals due to study termination and losses to follow-up. It will now be shown how, starting with these data, an unbiased estimate of the 4-year mortality in the example discussed above can be calculated. Table 9.6 lays out the data. Fourteen persons entered the study, and in the first interval there were 2 deaths (patients F and M — see Fig. 9.2) and 1 withdrawal (patient N). If there were no withdrawals, the probability of dying in the first interval would be just 2/14, but the single withdrawal must somehow be taken into account. If it can be assumed that any withdrawals occurred on average halfway into the interval, it could be argued that each withdrawal only contributes a 'half person' to the number at risk, and that the denominator of the probability of death should be reduced accordingly. Instead of 14 persons being at risk of death in the interval, there would be only 13·5 persons, and the probability of death would be calculated as $2/13\cdot5 = 0\cdot1481$. This is the total number of deaths in the interval, divided by what is called the adjusted number at risk. This is a central feature of the life table, that withdrawals alive due to study termination and losses to follow-up only contribute one-half to the number at risk required to calculate a mortality probability. The adjusted number at risk is denoted n_i' (in the ith interval) and

Table 9.5   Clinical life table notation.

Meaning	Symbol
Interval	i
End-points of interval i	$i-1$ $\quad i$
Numbers entering interval i	n_i
Numbers dying in interval i	d_i
Numbers withdrawn or lost to follow up in interval i	w_i
Adjusted number at risk at the start of interval i	n_i'
Conditional probability of death in interval i	q_i
Conditional probability of surviving interval i	p_i
Unconditional probability of surviving from time 0 to the end of interval i (i.e. to time i)	P_i
Unconditional probability of dying by the end of interval i (i.e. by time i)	Q_i

Table 9.6 Clinical life table for data of Fig. 9.2.

(1) Interval i $(i-1)-i$	(2) Numbers entering interval n_i	(3) Numbers with-drawn/ lost during interval w_i	(4) Adjusted number at risk n_i'	(5) Deaths during interval d_i	(6) Proba-bility of death during interval q_i	(7) Proba-bility of survival during interval p_i	(8) Cumula-tive proba-bility of survival to end of interval P_i	(9) Cumula-tive proba-bility of death by end of interval Q_i
1	14	1	13·5	2	0·1481	0·8519	0·8519	0·1481
2	11	2	10·0	2	0·2000	0·8000	0·6815	0·3185
3	7	0	7·0	1	0·1429	0·8571	0·5841	0·4159
4	6	1	5·5	1	0·1818	0·8182	0·4779	0·5221
5	4	2	3·0	1	0·3333	0·6667	0·3186	0·6814
6	1	1	—					

$$n_i' = n_i - 0.5w_i \tag{9.2}$$

$$q_i = d_i/n_i' \tag{9.3}$$

where q_i is the estimated probability of death in the interval. The (conditional) probability of surviving the interval is then

$$p_i = 1.0 - q_i \tag{9.4}$$

which is given in column 7 of Table 9.6 as 0·8519 for the first interval. Eqn. 9.1 is now used to calculate the cumulative probability of survival from the start of the study (time 0) to the end of interval 1. This is, of course, the same as the conditional probability for the first interval, so $P_1 = p_1 = 0.8519$. The cumulative probability of death is then obtained by subtracting this from 1

$$Q_i = 1.0 - P_i \tag{9.5}$$

which is 0·1481 or 14·81%.

Now move to the second row of Table 9.6 to calculate the same quantities for the second interval. The number entering the interval is given by the number entering the previous interval less all the withdrawals and deaths.

$$n_i = n_{i-1} - (w_{i-1} + d_{i-1}) \tag{9.6}$$

which gives a total of 11. Check this with Fig. 9.2. The calculations proceed as before. Since there were 2 withdrawals in this interval, the adjusted number at risk is $11.0 - 1 = 10.0$, and the conditional probability of surviving the interval is 0·8000. The cumulative probability of surviving to the end of the interval is again obtained using Eqn. 9.1, multiplying this conditional probability of 0.8000 by the cumulative probability of surviving to the end of the previous interval (0.8519). This gives $P_2 = 0.6815$ and a cumulative probability of death by the end of the second interval at 2 years as $1 - 0.6815 = 0.3185$ or 31.9%. This process is continued for the next three intervals, as shown in the table. The 4-year mortality, calculated in this way, turns out to be 0.5221 or 52.21%. This is the best estimate of 4-year mortality available from the data. Usually, the cumulative probabilities of survival or death would be displayed graphically, as already illustrated.

The main assumption underlying the clinical life table is that withdrawals due to study termination would have subsequently experienced a similar mortality rate as those actually followed for a longer period. Thus, the method does not allow for any secular changes in mortality and requires that all study participants, irrespective of when they entered the study in calendar time, are exposed to the same risks of death. It has been mentioned that losses to follow-up are treated in the same way as withdrawals, so it is also assumed that persons lost to follow-up are similar to persons with whom contact was maintained. This may not be so and the number of losses must be kept to a minimum.

As for any of the other descriptive statistics discussed in this book, standard errors of the cumulative proportions surviving or dying by any time-point can be estimated, and confidence intervals calculated. Simple significance tests are also available for the comparison of two life table curves at a fixed point in time. Often, however, life table curves comparing two groups may cross over each other, suggesting a survival advantage for one of the groups at one point of time, and a disadvantage at a later period. For this reason a statistical test to compare the complete life table curves in the groups being analysed is required. The logrank test is most commonly employed in this situation. Essentially, the logrank test involves the comparison of the observed number of deaths in each group (O) with the number of deaths that would be expected (E) if the groups had, in the population, similar survival experiences. The calculation of these expected values is performed separately in each interval, and then summed over all the intervals, thus taking account of the variable follow-up on each individual. The calculations are not, however, detailed here. The quantity O/E for a particular group is a relative risk type measure (often called a relative death rate), comparing the observed mortality in that group relative to the mortality in all groups included in the comparison. The ratio of 2 O/Es gives an average relative risk between the two groups involved, which is sometimes called the death rate ratio. The logrank significance test for comparing O/Es from different groups is a χ^2 statistic, similar in form to the χ^2 for a general contingency table. The logrank test may also be used to adjust a life table comparison for confounding qualitative variables that may have different distributions in the groups being compared (see the discussion of confounding in Chapter 7).

An alternative to the logrank test in comparing life table curves is to use *Cox's life table regression model* or, as it is sometimes called, *the proportional hazards model* (Cox, 1972). Essentially, this is a multiple regression type of approach which can allow for the problems of variable follow-up in longitudinal survival data; thus it also allows correction for quantitative confounders. Remember that logistic regression can be used for analysing survival or mortality at a fixed time point, when everyone is followed for the appropriate period (see Section 8.9). Survival analysis can also be performed by fitting the data to a parametric model in which a particular functional form is assumed to hold for the survival curve. Comparisons of the survival experiences of groups are then based on comparing the estimated parameters of the model.

9.9   The case-control study

One of the purposes of the prospective study is to determine associations between risk factors measured at the start of the study and subsequent morbidity or mortality. In essence, a prospective study goes forward from a risk factor to the development of the end-point of interest.* An alternative to the prospective study for the elucidation of associations between risk factors and disease is a case-control or retrospective study. As its name suggests, the retrospective study starts with the end-point and moves backwards in time to the identification of risk factors.

A group of persons with a particular disease (the cases) is studied as regards factors to which it was exposed in the past, and the results compared with those obtained in a comparison group (the controls) without the disease. If the factor is associated with the disease, then it should appear more commonly in the cases than in the controls. The investigation of Herity *et al.* (1981) into the association between smoking and drinking and the development of cancer of the head and neck will be taken as an example of this type of study. A case-control study divides into 4 stages: the selection of cases, the selection of controls, the measurement of the risk factor, and the analysis of the association. To avoid bias, cases in a case-control study should be newly diagnosed. Although this will always reduce the numbers available for a study, a group

---

* A prospective study must necessarily go forward in time. In very rare cases however with exceptionally good records on all individuals collected in the past, which have been kept completely up to date, a prospective study can be done 'retrospectively'. Such a study is however in essence still a prospective study.

containing a mixture of newly diagnosed cases and long-standing chronic cases can cause great difficulty in interpreting the results. The diagnostic criteria for defining a case must be explicit and clear. This will enable the study to be replicated elsewhere and avoid ambiguities of interpretation. Often persons with other concurrent disease will be excluded from the cases. Usually in a case-control study a presenting sample, to a particular hospital or unit, of newly diagnosed cases is taken. It must be remembered however that cases admitted to a hospital are not necessarily representative of all cases in the community at large. In the study of head and neck cancer, a presenting sample of 200 new patients attending a particular hospital over a two-year period for treatment of cancer of the head and neck formed the case group. The definition of head and neck cancer and its diagnostic subgroup is given in the original paper.

The selection of controls is, without any doubt, the most difficult part of a case-control study. Ideally, the controls should be representative of the general population without the disease, and thus be a random sample from the same population that gave rise to the cases. Practical considerations however usually dictate that controls are taken from a hospital population of patients who have neither the disease under investigation, nor a disease positively related to the risk factor being studied. One advantage of this approach is that the same factors that determined hospitalization of the cases in a particular hospital may also have been likely to determine the hospitalization of the controls. The problem is, of course, to what extent the controls may be judged representative of the general population.

Apart from the source of the controls, the next problem arises in their selection. A random sample from the hospital patients not affected by the disease in question could be taken, but it is then likely that cases and controls would differ as regards variables that might be related to exposure to the risk factors or development of the disease. Such variables, which would act as confounders of the association, could be controlled for in the analysis stage but are better adjusted for in the design of the study. Age and sex are two common confounders in case-control studies. To avoid the confounding effect of such variables, the controls are often chosen to have the same distribution as the cases in terms of characteristics such as age and sex. Two different methods are available to achieve this; the first has already been discussed and involves a paired sample (see Section 7.2). Typically, a control of the same sex and age (to within a specified number of years) is individually matched to each case, and the analysis proceeds as for paired comparisons discussed in Chapter 7. Some studies however use *frequency matching* whereby the distribution of, say, age and sex in the controls is fixed to be identical to that in the cases, but not by individual matching. Usually this is achieved by determining the age/sex distribution of the cases in, say, 10-year age groups. If there are 15 males aged 45–54 years in the cases, 15 males in the same age group would be chosen for the controls.* Although the overall distribution will be similar in the two groups, individual matching does not occur. What factors to match for in case-control studies often causes problems. Variables that are known to be associated with both the development of the disease and exposure to the risk factor are the prime candidates. As has been said, age and sex are two such factors. It should be noted, however, that to match for too many factors can, in practice, be a very tedious task and that any variables matched for cannot be analysed for a relationship with the disease. One can match on variables related to the disease but not to the risk factor of interest, if the influence of such variables is not to be analysed and a small effect of a different variable is being investigated. Matching must not take place on variables related to the risk factor only, since this will tend to ensure equal distribution of the risk factor in cases and controls, and hence no result.

Care must also be taken in the actual choosing of each individual control. Ideally, the person selecting the control should not know the nature of the risk factor being studied or subtle selection biases might occur. For instance, if cigarette smoking was one of the risk factors being studied, a potential control with a packet of cigarettes on his/her bedside locker might be deliberately avoided! In the study of head and neck cancer, the controls, frequency-matched to the cases for age (in 10-year age groups) and sex, were chosen from patients attending the same hospital 'for the treatment of non-smoking-related cancers and benign conditions' during the same period in which the cases were hospitalized.

Once cases and controls have been chosen, exposure to the risk factors must be determined. Unfortunately, this depends either on the patient's memory, or on available hospital records. It is important that cases and controls are interviewed in the same manner and by the same person. Ideally, that person should not know if the individual is a case or control in order to avoid a biased response as a result of leading questions or a more careful interviewing of cases. In practice, this is difficult to achieve. Also, if the case knows the purpose of the study, he or she might overemphasize or minimize exposure to the risk factors, thus biasing the results in this way. Some case-control studies are based on hospital charts and records only, and exposure information based on these may be quite dubious. Often such records are incomplete, and no mention of a particular factor either means that the factor was not present, or that exposure was never ascertained or recorded. In the head and neck cancer study, a predesigned questionnaire was administered by one of the investigators, and details of sex, age, occupation, education, tobacco and alcohol consumption and dental care were noted.

After collection of the data, the association between the risk factor and the

---

* Usually, in case-control studies, the numbers of cases and controls are taken to be equal.

Table 9.7 Relationship between smoking and head and neck cancer in a case-control study. Abbreviated from Herity, Moriarty, Bourke & Daly (1981) with permission.

	Cases	Controls	Total
Smokers	145 (72·5%)	107 (53·5%)	252 (63·0%)
Non- or ex-smokers	55 (27·5%)	93 (46·5%)	148 (37·0%)
	200 (100·0%)	200 (100·0%)	400 (100·0%)

$$\chi^2 = 15\cdot487; \, d.f. = 2; \, p < 0\cdot01$$

$$\text{Odds ratio} = \frac{145/107}{55/93} = \frac{145 \times 93}{55 \times 107} = 2\cdot29$$

disease must be examined. From the significance-testing point of view, the methods outlined in Chapter 7 for the comparison of two groups will be adequate for examining the relationship of a single risk factor and a disease. More advanced techniques, not detailed in this book, will have to be employed if frequency matching has been used, or if it is wished to adjust for confounding variables. It is important, also, to have a measure of the strength of the association between the risk factor and the disease. It has already been described how in a prospective study the absolute risks of disease in those exposed and not exposed to a risk factor can be calculated. Unfortunately, in a case-control study, no measure of absolute risk is available, since there is no group that was followed forward in time. Table 9.7 shows a 2×2 table with the smoking results in the head and neck cancer study. The result is significant by the chi-square test,* showing a predominance of smokers amongst the cases. It cannot however be said that the absolute risk of a smoker getting head and neck cancer is 145/252, since 252 smokers were not followed forward over a period of time; in fact, if 2 controls per case had been chosen, a totally different answer would have been obtained. Absolute risks cannot be determined in a case-control study. It is possible, however, to calculate an approximate estimate of the relative risk if it can be assumed that the incidence of the disease in the population is small, that cases and controls are random samples from their corresponding populations, and that only new cases are included. This approximation to the relative risk is called the *odds ratio*, and is calculated by dividing the 'odds' of a smoker getting head and neck cancer by the 'odds' of a non-smoker getting this cancer. The odds of an event are related to its probability; but the odds are defined as the number of persons who experience the event divided, not by the total number

---

* This illustrative analysis ignores the frequency matching, and treats cases and controls as independent samples.

of persons, but by the number of persons not experiencing the event. Now, an individual odd cannot be calculated directly from a case-control study either but, unlike the relative risk, the ratio of the two quantities ('odds') 145/107 and 55/93 = 2·29 estimates the true ratio of the odds, and is not dependent on the number of controls taken per case, being the same for any sampling fraction of cases and controls. 2·29 can then be interpreted as an estimate of the ratio of the odds, in the population, of a smoker developing head and neck cancer to the odds of a non-smoker developing this disease. Given the assumptions already mentioned, this odds ratio is a good approximation to the relative risk, and it can be said that a smoker has 2·29 times the risk of a non-smoker of developing head and neck cancer.

The above example dealt with (for illustrative purposes) two independent samples of cases and controls. If individually matched cases and controls were being analysed, the data in a 2×2 table would have to be laid out as described for the significance testing of paired proportions (Section 7.13). In this situation, an approximation to the relative risk is given by the ratio of

Table 9.8 Relative risks in case-control studies.

(a) Independent data

		Cases	Controls
Risk factor	Present	a	b
	Absent	c	d
		$a+c$	$b+d$

$$\text{Relative risk} \approx \frac{ad}{bc}$$

(b) Paired data

		Case	
		Risk factor present	Risk factor absent
Control	Risk factor present	a	b
	Risk factor absent	c	d

$$\text{Relative risk} \approx \frac{c}{b}$$

untied pairs. The number of pairs in which the case and not the control is exposed to the risk factor is divided by the number of pairs in which the control is exposed and the case is not. These approximate relative risk calculations are summarized in Table 9.8.

It was previously pointed out that the presence of a confounding variable such as age or sex, associated with both the disease and the risk factor, may distort an observed association between the risk factor itself and the disease. Such confounding can be controlled by study design through matching. Other confounding variables may exist, however, and if they have been measured, can be controlled in the analysis stage as indicated in Chapter 7. Essentially, the relative risk is examined at each level of a qualitative confounder, and an average of these relative risks is calculated. Methods for the analysis of frequency-matched data are also based on combining results obtained at each level of the matching variable(s). Sometimes one is also interested, not in controlling for a confounding variable, but in estimating the joint effect on disease occurrence of two variables acting together. The technique discussed in Section 9.6 for the measurement of synergistic effects can also be employed on relative risk measures obtained from a case-control study. If the confounding variables in a case-control study are quantitative rather than qualitative in nature, recently developed techniques allow the use of logistic regression in case-control studies to adjust results for such factors. A full discussion of these techniques is beyond the scope of this text.

9.10   Comparison of prospective and case-control studies

Both prospective and case-control (retrospective) studies can be utilized to examine associations between risk factors and disease, and each approach has its advantages and disadvantages. The prospective study generally will require large sample sizes and extensive periods of follow-up. This is due to the fact that the incidence of many conditions is low, even in an exposed group, and many persons must be studied over a long period to obtain even a few cases who develop the end-point of interest. The case-control study, on the other hand, utilizes existing cases with a large reduction in the required sample size. Case-control studies are thus cheaper to carry out and will provide results much faster. Such studies are especially useful in studying the aetiology of rare conditions.

Unlike the case-control study however, the prospective study is not as open to bias in the measurement of the risk factors, and allows complete ascertainment and uniformity of measurement for the relevant data. The case-control study relies on memory or previously recorded data, and has many problems in this area. Proper choice of adequate controls in a case-control study is perhaps its greatest weakness, and it is probably true to say that very few case-control studies, in practice, have controls that satisfy the most stringent criteria required for an unbiased comparison. The comparison groups in a prospective study however can usually be defined without bias, since they are formed without prior knowledge of which individuals will develop the disease being investigated. There is usually no predefined separate control group in a prospective study; comparisons are just made between groups with and without the risk factor present as determined at the baseline examination. The prospective study also allows the calculation of absolute risks of disease, whereas only relative risk measures are available with the case-control study. Further, the prospective study allows for the examination of the relationship of measured risk factors to many different end-points, whereas the case-control study is confined to one end-point and, usually, only a few risk factors.

Although the prospective study has many definite theoretical advantages over the case-control study in determining aetiology, the latter is more often encountered due to the sheer difficulty of setting up and following through the prospective study. Certainly, no prospective study should be started without a case-control study first, to check that a suspected association actually manifests itself. But, in many cases, the results of case-control studies only must be accepted as the method of determining disease aetiology.

9.11   Summary

In this chapter, the scope and application of the observational study in medical research have been outlined. The notion of risk was introduced and its estimation in different situations was considered. The design of cross-sectional, prospective and case-control studies was described, and appropriate analytical techniques introduced. The main purpose of observational studies in medicine is to identify risk factors for disease, or to determine factors related to prognosis in those who already have the disease. Results of observational studies relate, in the main, to prevention. The next chapter in this book considers studies of the treatment of disease, and is concerned not with the observational study, but with experimental trials.

CHAPTER 10
The Randomized Controlled Trial

10.1 Introduction

This chapter considers the design of the experimental trial in medical research. The purpose of the experimental trial is to evaluate the effectiveness of some intervention or therapy. What distinguishes the experimental trial from the observational study discussed in the last chapter is that the researcher has direct control over many aspects of the investigation, and in particular, over the allocation of individuals to different treatment groups. This chapter is not intended to be a handbook for the clinician wishing to undertake a trial, but merely a guideline to the principles and practices of such trials.

10.2 Treatment and control groups

One of the most important questions facing any practising physician or surgeon is 'What treatment shall I use?'. It is vital that the doctor (and patient) knows the effectiveness of the different treatments available, and thus what may be best in a particular situation. Advances in medicine require a detailed knowledge of treatment efficacy, and the experimental trial provides the only valid procedure to achieve this. Many therapeutic regimes, commonly used in the past, were seen to be worthless or even dangerous when evaluated in such a proper and scientific manner. Any proposed new therapy, be it medical or surgical, should be tested by means of a trial, unless the results are so startlingly obvious that a formal evaluation is not necessary, as for example a successful treatment for a condition that was 100% fatal.

'I have a wonder cure for the common cold. If you take this preparation for one day only, your symptoms will be cleared within a week.' Faced with a claim such as this, the most important question is 'What would happen to my cold symptoms if I did not take this preparation?'. The claim of effectiveness only stands up when a comparison can be made with the situation pertaining without the treatment. This is the foundation-stone for the evaluation of any therapy. Its effectiveness must be compared with the results of either no treatment, or the best treatment available before its introduction.

To evaluate a new therapy, then, requires comparing its results on a group of treated patients with the results on a group with the same disease not so treated. These two groups are usually called the treatment and control groups respectively. Many early evaluations of therapy used what are called *historical controls*. The results on a series of patients on the new treatment were compared to the results obtained on 'similar' patients in the past who did not have the 'benefits' of the newer approach. The word 'similar' is in quotations because the main problem with historical controls is that they are likely to be quite different from patients treated in the present. Historical controls may, in the first place, have had a better (or worse) outlook than the treatment group. Between the time when the historical controls were seen and treated and the present, there may have been changes in hospital admissions policy, general management may have improved, diagnostic criteria may have changed, and the historical controls may not have had as much attention and care as the treated group, who may be getting special attention because they are receiving the new therapy. For these reasons, a comparison between the results obtained on a treated group and a historical control group could be seriously biased, and any differences in outcome noted may not reflect a true treatment effect. A further problem with historical controls is that reliance is placed on past records to evaluate their prognosis, and missing or unrecorded information on some patients may further bias the results. In short, for a valid evaluation of therapy, a concurrent control group must be used. Also, by its very nature an experimental trial is prospective, in that individuals must be followed forward in time to determine the effect of a therapy, and usually individuals are entered into a trial over what is sometimes an extended period of time.

10.3   Types of trials

The experimental trial in medicine may be employed in three main situations, distinguished by the type of individual studied and the effect of the treatment or intervention involved. In the *clinical* or *therapeutic* trial, the study groups consist of persons with a particular disease or condition, and the treatment is therapeutic. The purpose of such trials is to determine if treatment can effect a 'cure' or remove manifestations of a disease already present in the patients. The total sample size for such trials is often in the region of 20 to 100 patients if the treatment is even moderately effective. Examples of such trials abound in the medical literature. Trials, for instance, of antihypertensive agents to reduce blood pressure, and analgesics to alleviate pain, fit into this category.

In *secondary* and *primary prevention trials*, the treatment or intervention under investigation is prophylactic, in that its purpose is the prevention of a particular manifestation of disease which is not present at the start of the trial. In secondary prevention trials, the subjects already have the disease in question, or have suffered one event, and it is hoped to prevent or delay recurrences or death. Examples are trials of chemotherapy regimes in patients with cancer, where the end-point is often cancer recurrence or death. Drug-treatment of patients who have had a heart attack, and coronary bypass surgery in patients with angina, also fit into this category.

The primary prevention trial, on the other hand, is performed on subjects free of disease, with a view to preventing the first occurrence of an event. Cholesterol-reducing drugs have been tested in this manner to evaluate their effectiveness in preventing coronary heart attacks, and trials evaluating the usefulness of risk factor modifications, such as the cessation of cigarette smoking, have also been carried out in this area.

Since both primary and secondary prevention trials are concerned with the prevention or delay of a particular event, rather than the elimination of a condition which is present, very large sample sizes and an extensive period of follow-up may often be required. This is because some events must occur in the study population before an evaluation of the intervention can be made, and often the rate of events which can be expected in the study group is so small that large numbers are needed to observe even a few events. Secondary prevention trials can require up to and over 1000 subjects, while primary prevention trials (the few there have been) may require 10 000 or more subjects in order to have any chance of detecting an important result. (Appendix D discusses the calculation of sample sizes in simple situations.)

Having examined the scope of the experimental trial, some of its salient features are now presented. Whether a clinical, a primary prevention or a secondary prevention trial is being conducted, the underlying requirements are the same, so that the discussion will, without loss of generality, be in the context of a secondary prevention trial evaluating a particular drug therapy (timolol — a beta blocker) in reducing mortality in patients who have had a heart attack (myocardial infarction). (The Norwegian Multicentre Study Group, 1981.)

Suppose now that a controlled trial has been performed with a treatment group and contemporaneous controls who did not receive the treatment, and suppose further that positive results (in terms of increased survival) in favour of the treatment are observed. What could explain these results? The first possible explanation is that there is really no difference between the two (population) groups* and that the observed difference is spurious, or due to chance (sampling variation). The whole purpose of statistical analysis is to answer this question at a specified probability level, so that either chance can be ruled out as the explanation (a significant result), or it can be accepted that it is a possible cause (a non-significant result).

---

* See Section 10.4 for an alternative and more correct interpretation of statistical significance in a controlled trial.

If the observed difference between the treatment and control groups cannot reasonably be ascribed to chance, three further possibilities remain, either singly or in combination, which might explain the difference. The treatment and control groups may themselves differ appreciably in factors related to their prognosis, or the two groups may have been handled and looked after in different ways. The third explanation, of course, is that the particular therapy being examined does indeed have a beneficial effect.

If chance is not the determining factor, the trial organizers will want to conclude that the action of the intervention explains the observed results, and to do so they must be sure that the groups were in fact similar in all respects except for the intervention given, and were handled in the same fashion. A properly run clinical trial is designed in such a way that biases due to group differences of any sort (aside from the intervention) can be excluded as an explanation of any observed differences in outcome that might be found. Note that it is the design of the trial and the implementation of that design, not the statistical analysis, that ensure avoidance of these biases. The next few sections discuss procedures utilized in a controlled trial to achieve these ends.

10.4   Randomization

How then can it be ensured that the treatment and control groups are as similar as possible, regarding factors that may influence their eventual outcome? (Assume that only one treatment is being tested, although trials with more than two groups are possible.) The best method is by a process of *randomization (random allocation)*. After a patient is deemed to be eligible for entering into the trial (see below), a coin is tossed. If it lands heads, the patient is allocated to the treatment group; if it lands tails, to the control group. This process is the essence of randomization, although admittedly, if used in practice, it would probably irrevocably damage any confidence the patient may have had in his physician (but see the discussion of informed consent in Section 10.8).

Randomization by the tossing of a coin (or any equivalent method) ensures that the physician running the trial is not consciously or unconsciously allocating certain patients to a particular group. Thus randomization can eliminate group differences due to selection bias. Without randomization for instance, trials of a surgical versus medical technique are wide open to this problem. Low-risk cases are much more likely to be assigned to the operation group, leaving high-risk patients to be managed by the physicians. Assigning volunteers to the treatment group, and those who do not volunteer to the control group, is also likely to result in a biased comparison — volunteers could be quite different in many respects from patients who do not volunteer.

Often it is suggested that patients be allocated to treatment or control groups alternately, or on alternate days. The problem with such methods is that referring doctors may know which day corresponds to which group allocation, and refer accordingly, or that the doctors running the trial may exclude certain patients if they know beforehand which group they are being assigned to. This latter problem can also arise if randomization according to birth date is employed (e.g. patients with an even birth year are assigned to one of the groups, and the remainder to the other). The process of randomization, embodied in the idea of tossing a coin (after patient eligibility has been determined), is the only way to ensure that there has been no bias in treatment allocation. Note that a bias may not necessarily be present with any of the other methods, but the problem is that it might be. The results of a controlled trial, based on a possibly biased method of group allocation, are always open to doubt.

It has been argued of course that the use of statistical methods to correct for group differences which could affect outcome (confounders) would obviate the necessity for randomization, and even allow for the use of historical controls. This is only true insofar as all the possible confounders are known and measured, and the statistical methodology is appropriate for the data being analysed. This leads to the second important reason for randomization: it ensures, in the long run, balance between the two groups as regards all factors, measured and unmeasured, that might confound the results.

Note it is not claimed that in practice balance will be actually achieved through randomization, but randomization does ensure that the two groups will differ only by chance. Significance testing, by its very nature, will allow for *chance* differences between the groups, and the p value allows for such differences when a significance level is assigned to a particular comparison. In a randomized controlled trial, it is necessary however to check whether the measured confounders have similar distributions in the treatment and control groups, and a more powerful comparison (more likely to detect differences between the effects of treatments if they exist) is obtained if statistical adjustment is made for any observed differences. However, if a treatment effect is only apparent after such statistical adjustment, the results of the trial may not be widely accepted. As long as patients are randomly allocated to the two groups, possible differences in unmeasured confounders are still allowed for.

In the trial of timolol which is being used as an example, randomization was employed to allocate the post-myocardial infarction patients to the timolol treatment or control groups. Several hundred comparisons were made between the two groups, and the researchers concluded that the differences between these measured factors tended to be small. The final analysis did however include adjustments for the largest differences and other factors considered prognostically important, and it was noted that these adjustments did not materially affect the conclusions based on the unadjusted analysis.

The third and perhaps more subtle reason for requiring randomization in a controlled trial pertains to the assumptions underlying significance testing. Most trials are based on a presenting, non-random sample and the difficulties regarding the assumption that the treated and control groups are random samples from specified (hypothetical) populations have already been mentioned in a previous chapter. This assumption is no longer required if the groups were formed through random allocation. Suppose, for example, that a randomized controlled trial resulted in 12 persons being allocated into one group, and 13 into the other. These particular two groups can be viewed as being one of the many possible allocations resulting from the randomization of 25 individuals into two groups of 12 and 13 respectively. There is a total of 5 200 300 possible different outcomes from such a randomization, and for significance testing it is sufficient to determine, under a null hypothesis of no treatment effect, the chances of obtaining differences in measured outcome between the two randomized groups as large or larger than that actually observed. The 'population' is, then, the 5 200 300 possible allocations and the 'sample' is the specific allocation obtained in the actual study. If the difference observed is larger than that expected by chance alone, the effect of the treatment is implicated as causing the difference, assuming no other biasing factors were present. Thus random allocation obviates the need for convoluted arguments concerning random sampling from larger populations. The statistical inference, however, relates only to the individuals entered into the study, and generalizing results to a larger population involves issues relating to the representativeness of the trial group to the general body of patients affected with the particular disease being studied. The generalizing of trial results is discussed in Section 10.6.

Having cited the reasons for randomization — avoidance of bias in allocation, ensuring balance, in the long run, between the groups, and compliance with statistical assumptions — the practice of randomization must be examined. Obviously, randomization by means of a coin is impractical, and as any conjurer will know, bias is even possible here! What is done is to make use of a table of random numbers to simulate the tossing of a coin. The use of such tables to take a random sample from a defined population (Chapter 3) has already been discussed and the tables are used in a different context here. Usually the total sample size of a trial is fixed beforehand (see below) and a randomization schedule is made out before the trial commences. In practice, a table of random numbers is entered at a random point. Start at the top of column 2 in Table B.1 for instance. Go down the column in order, assigning each consecutive patient to the treatment or control group according to whether the digit in the table is odd or even. Assigning even numbers to the treatment group, the first ten patients would be assigned as follows (in order, where T = treatment, C = control): T, T, T, C, C, T, C, T, C, T, since the first ten numbers in the column are 4, 4, 8, 3, 9, 6, 5, 4, 3, 6. Continue in this way until a schedule is made out for all the patients to be entered into the trial. Since even and odd numbers appear at random in the table, and since on average 50% of the digits are even, this satisfactorily simulates the tossing of a coin. (If there are more than two groups in the trial, or it is required, unusually, to allocate in a different ratio than 1 to 1, modifications of this procedure will have to be adopted.)

One problem immediately manifests itself: in randomizing the 10 patients, there are 6 in the treatment group and 4 in the control group. This type of result is to be expected with *unrestricted randomization* as described, and, using this method, it is not possible to ensure equal numbers in the two groups. This is not a major worry with large trials, but with a small total number of patients in a typical therapeutic trial such an imbalance of numbers is not desirable. A solution to this problem is to use a *restricted randomization* procedure. It is decided, beforehand, that of every *n* individuals randomized half will be in one group and half in the other. Suppose that of every 10 consecutive patients 5 are to be randomized to the treatment group and 5 to the control group. The tables of random numbers would be used as before, but after 5 persons are allocated to one group or the other the remaining patients in a block of 10 are assigned in such a way as to ensure that there are 5 in each group. Starting, for instance, at the top of column 5, the sequence C, T, T, C, C, C, C, is obtained from the numbers 7, 4, 8, 5, 9, 9, 3. Stop at this point, because 5 out of the 7 patients have been allocated to the control group, and allocate the remaining 3 patients out of this block of 10 to the treatment group, obtaining finally C, T, T, C, C, C, C, T, T, T. This procedure, if continued, ensures balance of patients in multiples of 10 and is advisable even for large sample sizes. The timolol study used restricted randomization in blocks of 10. As well as ensuring balance of numbers in the trial as a whole, restricted randomization ensures, when interim analyses are being performed before the end of the trial proper, that if only a portion of patients has been entered, the balance is still achieved. Restricted randomization also guards against imbalances due to a time-trend in the type of cases admitted to a trial.

It has already been mentioned that randomization, in the long run, ensures valid comparability of groups and that any imbalance of confounding variables can be adjusted for at the end of the trial. However it is preferable to employ a design that aids comparability on known confounders than to adjust for these in the analysis stage. *Stratified randomization* achieves this purpose. If a few variables are known to be related to prognosis, then prior to randomization patients can be stratified into groups according to the values of these variables. Randomization then takes place separately within each group. This ensures balance with regard to these factors. In many trials too, the required sample size is so large that many different centres may have to participate. Such *multicentre trials* randomize separately within each centre to avoid imbalance of patients allocated from different centres who may differ in various respects. Too many strata should not be used however in stratified randomization, because the trial may become administratively difficult to run and, paradoxically, with too many strata balance may be difficult to achieve. Restricted randomization should always be employed in each stratum to ensure that the numbers are balanced. In practice, stratified randomization is achieved by forming a separate randomization schedule for each stratum in the trial.

In the timolol trial, eligible patients were first assigned to one of three risk groups, and randomized separately within each group. In risk group I, 178 patients were allocated to timolol and 174 to the controls. In risk groups II and III, the numbers in the treated and control groups were 547 and 543, and 220 and 222 respectively, giving 945 patients on timolol and 939 in the control group. Thus the treatment and control groups were well-balanced as regards numbers, and the distribution of the three risk groups. The timolol trial was also multicentre, with 20 centres participating, and the above procedure was also carried out separately in each centre.

As has been stressed, the randomizing doctor must not know to which group the patient is to be allocated until after he/she has been judged eligible for entry into the trial. For this reason, the schedule of randomization should not be known beforehand. This is often achieved by a sealed envelope technique, where a separate pile of sealed opaque envelopes is prepared for each stratum within which randomization is to take place. The envelopes are marked consecutively, and inside each is a card, detailing the group to which each particular patient is to be allocated. Thus, in each centre of the timolol trial there were (presumably) 3 sets of envelopes for each of the three risk groups. If an eligible patient was in risk category I, the next envelope in the appropriate pile was opened and the patient's randomization group determined. As long as the size of the randomization block (for restricted randomization) is not known to the doctor, there is no way, without deliberate cheating, that the allocation group of a patient can be determined prior to the actual randomization. This implies, of course, that the randomization schedule is made out by an individual (usually the statistician or a member of the trial organizing committee) who is not directly involved in the actual process of the randomization. An alternative method of randomization, often employed in multicentre trials, is to telephone a central office once a patient is deemed eligible and to let them assign the patient from a prepared schedule. This has the advantage that at any time the actual number of patients entered into a trial is known by the central organizing committee.

The distinction between random sampling and randomization (random allocation) must be stressed. The purpose of the former is to choose a group which is representative of a larger population, and random sampling is not usually employed in controlled trials. The purpose of randomization, on the other hand, is to divide a single group into groups that differ only by chance. Randomization is the only way to ensure that individuals entered into a trial are not allocated to the treatment or control groups in a biased manner. (Although the above discussion has been in the context of randomizing individuals, it should be noted that some primary prevention trials have been based on the randomization of individual communities or factories into an intervention or control group.) The next section of this chapter dicusses how to ensure that subsequent biases, arising from how the groups are cared for and evaluated, do not affect the validity of the final comparison.

10.5   Single and double blind trials

Once an individual has been entered into a trial, biases can still occur subsequent to randomization. If a patient knows to which of the two groups he/she has been assigned this, in itself, may introduce subtle biases in evaluating the eventual outcome. For instance, patients who know that they are on a 'new wonder drug' may for that reason alone, apart from any real effect of the treatment, experience a good prognosis. This is known as the *placebo effect* — in essence, this is the effect that an intervention may have on an individual, totally independently of the true pharmacological or surgical effect of the particular intervention. In the last world war, injured soldiers injected with saline only (because of lack of availability of morphine), who thought they were being given morphine, experienced considerable relief of pain. Also, if a patient knows which group he/she is in, the stated response to the treatment may be biased one way or the other, due perhaps to the desire to 'please the nice doctor'! A *single blind* trial is one in which the patient does not know to which of the two groups he/she has been allocated.

In a trial of a drug for instance single blindness can be achieved by giving persons in the control group tablets of a similar size, colour, taste and smell as the active treatment but which contain an innocuous or inactive substance, such as starch or flour. Such a preparation is called a *placebo*. It should have no pharmacologically active ingredient related to the drug being studied, and its only purpose is to 'blind' the patients as to their allocated group.* A placebo treatment is easiest in a trial comparing a new treatment

---

* In a placebo drug trial, randomization can be carried out, not through a sealed envelope method, but by preparing bottles of tablets to be given to consecutive patients. The bottles would contain either the placebo or the active treatment, as the randomization schedule required.

with no treatment at all, and there have been trials carried out using placebo surgical procedures by making a small skin incision but not performing the operation. Needless to say, there would be many ethical problems using such an approach (see Section 10.8). If, as is often the case, a drug trial is designed to test a new treatment against the usual standard treatment, then if the trial is to be single blind, either the two drugs must be presented as similarly as possible, or a 'double placebo' procedure must be used, where each group receives one of the active drugs and a 'look-alike' placebo of the other. Single blindness, of course, should also mean that all the patients in a trial are managed similarly, with the same number of check-ups, out-patient visits and diagnostic procedures.

In some situations of course a single blind trial is not possible, as for instance in comparing a surgical and medical intervention. If a trial is not single blind however, biases may result. What is generally much more important however, is that a trial be *double blind*. In a double blind trial, neither the patient nor the doctor managing the patient or evaluating any response to treatment is aware of which group the patient has been randomized into. The purpose of the double blind trial is to eliminate the possible biases caused by one group receiving better overall care (because they are known to be in the treatment group) or by the doctor unconsciously evaluating the patients in one group more stringently than in the other. In trying to be 'fair', for instance, a doctor may over-compensate, and thus judge individuals in the treatment group more harshly than if they were in the control group. For end-points that are subjective, in that they require a judgement in their interpretation, a double blind trial is definitely required. Thus a trial of antidepressants, with an end-point evaluated by means of an interview concerning depressive symptoms, would need to be double blind to avoid possible biases in patient response, and doctors' evaluation of that response. It could be argued, if a trial had mortality as an end-point, that double blindness is not required. True, there is no room for bias in determining if an individual is dead or alive, but if a specific cause of death is the end-point there could be biases in assigning that cause to a decedent.

One obvious problem with a double blind trial arises if the doctor is worried about whether a particular symptom exhibited by the patient is a side-effect of the active treatment, and whether the treatment should be stopped and the patient withdrawn from the trial. In such cases, the doctor may have to break the blindness of the study for the individual patient's welfare, and a record of the randomization schedule should be available. The term 'breaking the code' is sometimes used when a patient's group is determined in this manner, and should always be allowed for in the planning stages of the trial. In fact, a full list of the criteria for withdrawing a patient should be made out beforehand, and once any patient exhibits one of these symptoms they should be withdrawn from the trial, even if it transpires that they were in the placebo group. In any placebo trial, there are likely to be more withdrawals from the active therapy.

In the timolol trial, the controls received a placebo tablet similar in shape, size and colour to timolol, but differing slightly in taste. Although the end-point being evaluated was death, this trial was also double blind and the cause of death was classified by a steering committee who were unaware of the randomization group of any individual. Very definite criteria for withdrawing a patient from the trial were laid down beforehand, and the trial was analysed using life table methods (see Sections 9.7 and 9.8), counting trial withdrawals as losses to follow-up 28 days following their withdrawal.* Thus, events in withdrawals occurring a month later than the actual withdrawal were not included in the major analysis. A further analysis was performed, however, including all end-points observed in withdrawals, to check for biases due to different withdrawal rates in the two groups. Reasons for withdrawals, and the timing of these withdrawals were given in the trial report. This analysis did not materially affect the results.

The description of the design of the randomized double blind controlled trial in medicine is now completed and other aspects of experimental trials which deserve mention, particularly relating to patient selection and follow-up, are now discussed.

10.6   Applicability versus validity

The *validity* of trial results relates to whether or not the observed results of the trial are true, or whether bias of one form or another affected these results. Double blindness with stratified randomization is vital to achieving this end, but other factors are also relevant.

The sample size of the trial should be adequate to detect an important treatment effect at a given significance level. This question was discussed in Section 6.7 but its importance cannot be over-stressed. The sample size required for a trial must be estimated beforehand. Appendix D gives some sample size formulae that will suffice in certain simple situations, but a statistician should be consulted, concerning this and other aspects of a trial, at its planning stages. A note of warning to those planning a trial: the version of Murphy's law for the controlled trial states 'if bias can occur, it will', but another law also holds; 'if the annual supply of suitable patients when the trial is being designed is n, when the trial commences it will reduce to $n/10$' (Lasagna's law). The trial organizers are invariably over-optimistic about how many patients will be available for a study.

---

* In this chapter the term withdrawal is used to indicate patient non-participation resulting from cessation of therapy, and not in the sense of Sections 9.7 and 9.8.

Many trials are undertaken with sample sizes which are too small to detect even an enormous treatment effect, and such trials result in non-significant differences between the comparison groups. Again it must be stressed that statistical non-significance does not imply a lack of medical importance. If the confidence interval of the difference between the treatment and control groups is calculated in such trials, although overlapping zero, it will often include at its extremes the possibility of large treatment effects. The treatment may have no effect, but it could have a large effect that has been missed, due to a small sample size. Often, sample sizes required for trials may seem excessive and in many cases will require many centres to enter patients. As already mentioned, the timolol trial entered a total of 1884 patients (945 on timolol and 939 on placebo) but the original report does not give details of how this figure was arrived at. The fact that the trial did however produce significant results suggests that care had gone into prior sample size calculations.

In any trial, the end-points on which the effect of treatment is to be judged must be stated clearly, or the trial's validity may be suspect. These end-points, and there may be more than one, should be specified at the start of the trial; a particular end-point not considered at the start of the trial but which subsequently turns out to be greatly affected by treatment could relate to a chance occurrence, and positive results for such sought-for end-points are always a little suspect. The more objective an end-point is, the better, but when necessary subjective end-points have few disadvantages provided that the study is double blind. (See also discussion of measurement accuracy and validity in Chapter 13.) As mentioned above, the major end-point for the timolol trial was mortality, both cause-specific and total, and non-fatal reinfarction. Events occurring when the patient was on therapy (active or placebo) or within 28 days of withdrawal from the study formed the basic end-points, although events in withdrawals were recorded up to the end of the study.

The validity of any trial is seriously compromised by inadequate follow-up of any of the patients entered. Many trials may run into years of patient entry and subsequent follow-up, and losses to follow-up can seriously bias the results. The follow-up of patients however is not an easy task, and its difficulty should not be underestimated. What happens to patients during follow-up is also very important. Withdrawals from the study due to adverse effects of treatment must be followed up as stringently as those who remain in the trial (see below). Treatments and interventions during follow-up, other than that being evaluated, should also be recorded. Some measure of patient compliance with the treatment (and placebo) regime is also required if treatment is long-term. Definite decisions as to what information is required at each follow-up must be made at the planning stage of the trial and, if a mortality end-point is included, cause and date of death must be ascertained from the appropriate sources. In the timolol trial, patients were seen at one, three and six months following discharge from hospital, and thereafter every six months until the trial completion date. Patients were entered between January 1978 and October 1979, and analysis was based on a variable follow-up of all patients until October 1980. Thus all participants had at least one year of follow-up with early entrants having just under three years. The withdrawal criteria were carefully determined beforehand and reasons for individual withdrawals completely documented. Compliance with the treatment regime was based on a count of remaining tablets in the supply given regularly to each patient.

Appropriate statistical analysis of trial data is a *sine qua non* for the validity of results. Many trials will necessarily involve a variable length of follow-up of trial participants, and thus life table methods or a survival model such as that of Cox will be appropriate for an end-point such as death, or other definite event. (See Section 9.7). In trials where the end-point may occur within a short period of time, each participant can be followed up for the same period, and more standard analytic techniques applied. Great care must however be taken in the analysis of data based on variable follow-up.

Even though the trial may have included stratified randomization, the two groups must be assessed in terms of comparability with regard to prognostic factors and, if necessary, statistical adjustment techniques used in the analysis. One must however be wary of over-analysing a clinical trial. By searching hard enough, subgroups of patients in whom the treatment appears to work well will always be found. Unless these subgroups are defined beforehand, and a stratified randomization made within each subgroup, such treatment differences could easily be chance occurrences, or due to imbalances of other prognostic factors. Little credence can be placed on results in subsets of patients when the groups are retrospectively determined, even if such results are statistically significant. As mentioned, the timolol trial employed Cox's regression model to correct for possible confounding variables, but presented the final results in terms of unadjusted clinical life tables, since the adjustment did not materially affect the results.

In nearly all trials there will be individuals who, for one reason or another, did not receive any or all of the treatment required, in the group to which they were randomized. Patient withdrawals due to side-effects, poor compliance, and losses to follow-up all fit into this category. Should such persons, for analysis purposes, be included or excluded, or even changed from the treatment to the control group? The answer to this question depends on the purpose of the trial. If the purpose of the trial is to determine if the treatment can work or has an effect (an 'explanatory' trial), then non-compliers and withdrawals can be excluded from the analysis, and end-points counted only in the patients on active therapy or placebo. Although answering the specific question as to whether or not the treatment can work, the explanatory trial will not answer the perhaps more important question: 'Will this treatment work if employed in practice on a group of patients?' The analysis of such a 'management' trial requires that the groups be analysed as randomized (i.e. according to the intention to treat, rather than what actually happened) with all events in each group counted. This is the more true-to-life situation, where in any group of patients there will be drop-outs and withdrawals from treatment. The management trial is thus far more relevant to clinical practice. In the timolol trial, both methods of analysis were employed. The main analysis presented in the report only included end-points occurring when the patients were actually on treatment, or within 28 days of withdrawal from treatment; an analysis including all end-points, however, was also performed on the intention-to-treat basis, showing only a slightly smaller effect of timolol on survival. The results of the trial showed that timolol reduced total (cumulative life table) mortality at 33 months from 17·5% in the placebo to 10·6% in the timolol group — a reduction of 39·4% ($p < 0.001$). This effect of timolol was also significant in risk group II alone. When total deaths were analysed on an 'intention-to-treat basis', including all mortality end-points in those withdrawing from treatment, the mortality reduction was from 21·9 to 13·3% ($p < 0.001$) showing that there seemed to be no bias in the results due to selective withdrawals from treatment.

The most important of the factors that determine the validity of a controlled trial (whether the results are true) have now been covered. These factors include double blindness, stratified randomization, adequate sample size, and clearly defined end-points. Completeness of follow-up is essential in terms of the end-points being analysed and other factors which may relate to them. Finally, an appropriate statistical analysis must be performed. In all of this, only the suspicion of bias is enough to put a question mark on the results. The onus is on the investigator to show that bias was as far as possible avoided, not on the reader of the trial report to show that it actually existed.

The question now arises of the applicability of trial results, which relates to whether or not the results of the trial can be judged useful in clinical practice. This is determined almost totally by the type of patients selected for inclusion in the trial, and the type of treatment tested, although obviously it also relates to which end-points were studied. Many explanatory trials restrict patients studied to those at high risk of experiencing the end-points. This has obvious advantages in reducing the required sample size (end-points would be more numerous), but the generalization of results to subjects who are not high-risk is questionable. Explanatory trials can show that the treatment works for some, but will not show that adopting this policy of treatment will have any real effect on the patient population at large. A management trial on the other hand is, as has been said, designed to see how the treatment works in practice, and thus low-risk cases should not generally be excluded. In a trial, the patients entered are not a random sample of all patients. They are usually a small subset of such patients. The generalization of results to the patient population at large requires knowledge of how the patients were actually chosen for trial participation. Many trials will exclude patients with serious diseases other than that being studied, thus reducing the applicability of the end results, while ensuring on the other hand that imbalance of groups with 'awkward' cases is avoided. Diagnostic inclusion and exclusion criteria should however be clearly defined for any trial. The careful reading of a trial report may be a guide as to what kind of patient the trial may be generalized to. Trials based on volunteers are always suspect, because volunteers with a particular condition are likely to be quite unrepresentative of the full patient population.

Ideally a trial should carefully present the sources of the patients studied; if they are hospital cases or cases in a specialized centre, results may be hard to generalize. The presentation of the timolol trial is exemplary as regards this point. Male and female patients, aged between 20 and 75 years, who were admitted to one of the participating centres with a suspected myocardial infarct, were registered as potential trial entrants. 11 125 patients were registered, of whom 4155 (37·3%) were diagnosed as having a definite myocardial infarction according to the defined criteria. Of these, 1884 (35·3% or 16·9% of the total registered) were eventually entered into the trial. Exclusions were due to early deaths, contra-indications to timolol treatment, requirements for concomitant treatment or other factors which could have caused problems in randomizing to a placebo group, together with likely difficulties with successful follow-up. It should be noted that the entry criteria should be satisfied prior to randomization, and exclusions made before this takes place. If this is not done, serious imbalance of the groups may result. In the timolol trial, even ignoring selection biases causing admission to the particular centres, only 17 patients out of every 100 with a suspected myocardial infarction could be judged suitable for timolol, and survive long enough to take it. The results must be interpreted in this light. Mitchell (1981) discusses this aspect of the timolol trial in great detail.

Another aspect of trials relating to their applicability or generalizability is the question of the actual treatment regime studied. Most trials use a fixed treatment dosage when drug therapy is in question, but to what extent this mirrors real clinical practice is a moot point. Often, in real life, the dose of a drug is adjusted to meet the individual patient's requirements or condition. Thus, a trial of a fixed dose of an antihypertensive drug may not prove instantly generalizable to clinical practice. On the other hand, it must be said that trials allowing variable dosage are administratively difficult, and cause problems in determining the validity of the results. It is impossible for instance to adjust the dose of a placebo, so blindness is lost to a large extent. The timolol trial employed a fixed dosage of timolol versus placebo, with treatment started immediately after randomization (half a ten milligram tablet, twice daily for two days, and then one tablet twice daily until trial completion).

The timolol trial was, without any doubt, well-designed, well-executed, and well-presented. Many trials do not fit into this category, or are so poorly presented when published that it is impossible to judge their validity or applicability. A clear and concise presentation of all the factors discussed so far in this chapter is required if the results of clinical trials are to be correctly interpreted, and needless to say, all the factors need to be considered when a trial is being designed in the first place.

10.7   Alternative trial designs

The secondary prevention trial of timolol described and discussed in the previous sections was based on a fixed sample size design, to compare a single treatment and placebo in two separate groups of patients. Other designs for randomized controlled trials can be used, and three of the most common are described below.

The *sequential trial* design avoids the sample size being fixed beforehand in the comparison of two groups, and in general enables the trial to be completed with a minimum of patients consistent with a statistically significant result. The fixed sample size trial, on the other hand, cannot be evaluated until all patients have been entered, unless allowances have been made in the sample size calculation for interim analyses (see Section 13.6). Keeping the sample size in a medical trial at a minimum may be desirable on ethical grounds, but unfortunately a sequential trial can only be employed in certain situations. The more commonly used sequential trial design is described below. The basic idea behind the sequential trial is that patients enter in matched pairs, one member in each pair receiving (at random) the treatment to be tested and the other a placebo (or comparative treatment). Success or failure of the treatment is determined on each pair of patients sequentially as soon as the results become available and eventually, when a sufficient number of pairs have been entered into the study and evaluated, a statistically significant or non-significant result is obtained. At this stage, the patient entry is terminated with no greater number entering the trial than is required to achieve a definite result. Analysis of the data takes place continually throughout the period of the trial, instead of being contingent upon the entry of a fixed number of patients.

The usual sequential trial however can only be used to compare two groups, and one end-point only can be evaluated. This end-point is usually defined in terms of treatment success or failure, or in such a way that one of the treatments can be judged superior to the other in each patient pair. The sequential trial also will only achieve its aim of reducing the number of patients required if patient response to treatment can be determined fairly quickly after the commencement of therapy. If there is a long delay, many pairs of patients may already have been entered into the study unnecessarily when the trial is stopped. The statistical techniques involved in a sequential trial (sequential analysis) are somewhat complex and are not discussed here, but a brief outline of the method is given. Suppose it is wished to compare the effects of treatments A and B. As pairs of patients, suitably matched,* become available, one of the pair receives (at random) treatment A and the other treatment B. For each pair of patients, four outcomes are possible: both treatments a success; both treatments a failure; treatment A a success and treatment B a failure; treatment A a failure and treatment B a success. For the purpose of the sequential trial, the first two outcomes are described as 'tied pairs' and are discarded from analysis. Only the 'untied pairs' are used in the comparison of the two treatments†. Now, suppose a score of $+1$ is given to an outcome in which treatment A is a success and treatment B a failure, and a score of -1 to an outcome in which B is a success and A is a failure. As the trial proceeds, a cumulative score is kept. It is evident that if treatment A is markedly superior to treatment B, an increasing positive score will be cumulated, whilst an increasing negative score will cumulate in the reverse case. If there is no marked difference between A and B, then scores of $+1$ and -1 will occur in a random fashion, so that the total score will oscillate around zero. These three possible outcomes are then used to make a decision about the relative efficacy of the two treatments.

The application of sequential analysis makes use of a *sequential analysis chart*, and such a chart is shown in Fig. 10.1. This chart was used in the analysis of a clinical trial, set up to determine if the occurrence of a particular complication of a disease was increased when a particular therapy was employed. The end-point of the trial was, unusually enough, an unwanted treatment effect. The study was performed on premature infants with the respiratory distress syndrome. Diuretic treatment of such infants to reduce fluid retention and help alleviate their symptoms is often used. It had been suggested that a particular diuretic, furosemide — which shall be called treatment A — seemed to increase the incidence of a particular heart condition (patent ductus arteriosus), a complication in premature infants with the respiratory distress syndrome. It was decided to compare the heart functions of infants under treatment and infants on an alternative diuretic (chloro-thiazide) which, for simplicity, shall be called treatment B. One of each member of consecutively admitted pairs of infants was assigned randomly to

---

* On the basis of prognostic variables, or using each two consecutive eligible patients to form a pair.

† Note the similarity to McNemar's χ^2 test (Section 7.13).

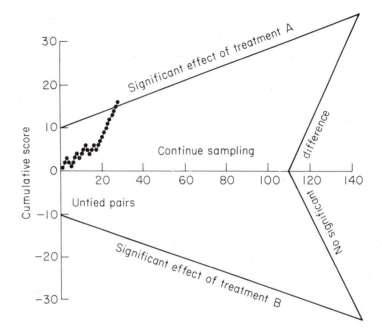

FIG. 10.1. Sequential analysis chart for comparing the effect of furosemide (A) and chlorothiazide (B) on a heart score in premature infants. Green, Thompson, Johnson & Lock (1983) with permission.

treatment A and the other to treatment B. After a specified period, the heart score, ranging from 0 to 6 (6 being a severe grading), was determined blindly on each infant and each pair was classified as 'favouring' treatment A or B (if not tied) according to which infant had the highest score. Whenever a pair of infants did not have an identical score (untied pairs), the results were entered into the chart in Fig. 10.1. The horizontal axis on the sequential analysis chart records the number of untied pairs included in the trial. The vertical axis records the cumulative score as the trial proceeds (a positive score indicating, in the example, that the treatment A infant had a higher heart score than the treatment B infant). In the figure, the cumulative score is shown by the zig-zag line. It is now necessary to explain the meaning of the four 'boundary lines' marked on the chart. A trial may be terminated as soon as the score line reaches one of the boundary lines. If the score line crosses the upper boundary line, this is interpreted to mean that treatment A resulted in a significantly higher heart score than treatment B. The opposite interpretation applies if the score line crosses the lower boundary line. Of course, the score line will not cross either boundary line unless a relatively high score has accumulated in favour of one or other of the treatments. If, on the other hand, the score line crosses either of the end boundary lines, this is interpreted to mean that there appears to be no significant difference between the two methods of treatment; the score is not high enough in relation to the number of untied pairs tested to indicate a significant advantage of one treatment over the other.

The trial continues until the score line reaches one of the boundary lines, at which point a decision can be reached, at a predetermined level of significance and power, about the relative advantages of the two methods of treatment. In the example, the score line reached the upper boundary line after 28 untied pairs had been recorded. When the heart score was higher on an infant on treatment B, the score line would move downwards. When the score was higher in a treatment A infant, it moved upwards. Twenty-two of the untied pairs favoured treatment A, 6 favoured B, and, eventually, the cumulative score of 16 in favour of A was reached. This was sufficient to cause a rejection of the null hypothesis that there was no difference in treatment effects, and to declare that treatment A significantly increased the heart score in these infants. It can be seen that once the boundary lines have been fixed, plotting and analysing the results of the trial as they become available is quite simple. The complexity of the technique lies in fixing the boundary lines for the particular experiment being conducted, and details of this are not given here. The chart is set up, however, based on the same criteria for determining a fixed sample size in the more usual type of experiment. The chart in the trial discussed was based on a β error of 0·05 in detecting a twofold preference for one of the treatments at a two-sided significance level, α, of 0·05. If a fixed sample size trial design had been used, the sign test for paired data (Section 7.7) or McNemar's test for paired proportions (Section 7.13) could have been employed.

While the sequential trial uses matched pairs to avoid the fixed sample size approach of the usual controlled trial, the *cross-over trial* uses a matched design with each patient as his own control. Treatments are compared on the same patients in different time-periods. Self-paired experiments such as this ensure that the treatment or control groups are identical as regards patient characteristics, and thus require a smaller total sample size than an independent two-group comparison. In a comparison of two treatments (A and B again) the patient is first randomly assigned to, say, treatment A for a specified period. The effect of treatment is evaluated, and the patient is withdrawn from the treatment for a time until any residual effect disappears. After this washout period, the patient is 'crossed over' to receive treatment B, and again the treatment effect is evaluated after a second period. Patients entering the trial are thus randomized to A and then B, or B and then A. The basic analysis is, of course, by means of a paired comparison of the two treatments.

Unfortunately, the cross-over trial can only be used in situations where the treatment effect is fairly immediate, and also disappears after the withdrawal of treatment. The cross-over trial can be used, for example, in testing antihypertensive therapy, or anti-inflammatory drugs for arthritis. In both these examples, the 'symptom' returns after treatment withdrawal, so that a second treatment can be applied after the first. It is sometimes difficult however, in the cross-over trial, to disentangle real treatment effects from a possible carry-over effect from the last treatment, even with a long washout period, or from changes in response with the passage of time.

The third trial design which is considered in this section in a sense answers two questions for the price of one. If it is wished to compare the separate effects of two different treatments (A and B) against a placebo, a *factorial design* should be considered. It might be tempting to design a three-group trial with, perhaps, randomization to A, B or the placebo, but it can be far more efficient to have four groups in such a comparison. Patients would first be randomized to receive either treatment A or the placebo. Within each of these groups, a second randomization would be made to either treatment B or placebo. Four groups would result: A and B; A only; B only, and neither A nor B. In the first International Urokinase/Warfarin Trial in Colorectal Cancer* patients with operable colorectal cancer are randomized into receiving post-operatively either an intravenous drip containing urokinase, or a saline drip (the placebo). Within each of these groups, patients are again randomized to receive either long-term warfarin therapy, or no such treatment. The trial design requires 100 patients in each of the four groups, and the end-points being examined are survival and recurrence-free interval. Table 10.1 shows the patients in their randomized groups. A factorial design, such as this, is analysed for the effects of the two treatments separately. The effect of urokinase, for example, is determined by comparing the 200 persons on urokinase with the 200 persons not on this treatment, irrespective of their warfarin therapy. The comparison is not biased by the warfarin therapy, because half of each group is on this drug so that it cannot act as a confounder. Similarly, the effect of warfarin is analysed without reference to the allocation to urokinase. The sample size requirements for a factorial

Table 10.1 A factorial design for evaluating the effects of urokinase and warfarin in colorectal cancer.

	Urokinase	No urokinase	Total
Warfarin	100	100	200
No warfarin	100	100	200
Total	200	200	400

* Trial results to appear in late 1986.

design like this are the same as for a normal two-group comparison, so in essence the extra result is free. The only problem arises if there is a synergistic effect (see Section 9.6) between the two treatments, and the group randomized to receive both has a better result than expected on the basis of either therapy in isolation. Apart from this, the factorial design provides a useful adjunct to the usual two-group trial.

10.8   Ethical considerations

Many ethical problems are raised in the context of the randomized controlled trial in medicine, and in this section some of the issues involved are indicated. Such ethical issues are still hotly debated in the medical literature and there are no hard and fast answers to many of the problems raised. However, ethical questions are distinct from medico-legal ones, and no attempt to consider the latter is made. To turn the basic question on its head, it might be asked whether it is ethical not to perform randomized controlled trials on proposed new therapies. In the history of medicine, many therapies commonly employed simply did not work or resulted in more harm than good. Most of these therapies could have been determined as useless far sooner if subjected to a formal trial and indeed many such therapies were abandoned as a result of their being tested scientifically. It is essential to know if a particular treatment is beneficial and the randomized controlled trial is, in essence, the only way by which this knowledge can be obtained. Clinical judgement on a haphazardly selected group with partial follow-up is not a firm basis for the evaluation of treatment. If the randomized controlled trial were to be considered unethical in all cases, then many patients would be condemned to unproven and worthless interventions and the advance of medical science would be halted almost completely.

Although one hopefully agrees with the above point, dilemmas still remain in accepting the existence of experimental trials in medicine. There are conflicts between an individual patient's welfare in the trial itself and the welfare of all patients with the particular condition in the future. There are conflicts between the doctor as healer and the doctor as investigator. In a trial patients are allocated into two groups, one of which will receive the new treatment under investigation, while the other will receive the best treatment available or, in certain instances, no treatment at all. The first question that is asked is whether it is ethical to withhold a potentially good treatment from some individual patients for the eventual good of a larger group. Herein lies the crux of the controlled trial; if the treatment is *known* to be good, a trial cannot ethically take place, but on the other hand, a trial cannot take place either without there being some suspicion that the treatment may be good. This leads to the conflict between knowledge and possibilities, and what may be firm 'knowledge' in one doctor's mind may be just a vague hope in another's. From the doctors' point of view, the individual patient's welfare must be of paramount importance, and if doctors have evidence that a new therapy is beneficial, they are not justified ethically in involving themselves in a trial of that treatment. Other doctors however may view the same evidence differently.

It would seem to be impossible to define universal criteria for what could be considered as evidence in favour of employing a particular therapy, apart from a well-designed and well-executed randomized controlled trial. On the other hand, there is no real argument against the doctor who says 'I tried it out on 10 of my patients, and it really worked. I won't allow any of my patients to be entered into a trial'. It is interesting, however, that some doctors may feel far less uneasy using a possibly inferior therapy through ignorance than they do in submitting a possibly beneficial treatment to the rigours of a controlled trial.

The subjective nature of what evidence is required to form knowledge is thus a major problem in determining whether or not a particular trial is ethical. As healers, doctors must do what they think best for the individual patient; as investigators, they also have a responsibility to that individual patient to determine what indeed is the best therapy. It would seem then that from the point of view of participating doctors a trial is only ethical insofar as those doctors accept that they do not know which of the two treatments is better, and have no preference for either.*

The question of exactly when a trial should be undertaken is relevant to this whole question. It is ethically easier to commence a trial at the introductory stages of a new therapy, since there would be little or no knowledge about its effects. However, a trial at the early stages of a new intervention is more likely to miss its full usefulness if it takes time (as with a new surgical procedure say) to get the treatment 'just right'. If on the other hand one waits too long, the procedure may become generally accepted as worthwhile (without formal evaluation), making a trial ethically difficult to perform.

A similar problem arises once a trial is underway. If particular doctors see the results as they accrue, and a trend in favour of one of the treatments becomes apparent, some may wish to change all their patients to that treatment because of their 'knowledge' of its better effect. Early trends in a trial, which will generally be statistically non-significant, may be very misleading; often an early trend will settle itself out after a time to give an entirely different result at the end of the trial when the validity and statistical

---

* One criterion for making this judgement has been suggested and that is the answer to the question 'Would I allow a member of my family enter the trial and be randomized to one or other of the treatments?'.

significance of the results can be determined. It may in fact be unethical to stop a trial on the basis of early positive results which do not achieve significance, since the trial would not then have achieved its purpose. It must be stressed, however, that the patient's welfare comes first, and that if a doctor for any reason feels it better to withdraw a patient or change treatment, ethical considerations demand that this be done, irrespective of trial requirements.

In multicentre trials, this dilemma of early trends is often overcome by letting a steering committee, only, examine results as they come in. Trial participants will not be informed of results until the study has been completed, unless very definite trends are apparent. The ethical problem is thus switched from the participating doctors to a steering committee.

Patients have the right to expect individual and personal treatment from their doctors and it must be asked if this individual right can be sacrificed for the benefit of humanity and the progress of knowledge. This right of the individual patient seems to be sacrificed if the doctor has no choice over which therapy is to be given, which, of course, would be determined by 'the toss of a coin'. However, when there is an honest lack of knowledge about which is the better treatment, the patients do not lose out. Outside of the trial, the chosen therapy would be, necessarily, at the whim of the doctor, and the fact that the treatment is chosen at the whim of a coin instead surely does not make a difference.

The question then of whether a randomized controlled trial is in itself ethical relates to the nature of evidence required to form knowledge. In most cases, a large body of doctors will agree on the necessity for a trial, although there will always be dissidents. As long as particular doctors are sure of their 'ignorance', the trial is, for them, ethically justified and patients' rights would not seem to be abrogated if they enter a trial. Indeed, rather than querying whether it is ethical to withhold a potentially good treatment from patients in the control group, it should perhaps be asked whether it is ethical to withhold the standard treatment from patients in the treatment group.

Once the hurdle of determining whether it is ethical to undertake a particular controlled trial in the first place is overcome, ethical problems still remain, relating to the design and conduct of the trial itself. Firstly, the treatment to be investigated must be safe. Safe, however, is a relative term, since no therapy is without risk. The right balance must be struck between potential benefit and possible harm. Nor can the design and analysis of the trial be divorced from ethical questions. It is not ethical to enter patients into a trial whose eventual results may never be accepted because of failure to avoid bias in the setting up and execution of the trial. Also, if the sample size of a trial is too small to detect important results, it should probably not have been started in the first place. Nor of course should more patients than necessary be entered into a trial. The sequential trial is designed to avoid some of these problems, but as already noted, its applicability is limited. Other little-used designs have also been proposed to reduce the number of patients on an inferior treatment. These *adaptive designs* require that a greater proportion of patients be randomized into the group showing the more favourable result at any time. Such trials, however, are limited in applicability and are in fact less appealing than they appear to be at first sight.

From the point of view of patient selection, ethical considerations will often demand certain exclusion criteria. The exclusion of pregnant women from most drug trials is universal, and ethical considerations must take precedence over the requirement of applicability of trial results.

The use of placebos and double blind procedures in a trial also raises ethical problems. Unless the condition being studied is fairly innocuous, like the common cold for instance, or no proven therapy is available, the control group should receive a standard therapy. Single blindness can still be achieved by using the double placebo procedure, and no control with a serious condition for which treatment is available should be given a placebo only. How far one should go with placebos is a moot question. There are some examples in the early literature of placebo surgery. Ligation of the internal mammary arteries, for instance, used to be a common procedure for the relief of angina, but a clinical trial showed this treatment to be useless. Those in the control group had a placebo surgical skin incision made, but without further operative intervention. Would the results of this trial have been accepted without the placebo procedure?

In general, blinding of patients to their particular treatment does not seem to raise serious ethical problems so long as informed consent has been obtained. As discussed previously, the double blind trial refers to the blindness of the patient and of the doctor managing the patient and evaluating any responses to treatment. There is no problem, however, in allowing the doctor who is managing the patients know to which treatment they have been allocated, so long as patients in the treatment and control groups are looked after similarly. In any case, if the patients' doctor is 'blind', the treatment code should always be easily available. The doctor evaluating the patients' response should, however, be 'blind'. Again it must be stressed that doctors have the right and duty to withdraw a patient from a trial if they see fit.

The largest ethical problem with the randomized controlled trial today is, however, that of informed consent. In the United States, informed consent is a legal requirement of any trial in medicine, but there are no such restrictions in Ireland or the United Kingdom. As with all ethical questions, that of informed consent does not have a simple 'yes' or 'no' answer. There is no doubt that patients have a right to know that they are participating in an experimental trial, and that the therapy being tested is unproven. The problem is however that many patients may not wish to exercise this right. Informed consent may demand that some patients know more about their illness and their prognosis than they wish to; many prefer to put trust in their doctor that the best possible care will be given them. Is it ethical to burden such patients with the knowledge that in fact it is not known what is the best treatment, and with all the ancillary information that would be required for them to give an informed consent? Seeking consent and the extent of it is a major question that must be decided by trial organizers in the context of the particular situation. The ever-present possibility of legal action by a patient in a trial usually decides investigators in favour of seeking consent, but this is not why informed consent should be obtained. The patient's right to know what is happening is, surely, far more important than the doctor's legal protection.

If informed consent is to be obtained, what should it include?* This again is a debatable issue. Patients cannot be expected to understand everything about their disease, and in fact one of the reasons for the trial in the first place is that doctors do not know the best therapy themselves. Informed consent however does demand that the relevant facts concerning the trial and its purpose be explained as fully and clearly as possible. The two treatments should be described, as should also their possible benefits and side-effects. If the study is blind, this should be explained also. Most doctors however balk at explaining that they will not be choosing the treatment, but that the patient will be randomized. This is of course central to the trial itself, but it may result in destroying the doctor–patient relationship. Whether randomization is to be included in the description of a trial, for the purposes of informed consent, must also be left to the individual trial organizers to decide.

An important element in the process of seeking informed consent is the pressure that the doctor may, unconsciously, place on the patient to participate. Patients must fully realize that they are under no obligation to do so, and that failure to become involved in the trial will not compromise their position with the doctor in any way whatsoever.

Recently, a trial design has been proposed by Zelen (1979) which neatly avoids the problem of obtaining informed consent to randomization and the consequent reduction of patient participation due to refusals. The resulting trial is controlled and (partially) randomized but its value is yet to be proven.

As has been seen, the randomized controlled trial poses many ethical questions, all of which are related to holding sacrosanct the welfare of

---

* It would seem that from the ethical point of view verbal informed consent is just as good as a written and signed statement. Written informed consent is often obtained for legal purposes only, though it does help to ensure that all points have been explained to the individual patient.

individual patients and recognition of their rights. A very general principle could be proposed — that no patients in a trial be worse off than if they were not in the trial in the first place. The interesting fact is, however, that patients in a clinical trial often get better overall care and much more careful assessment and follow-up than the ordinary patient on standard therapy.

10.9   Summary

In this chapter the purpose, design, implementation and analysis of the randomized controlled trial in medicine have been discussed. The necessity of treatment evaluation with concurrent controls and the avoidance of bias with the randomization and blinding of trial patients and doctors were stressed; the distinction between therapeutic (clinical), primary prevention and secondary prevention trials was made, and designs other than the usual two-group comparative trials were discussed. Criteria were given for evaluating the validity (are the results true?) and applicability (are the results useful in clinical practice?) of trials, and the chapter concluded with a brief foray into the ethical problems raised by the randomized controlled trial.

CHAPTER 11
Vital Statistics

11.1 Introduction

A branch of statistics which is of particular interest to medical and social scientists is that concerned with the study of human populations, often described as *demography*. Demographic studies involve *vital statistics* which are now briefly considered.

Vital statistics are important in medicine and this chapter outlines and explains a number of the more common measures in use. They are concerned with quantitative aspects of deaths, births and fertility, marriage, ill-health and similar characteristics. Such descriptive measures are commonly expressed in the form of *rates*; thus it is usual to speak of death rates, birth rates, bed occupancy rates, and so on. This is because absolute numbers are not very informative when, as is often the case, it is wished to compare, say, mortality conditions in two or more different countries or areas, or in the same area at different points in time. The larger the population of an area, the larger will be the expected number of deaths in any given interval of time. If, therefore, the mortality conditions of areas of different populations are to be compared it is necessary to use a measure such as the annual number of deaths per thousand population, which is independent of the absolute size of the population.

11.2 Measures of mortality

The simplest measure of mortality is the *crude death rate*, defined as the number of deaths in a particular time period (usually a year) per thousand population. The annual crude death rate can be expressed as

$$\frac{\text{Annual number of deaths}}{\text{Mean population during the year}} \times 1000$$

Note that since the population typically varies slightly during the year, the denominator is an estimate of the 'mid-year' population (often, however, this is difficult to estimate accurately unless there are regular and up-to-date population census data available).

Separate crude death rates can be calculated for males and females, for particular areas of a country, and for other subgroups in the total population, including particular age groups, to which reference is made below. The denominator would then refer to the mean population of the particular subgroup or area of interest.

For analytical purposes, crude death rates are of limited usefulness and may be misleading if used for comparisons. For example, country A may have a higher crude death rate than country B simply because, at the time of the comparison, the former had a higher proportion of elderly people. The death rate at every age may be lower, and the expectation of life higher, in A and it would therefore be misleading to conclude, on the basis of a comparison of crude death rates, that country B's population is healthier or enjoys a higher level of medical care than that of country A. Comparisons must take into account the age distribution of the population. In addition, the overall crude death rate is also affected by the sex ratio in the population, since females generally have a longer expectation of life than males and, usually, separate death rates for females and males are calculated. Crude death rates for a number of countries are illustrated in Table 11.1.

A way of neutralizing the effect of age distribution on the crude death rate is to calculate separate death rates for each age group in the population. These are called *age-specific death rates*, defined as

$$\frac{\text{Number of deaths in a specific age group}}{\text{Mean population of that age group}} \times 1000$$

(Deaths and mean population relate to a specific calendar period, usually a year, although some rates are calculated at quarterly or even monthly intervals.)

Table 11.1   Crude death rates for various countries (deaths per 1000 mean population).

Country	Year	Crude death rate
Argentina	1978	8·9
Egypt	1981	10·1
France	1981	10·3
Hong Kong	1981	4·8
Ireland*	1980	9·7
Japan	1981	6·2
Spain	1981	7·6
Sweden	1981	11·1
United Kingdom	1980	11·8
United States	1981	8·7

Source: *UN Demographic Yearbook.*

* In this and subsequent references, Ireland means the Republic of Ireland.

Corresponding age-specific death rates for different populations can then be compared. The comparability of these rates is also affected by the age distribution *within* each age group but, provided the age group class intervals are fairly narrow, the influence of the within-group age distribution can be considered negligible. Five-year and ten-year age group intervals are commonly used. As an example, age-specific death rates for Scotland and for England and Wales are recorded in Table 11.2.

Note that male mortality rates exceed female mortality rates in every age group, a characteristic common to all developed and most developing countries. Note also, the relatively high mortality rates in the age group under 1 year (infant mortality) compared with subsequent age groups. This is further discussed below.

Although age-specific death rates provide the most appropriate basis for comparing the mortality experience of different populations, it is useful to have a single overall measure of mortality which, unlike the crude death rate, allows for the effects of age distribution (assume throughout that males and females are considered separately). This is achieved by the calculation of one or more of a number of *standardized* mortality measures, the best-known of which are now briefly described.

As an example, suppose it is desired to compare the mortality experience of the populations of two different regions in a country. The *direct method* of

Table 11.2   Age-specific death rates for males (1982).

| | Death rates per 1000 mean population | | | |
| | Scotland | | England & Wales | |
Age group	Females	Males	Females	Males
Under 1 year	9·7	12·8	9·4	12·2
1–4	0·4	0·6	0·4	0·5
5–9	0·2	0·3	0·2	0·3
10–14	0·2	0·3	0·2	0·3
15–19	0·3	0·9	0·3	0·8
20–24	0·3	1·0	0·4	0·9
25–34	0·6	1·1	0·5	0·9
35–44	1·5	2·4	1·2	1·8
45–54	4·8	7·8	3·6	5·9
55–64	11·9	21·8	9·7	17·5
65–74	29·9	53·1	24·3	45·8
85–84	76·0	116·2	65·8	105·2
85 and over	192·6	240·2	178·2	232·2
All ages	12·4	12·8	11·5	12·0

Sources: *Population Trends*, Autumn 1983; Registrar General, Scotland. Annual Report 1982.

standardization is as follows: the age-specific mortality rates of the first region, and then of the second region, are successively applied to the corresponding age groups of a *standard population*, yielding the number of deaths which would occur in that standard population if it were subject to the mortality rates prevailing in each region. Denote the hypothetical number of deaths resulting from these calculations as D_1 and D_2 respectively. Any difference between these two figures can be attributed to differences in the mortality rates of the two regions, since the effect of age distribution has been eliminated by the use of a standard (common) population.

The hypothetical numbers of deaths, D_1 and D_2, can be expressed as a rate. If the size (number) of the standard population is denoted P, then the expression $(D_1 \times 1000)/P$ is called the *direct age-standardized death rate* for region 1, while $(D_2 \times 1000)/P$ is the direct age-standardized death rate for region 2. These statistics give the overall death rates which would occur in the standard population, if that population were subject to the age-specific mortality rates of regions 1 and 2 respectively.

An alternative, although equivalent, mortality measure is the *comparative mortality figure* (CMF). Denote the actual or observed total deaths in the standard population as D. Then for region 1 the CMF is $(D_1 \times 100)/D$ and for region 2 it is $(D_2 \times 100)/D$. The CMF is thus the ratio of 'expected' (i.e. the number which would occur if the standard population were subject to the mortality conditions of regions 1 and 2 respectively) to observed deaths, multiplied by 100 to express it in percentage terms. A CMF less than 100 indicates that mortality conditions are 'better' in a particular region compared with the standard population, while a CMF greater than 100 indicates they are 'worse'. Moreover, the CMFs for different regions can be compared.

The direct age-standardized death rate and the CMF are related. Defining the observed death rate for the standard population as $(D \times 1000)/P$, it is easily shown that

$$\text{CMF} = \frac{\text{Direct age-standardized death rate for the region}}{\text{Observed death rate for standard population}} \times 100$$

The thoughtful reader may remark that while the measures explained above have been standardized with respect to age, the numerical values of the measures will depend upon the standard population selected. In the example above, and in similar cases, the normal practice is to select as standard the national population, of which the populations of the different regions (or occupations, or socio-economic groups) form a part. For comparisons over time, however, there is a choice of standard populations, and the numerical values of the CMFs will vary, depending on which year is selected as the population standard. If the age structure of the standard population remains relatively stable over time, which year is chosen as standard will not make a great deal of difference, particularly since it is the relative rather than the absolute values of the CMF which are of interest. Nevertheless, this is a potential limitation of the CMF. Another feature of direct standardization which may cause problems is where the population of interest (of a region, or occupational group, or whatever) is small, or contains small numbers in particular age groups. In these circumstances, the chance occurrence of one or two individual deaths in a particular year may give rise to a much greater than normal age-specific mortality rate and hence distort the CMF. The converse (i.e. an atypically low mortality rate in a particular age group) may also occur.

In the *indirect method* of standardization, the age-specific mortality rates of a standard population are applied to the corresponding age groups of the populations of interest (in the example, regions 1 and 2), to yield the number of deaths 'expected' if each region had experienced the mortality conditions of the standard population. Denote the number of expected deaths in each region as $D_1{}^E$ and $D_2{}^E$ respectively, and the observed or actual number of deaths in each region as $D_1{}^O$ and $D_2{}^O$. The ratio of observed to expected deaths, multiplied by 100, is called the *standardized mortality ratio* (SMR), i.e. for region 1

$$ \mathrm{SMR} = \frac{\text{Observed deaths in region 1}}{\text{Expected deaths in region 1}} \times 100 = \frac{D_1{}^O}{D_1{}^E} \times 100 $$

and a similar equation holds for region 2.

Like the CMF, the SMR is based on a comparison of observed and expected deaths and is similarly interpreted. The former compares observed deaths in the standard population with the number which would have occurred if that population had been subject to the age-specific mortality rates of a particular region (or occupation). The latter compares the observed deaths in a particular region (or occupation) with the number which would have occurred if that region had been subject to the age-specific mortality rates of the standard population. As with the method of direct standardization, the calculations involved in indirect standardization also permit the calculation of age-standardized death rates, but this is not elaborated here.

In many applications, the CMF and the SMR will be equal or very close in value, but this is by no means always the case. Like the CMF, the SMR has a number of limitations, but it requires less information to calculate. In particular, it is not necessary to know the age distribution of deaths in the regions or occupations of interest.

The most common applications of SMRs are comparisons of mortality between different occupations or socio-economic groups, and the analysis of trends in mortality.

As an example of the latter, Table 11.3 records standardized mortality ratios for respiratory tuberculosis for males and females in various years in England and Wales. The figures in this table are calculated as follows: the

Table 11.3 Standardized mortality ratios for respiratory tuberculosis
(1968 = 100).

	1962	1967	1972
Males	178	108	66
Females	164	115	63

Source: Registrar General's Statistical Review of England & Wales,
1972, Part 1, HMSO.

actual male and female age-specific mortality rates for this disease in 1968 are
applied to the male and female populations of 1962, 1967 and 1972 to yield
'expected' deaths from respiratory tuberculosis in those years, i.e. the
number of deaths which would have occurred if mortality rates in those years
were identical to those prevailing in 1968. The ratio of *actual* (observed)
deaths to 'expected deaths' in each year, multiplied by 100, is the standardized
mortality ratio. With 1968 as the standard, SMRs in excess of 100 indicate
that deaths were higher than 'expected' (i.e. that mortality conditions were
less favourable than in the standard year), and SMRs less than 100 indicate
that mortality conditions were more favourable. (For 1968, the ratio is 100
since observed and expected deaths are identical.) Calculated for a series of
years, the SMRs illustrate the trend in mortality conditions for a particular
disease.

Two other ways of using standardized mortality ratios are illustrated in
Tables 11.4 and 11.5. Table 11.4 shows SMRs for all causes for different socio-
economic groups of males aged 15–64. These are calculated by applying the
age-specific mortality rates for all *males* aged 15–64 to the population of each
socio-economic group, calculating the 'expected' number of deaths, and
comparing the observed and expected deaths. Thus, for example, observed
deaths for members of the armed forces (SMR = 147) and unskilled manual
workers (SMR = 139) were noticeably higher than the number 'expected' on
the basis of mortality rates for all males. Note, in contrast, that the crude
death rate for members of the armed forces is substantially less than the
overall crude death rate, due to the fact that most armed forces personnel will
be in age groups with very low age-specific mortality rates.

Table 11.5 records SMRs for different occupations for a particular cause of
death, in this case circulatory diseases. Age-specific mortality rates of deaths
from circulatory diseases, for the whole population of males aged 15–64, are
applied to the population of each occupation, to yield the number of deaths
'expected' in each occupation if its mortality experience was the same as the
total population of males aged 15–64. The ratio of actual to expected deaths
yields the SMR. From the sample of occupations included in the table, it will
be noted that fishermen, publicans and pharmacists appear to suffer much

Table 11.4   Mortality by socio-economic group: males aged 15–64, England & Wales 1970–72.

Socio-economic group	Crude death rate per 100 000	Standardized mortality ratio (SMR)
Employers in industry	805	102
Managers in industry	566	80
Professional workers — self-employed	546	69
Professional workers — employees	370	79
Ancillary workers and artists	402	75
Foremen and supervisors non-manual	460	67
Junior non-manual workers	663	106
Personal service workers	735	134
Foremen and supervisors manual	625	79
Skilled manual workers	619	113
Semi-skilled manual workers	792	115
Unskilled manual workers	1020	139
Own account workers (other than professional)	464	77
Farmers — employers and managers	779	99
Farmers — own account	464	61
Agricultural workers	597	103
Members of armed forces	277	147
Inadequately described occupations	449	86
All men	597	100

Source: OPCS Series OS No. 1 Occupational Mortality, England & Wales 1970–72.

Table 11.5   Standardized mortality ratios for selected occupations for circulatory diseases: men aged 15–64, England & Wales, 1970–72.

Occupation	Standardized mortality ratios
Fishermen	137
Motor mechanics	113
Carpenters	97
Railway guards	118
Typists and secretaries	63
Publicans	151
Athletes, sportsmen	82
Medical practitioners	85
Pharmacists	138
University teachers	47

Source: OPCS, Series OS No. 1, Occupational Mortality, England & Wales 1970–72.

higher than average mortality from circulatory diseases, while typists and university teachers record a much lower than average mortality from these causes.

Pursuing this a little further, Table 11.6 records SMRs for various causes of death for some of the occupational groups included in Table 11.5. Fishing and running a public house appear as high-risk occupations, while typing emerges as a very safe occupation. Athletes enjoy lower than average mortality from most diseases, but are more vulnerable to death through accidents. University teaching is even safer than typing, except for being more liable to death by accident than typists (either through absent-mindedness, or assaults by students!).

In concluding this discussion of standardization, it is worth repeating that some caution should be exercised regarding the interpretation of standardized mortality ratios for particular occupations or social groups. Firstly, in some cases quite small populations are being considered, and SMRs can change significantly from one period to the next, just through chance. Secondly, SMRs do not necessarily indicate the mortality risk of a particular occupation; in a pure experiment, individuals would be randomly allocated to particular occupations and their mortality experience then examined, but of course in reality the choice of occupation is not a random process. Professional athletes, for example, need talent and specific physical characteristics to make a success of such a career, while fishermen will usually be found amongst people who live on or near a sea coast with an established fishing industry. Occupational mortality may, therefore, be influenced not so much by the nature of the occupation as by other factors (education, area of work or residence, specific employment requirements and so on) which are associated with individuals who work in that occupation. In principle these factors, like age and sex, should also be standardized before valid comparisons of occupational mortality risk can be made, and more complex standardization techniques do take account of this.

Table 11.6 Standardized mortality ratios for selected causes for selected occupations: men aged 15–64, England & Wales 1970–72.

Occupation	All neoplasms	Circulatory diseases	Respiratory diseases	Accidents
Fishermen	183	137	235	253
Typists and secretaries	59	63	45	30
Publicans	146	151	148	103
Athletes, sportsmen	95	82	93	148
University teachers	49	47	17	63

Source: OPCS (*op. cit.*).

The discussion of standardized mortality ratios began with age-specific mortality rates, and this section is concluded with a description of a number of age-specific and other mortality rates which are regarded as standard 'vital statistics'.

An age-specific death rate of particular interest is the *infant mortality rate*, which is often taken as an indicator of the level of medical and social standards in a community. It is defined as the number of deaths of infants under 1 year of age during a calendar period per 1000 live births during the same period.

$$\frac{\text{Number of deaths of infants under 1 year of age during a calendar period}}{\text{Live births during the same period}} \times 1000$$

(Infant mortality rate, 1981: England & Wales, 11·1; Ireland, 10·6; Japan, 7·1; United States, 11·7.)

The infant mortality rate can be subdivided into two further rates, the *neonatal mortality rate* and the *post-neonatal mortality rate*. The neonatal mortality rate is defined as the number of deaths of infants under 28 days during a calendar period per 1000 live births during the same period.

$$\frac{\text{Number of deaths of infants under 28 days during a calendar period}}{\text{Live births during the same period}} \times 1000$$

(Neonatal mortality rate, 1981: England & Wales, 6·6; Ireland, 6·7.)

The post-neonatal mortality rate is defined as the number of deaths of infants 28 days and over and under 1 year during a calendar period per 1000 live births during the same period.

$$\frac{\text{Number of deaths of infants 28 days and over and under 1 year during a calendar period}}{\text{Live births during the same period}} \times 1000$$

(Post-neonatal mortality rate, 1981: England & Wales, 4·5; Ireland, 3·9.)

It is immediately obvious, as would be expected, that the sum of the neonatal and post-neonatal mortality rates provides the figure for the infant mortality rate. The reason for this subdivision of the infant mortality rate is because death in the early part of any infant's life is governed mainly by prenatal influences (e.g. congenital malformation, immaturity), while death in the later part of the first year is more generally environmental in origin (e.g. pneumonia, bronchitis). It is important then to calculate different rates for these periods of an infant's life.

A *stillbirth rate* may also be calculated. This is defined as the number of stillbirths during a calendar period per 1000 total (live and still) births during the same period.

$$\frac{\text{Number of stillbirths during a calendar period}}{\text{Total (live and still) births during the same period}} \times 1000$$

(Stillbirth rate, 1981: England & Wales, 6·6; Ireland, 8·2.)

The *perinatal mortality rate* has received increased attention in recent years. It is defined as the number of stillbirths, together with the number of deaths within the first seven days of life, during a calendar period per 1000 total (live and still) births in the same period.

$$\frac{\begin{array}{c}\text{Number of stillbirths} + \text{deaths within the} \\ \text{first 7 days of life during a calendar period}\end{array}}{\text{Total (live and still) births during the same period}} \times 1000$$

(Perinatal mortality rate, 1981: England & Wales, 11·8; Ireland, 13·6.)

There are several reasons for creating a perinatal mortality rate. Stillbirths and early neonatal deaths commonly have a similar aetiology, and the rate is regarded as an important index of the quality of obstetrical care. Further, since an infant who shows *any* sign of life is not regarded as being a stillbirth, the perinatal mortality rate overcomes the difficulty of deciding whether or not an infant is stillborn.

A *maternal mortality rate* is defined as the deaths ascribed to puerperal causes during a calendar period per 1000 total (live and still) births during the same period.

$$\frac{\text{Deaths ascribed to puerperal causes during a calendar period}}{\text{Total (live and still) births during the same period}} \times 1000$$

(Maternal mortality rate, 1981: England & Wales, 0·09; Ireland, 0·04.)

The *case fatality (mortality) rate* is often of interest if it is desired to determine the proportion of patients with a particular disease or condition who die, e.g. in a pertussis outbreak. It is defined as the number of deaths from a particular disease or condition as a percentage of the total numbers suffering from the disease or condition.

$$\frac{\text{Number of deaths from a particular disease or condition}}{\text{Total numbers suffering from the disease or condition}} \times 100$$

In concluding this section on the measurement of mortality it is pertinent to refer to the accuracy of death certification. A variety of studies on the accuracy of certified cause of death have been conducted. These include: international comparisons of medical certificates of cause of death; comparisons of clinical findings with those found at autopsy; assessment, by means of a survey of certifiers, of the diagnostic evidence recorded on the certificate; comparison of the wording on the death certificate with the clinical diagnosis obtained from clinical case notes; and examination of the relation between certified cause of death and the age of the certifying doctor. All of these studies, using different approaches, have demonstrated considerable inaccuracies in certification and have shown it to be subject to various errors. There are three important reasons why accurate statistics of mortality are required: firstly, mortality data are frequently used to identify associated factors, e.g. occupation; secondly, mortality data are necessary to plan health services and later to evaluate these services, e.g. screening for cervical cancer; and finally, such data are of importance in research studies of an epidemiological type. For these reasons then, the medical profession must endeavour to determine accurately the condition from which a patient has died. It is not possible here to enter into a discussion of methods of improving accuracy of death certification but increasing autopsy rates would help considerably, although it should be emphasized that autopsies are not a complete answer. There is, among other things, a great need for education of medical graduates and undergraduates in the correct method of death certification and of the importance of determining the true cause of death.

11.3   Measures of fertility

The *birth rate*, or *crude birth rate*, is defined as the number of live births occurring during a calendar period per 1000 of the mean population during the same period.

$$\frac{\text{Number of live births occurring during a calendar period}}{\text{Mean population during the same period}} \times 1000$$

(Birth rate, 1981: England & Wales, 12·8; Ireland, 21·0.)

The crude birth rate, like the crude death rate, is of limited value since it depends on the age and sex composition of the population. Specifically, the rate is influenced by the number of women of child-bearing age in that population, and because it relates to the total population it does not necessarily indicate the relative fertility of that population. For this reason, a *general fertility rate* is calculated. This is defined as the number of live births occurring during a calendar period per 1000 women of child-bearing age in the population during the same period of time.

Since the general fertility rate is based only upon the number of women of child-bearing age in the population (usually taken to be the age range 15–45), it is, clearly, a better measure of fertility than the crude birth rate. However, the general fertility rate is also limited, because it does not take into account the age distribution of women of child-bearing age within the population of females 15–45. For this reason *age-specific fertility rates* (similar to age-specific mortality rates) are calculated, from which a further measure called the *total fertility rate* is calculated. The total fertility rate represents an estimate of the average number of children born to a woman throughout her child-bearing period, subject to prevailing age-specific fertility rates. Thus, a total fertility rate of 3700 per 1000 implies that, on average, 1000 women would be expected to bear a total of 3700 children throughout their child-bearing age span.

The concept of the total fertility rate is closely related to analysis of population trends. In analysis of population trends, the important factor to be determined is whether or not the female population is replacing itself from one generation to the next, for in the long run this determines the trend in total population. For this purpose, *gross* and *net reproduction rates* are calculated. The gross reproduction rate is similar to the total fertility rate, except that it refers to *female* births only; thus, if it happened that males and females were born in equal numbers,* a total fertility rate of 3700 per 1000 would give rise to a gross reproduction rate of 1850 per 1000. The net reproduction rate is derived from, and is slightly less than, the gross rate — it takes account of mortality conditions as they affect women throughout the child-bearing span. In summary, the net rate measures the average number of female children born to a woman during her child-bearing life, subject to prevailing specific fertility and specific mortality rates.

11.4   Measures of morbidity

Morbidity, which is ill-health or sickness, poses a variety of measurement difficulties. While death is an event which occurs at a point in time, sickness may last for a period of time, may recur within one period of time, and may be present with different degrees of severity. A person may have more than one illness; moreover, except for certain infectious diseases most illnesses are not subject to notification, and sources of information on illness are necessarily partial and not recorded in such a way as to permit the derivation of measures of morbidity with the same degree of convenience and accuracy as mortality. Sources include hospital in-patient and out-patient records, general practitioner records and, in many countries, information on illness or absence from work, collected as part of the administrative procedures of social security systems. The development of comprehensive systems of social security, the increased use of computers for processing and filing data, and the growing importance of preventive medicine are greatly improving the range of available data on morbidity, but much remains to be done.

---

* In fact, the ratio of female to total live births is slightly less than half.

It is not intended here to discuss morbidity statistics (which include virtually any information connected with health or ill-health) in any detail, but there are two types of measure of morbidity which are in common use and will be explained. These are the *incidence rate* and the *prevalence rate* and they are often confused*. An incidence rate is defined as the number of cases of a particular disease or condition *commencing* during a specified time per 100 of the average population at risk during the same period of time.

$$\frac{\text{Number of cases of a particular disease or condition } commencing \text{ during a specified time}}{\text{Average population at risk during the same period of time}} \times 100$$

The prevalence rate which is commonly used is known as the *point prevalence rate*. The point prevalence rate is defined as the number of cases of a particular disease or condition *existing in* a population at a specified time per 100 of the population at risk at that time.

$$\frac{\text{Number of cases of a particular disease or condition } existing\ in \text{ a population at a specified time}}{\text{Population at risk at that time}} \times 100$$

Less commonly used is the *period* prevalence rate, which is the number of cases existing within a specified time period per 100 of the average population in that period. Incidence and prevalence rates are usually expressed as a percentage although other multiplying factors may be used. This of course presents no difficulty provided it is stated clearly what the multiplying factor is. Incidence is concerned with the number of *new* cases of a disease or condition occurring, while prevalence is concerned with the total number of *existing* cases in a population.

Finally, reference may be made to *average duration of illness*, often in connection with the economic and social consequences of absence from work through illness. Average duration of illness (for specific, or for all illnesses) may be expressed in terms of the total population (at risk), or of persons who were actually ill during the period of time to which the measure refers. In the former case, the denominator of the measure is the total population at risk in a particular time period, while in the latter case the denominator is the number of persons who were ill during the particular time period. (If a particular individual was ill more than once during the period, he or she will be counted as a separate 'person' for each illness.) The numerator of the ratio in each case is the total number of days of recorded illness, which may be measured in calendar days, or in working days only. Data for these calculations derive mainly from social security statistics.

---

*   See also Sections 9.4 and 9.6.

11.5 Hospital statistics

For legal, administrative and other purposes, hospitals maintain a considerable volume of statistical information relating to patients. In this section, a
number of measures related to the utilization of hospital resources, which are
commonly used for management and administrative purposes, are briefly
discussed.

The *average length of stay* is designed to measure the average number of
days spent (continuously) in hospital by a given group of patients. The
arithmetic mean is typically used as the measure of the average. The simplest
way of calculating the arithmetic mean length of stay is to record the length of
stay of each patient registered in the hospital over a particular period of time,
add these together and divide by the number of patients. An alternative, less
direct measure is to calculate the total number of 'occupied bed-days' over a
specific time period (say, a calendar month), and then to divide this total by
the number of patients leaving hospital (by discharge, transfer or death) in the
same period. This is not as precise a measure of the mean, since bed-days
taken in earlier months by patients discharged in the current month will not
be included in the numerator of the measure, and patients in hospital but not
leaving during the current month will not be included in the denominator.
The longer the period of time used for the calculation, the closer will this
indirect measure be to the (true) average length of stay. The direct measure is
to be preferred, since it is not only more accurate but also permits calculation
of the standard deviation length of stay, which indicates the variability of
length of stay around the mean; however, the form in which hospital records
are maintained usually necessitates the use of the alternative, indirect method
of calculation.

The *bed occupancy rate* is a measure of the degree of utilization of available
beds over an interval of time. This is often calculated as the ratio of the
number of occupied bed-days in a particular period to the number of
available bed-days over the same period, and multiplied by 100 to express it
in percentage terms. Thus, if there are 100 beds, over a 30-day calendar period
this gives 3000 available bed-days. If the number of occupied bed-days over
that period is 2400, the bed occupancy rate is $(2400/3000) \times 100 = 80\%$.
Occupancy rates over 100% can occur if extra beds, over and above those
usually available, have to be provided.

An alternative approach is to calculate the *daily* bed occupancy rate, and
then to calculate the average daily rate for the particular period. This will give
the same average occupancy rate for a given period as the method described
above (provided the number of available beds remains constant over the
period), but has the added advantage that the standard deviation can also be
calculated. The variability in the occupancy rate may be just as important as
its mean.

The difference between the total available bed-days and the number of occupied bed-days in any period represents unoccupied bed-days and can be used to calculate what is called the *turnover interval*. This is defined as the number of unoccupied bed-days divided by the number of patients leaving hospital (by discharge, transfer or death) in a particular period. In the hypothetical example above, there were 3000 available bed-days in a 30-day period, and 2400 occupied bed-days. The number of unoccupied bed-days is, therefore, 600. If, during this period, there had been, say, 150 'bed departures' (discharges, transfers or deaths), the turnover interval can be calculated as $600/150 = 4$ days. A truer measure of the turnover interval would be to calculate, for each of the 150 departures noted during the period, the actual time interval for which the bed is empty, and then to estimate the mean of these 150 time intervals. (This would also permit calculation of the standard deviation.) Usually, however, this method is not feasible, and the more indirect method is used. Like the measures of average length of stay, the longer the time period concerned, the closer will the indirect measure be to the true mean.

Another measure of resource utilization is the 'turnover' or *throughput* of patients per bed in any interval of time. Following the example quoted above, the average (daily) number of available beds in a 30-day period can be calculated as $3000/30 = 100$. The number of patients departing during this period was 150, so that the average throughput of patients per available bed is calculated as $150/100 = 1.5$.

11.6   Life tables and cohort analysis

In an earlier section, a number of measures of mortality were described. One measure not covered in that section is the *mean expectation of life at birth*. The calculation of life expectancy involves what are called *life tables*, and is a special example of a form of statistical analysis termed *cohort analysis*. Other applications of cohort analysis involving so-called clinical life tables were discussed in Chapter 9 (Sections 9.7 and 9.8). The life tables discussed in this section are often referred to as population life tables.

The disadvantages of the crude death rate as a measure of comparative mortality have already been pointed out. A comparison of crude death rates between countries A and B, or within the same country at different periods of time, may not be very meaningful because of differences in the age and sex compositions of the two populations. Ideally, it would be asked — 'What would the crude death rates be if the two countries had identical populations?' Another way of expressing this is to ask — 'What is the average expectation of life of an individual in each country?' It is to answer this question that life tables are constructed. To the extent that their purpose is to eliminate the effects of age distribution on measures of mortality, they have something in common with the standardized mortality measures described in Section 11.2.

The construction of life tables will now be explained with reference to Table 11.7. Suppose a *cohort* of 100 000 male births in a particular year is postulated. A number of the cohort will die during the first year of life (infant mortality). In Ireland, the number who die could be estimated by means of the current infant mortality rate. In the period 1970–72, the average male infant mortality rate for Ireland was 20·78 per 1000, so that out of 100 000 male births the 'expected' number of deaths can be estimated as 2078. Thus, of the original cohort, 97 922 may be expected to survive to age 1. These figures are shown in the columns headed l_x and d_x in the table.

How many of the hypothetical cohort will survive to age 2? This can be estimated by using the actual (1970–72) specific mortality rates for Ireland for the age group 1 and under 2 years of age. Thus, it is estimated that 136 of the cohort will die between the ages of 1 and 2, leaving 97 786 to survive until age 2.

The general procedure will now be clear. At each age, the cohort is subjected to the specific mortality rates for that age group. Eventually, of course, the cohort will 'die off'. The number who die at each age is determined by the specific mortality rates, and these are usually based on the average mortality rates for the most recent period for which accurate statistics are available.

Consider now the column headed L_x. The figures in this column measure the estimated total number of years lived by the cohort at each age. To explain this, suppose the whole cohort had survived to age 1 (the infant mortality rate was zero). In this case, the total number of years lived by the cohort, between birth and age 1, would be 100 000 — each member of the cohort would have lived for 1 year.

However, it is estimated that only 97 922 of the cohort live for a year, while 2078 live for only part of a year. Thus, the total number of years lived by the cohort is 97 922 plus some fraction of 2078. The precise method of calculation

Table 11.7   Irish life table no. 8 1970–72 — males.

Age x	l_x	d_x	L_x	T_x	e_x^0	Age x
0	100 000	2078	98 198	6 876 850	68·77	0
1	97 922	136	97 854	6 778 652	69·22	1
2	97 786	87	97 743	6 680 798	68·32	2
3	97 699	59	97 670	6 583 055	67·38	3
4	97 640	57	97 611	6 485 386	66·42	4

Source: *Irish Statistical Bulletin*. Vol. LI, No. 1, March 1976. (Table abbreviated.)

will not be explained here* — in summary, it is estimated that the total number of years lived by the cohort, between the ages of 0 and 1, is 98 198.

Similarly, the total number of years lived by the cohort between the ages of 1 and 2 is 97 786 (the number of years lived by the survivors to age 2) plus a half of 136 (those who die before reaching the age of 2). This is estimated to be 97 854. The interpretation of the L_x column should now be clear.

Turning now to the T_x column; the first figure in this column is the total number of years lived by the cohort at all ages — in fact, the sum of *all* the figures in the L_x column when the complete life table for all ages is constructed. Thus, the life span of all the members of the cohort is estimated to account for a total of 6 876 850 years. Since there were, originally, 100 000 persons in the cohort, the average number of years lived by the cohort is 6 876 850/100 000 = 68·77 years. This average, recorded in the last column of the table, is the mean expectation of life at birth of an Irish male. It indicates how many years an Irish male may be expected to live — or, alternatively, the average age of an Irish male at death — subject to certain specific mortality conditions.

The other entries in columns T_x and e_x^0 are also of interest. For example, the second figure in the T_x column measures the total number of years lived by the cohort from the age of 1 onwards; the second figure (69·22) in the e_x^0 column is derived from this, and measures the *mean expectation of life* at age 1. That is, a male who has survived to age 1 may expect, on average, to live a further 69·22 years. Thus, the figures in the e_x^0 column measure the average expectation of life at each age.

The reader may be surprised to note that the mean expectation of life at 1 (69·22) exceeds the mean expectation of life at birth (68·77), though on *a priori* reasoning it would be expected that the mean expectation of life would fall with increasing age. This apparently perverse result is due to the effect of infant mortality on the life expectancy of the cohort at birth. From age 1, however, the expectation of life declines with age as expected (see Table 11.7).

There are many other features of life tables which could be discussed, but sufficient has been explained to demonstrate their relevance in analysis of mortality, despite their limitations.

Life tables can be constructed for different populations and comparisons made on the basis of life expectancy. Separate tables can be constructed for males and females, for different areas of the country (e.g. urban and rural) and for different occupations. Comparisons can be made which are independent

---

* The simplest assumption would be that those who die live on average six months each, so that the 2078 of the cohort who die before reaching age 1 would live for a total of 2078/2 = 1039 years. This assumption is made for all age groups *except* the age group 0 to 1, since most deaths in this group occur in the first month of life.

of the effects of age and sex composition, and the mean expectation of life is a useful and simple concept to understand.

The most obvious limitation of life tables as described above is the use of *prevailing* age-specific mortality rates to calculate the *expected* mortality experience of the cohort. In the example above, age-specific mortality rates for 1970–72 were used. (There was a population census in 1971, so that the population of each age group could be ascertained with a high degree of accuracy, and this enabled firm estimates to be made of age-specific death rates.) If these are used to calculate the mortality experience of a cohort of 100 000 male births commencing, say, in 1971, then in the period 2001–2005, the figures which will be applied to the survivors of the cohort are the age-specific death rates for males aged 30–34 which prevailed in 1970–72. As the cohort ages, the applicability of the 1970–72 age-specific death rates becomes increasingly open to question. In this respect, the concept of the mean expectation of life at birth (or indeed at any other age) must be heavily qualified, since the actual mortality experience of a cohort of male births in 1971 (and hence their life expectancy) is not known. Thus, the mean expectation of life and other measures* derived from a life table are purely hypothetical measures based upon prevailing (recent) age-specific mortality rates. It is, of course, possible to attempt to anticipate changes in mortality conditions by *predicting* changes in age-specific mortality rates, based perhaps on an extrapolation of past trends, but in certain respects this introduces a greater degree of ambiguity in the interpretation of the life table statistics.

11.7 Summary

This chapter has described a number of vital statistics which are particularly important in medicine. Different measures of mortality were defined, and it was explained how the mortality experience of different populations could be compared by means of so-called standardized mortality measures, which neutralize the influence of age distribution on mortality. In a later section of the chapter, the use of population life tables in analysis of mortality was also explained.

Other sections of the chapter covered measures of fertility (birth rates and

---

* It is possible to calculate, from the life table, a death rate called the *true death rate*, which is actually the reciprocal of the mean expectation of life at birth. In this example the so-called true death rate is

$$\frac{1}{68\cdot77} \times 1000 = 14\cdot54.$$

reproduction rates), morbidity statistics and a variety of measures such as bed occupancy rates which relate to the use of health care resources. Such measures can help in assessing the efficiency with which scarce health care resources are used, although they must be interpreted with care. With increased computerization, there is a growing availability of data on morbidity and on the utilization of health care resources, and the use of computers in medicine is the subject of the next chapter.

CHAPTER 12
Computers in Medicine

12.1 Introduction

The development of microprocessors has been the most significant technological advance in this half of the twentieth century and their application has
profoundly affected — and will continue to affect — virtually every field of
human activity, from grocery shops to space exploration. In recent years,
computers have proved an invaluable aid to many aspects of medical
research work (although in a very limited way in relation to their full
potential), and are also extensively used for administrative purposes in
hospitals. Although, in principle, the functions performed by a computer
could be performed 'manually', in practice the immense amount of sorting
and analysis which is involved in many applications would not be feasible
without the aid of a computer. This is not simply because of the volume of
manual labour required to replace the computer; in many applications no
amount of manual labour could carry out the complex and interrelated
calculations required in the time necessary. In speeding up calculations by a
factor of millions, microprocessors permit the introduction of more sophis-
ticated process equipment.

The following section describes, briefly, the basic functions and configuration of a typical digital* computer system, while the next section outlines the
principal types of application of computers in medicine and health care.

12.2 Computer systems

In the simplest terms, a computer is a calculating machine which can perform
a wide variety of basic arithmetic and logical functions very rapidly. There is,
however, a considerable — and growing — variety in the design functions of
these machines, which range from highly specialized systems to carry out
one or a limited number of functions very efficiently, to general purpose

---

* The other main type of computer is the analogue computer, which is used in automated
  control systems. For most of the applications discussed here, the digital computer is used,
  although analogue computers are also used in clinical laboratories.

(usually large) machines which can carry out a great range of operations. Basic to all these machine types is the microprocessor, comprising thousands of transistors on a silicon chip. It is technical developments in the production of microprocessing components which have been responsible for the fall in price of computing equipment in recent years and the huge expansion in its range of applications.

Although a computer is capable of carrying out extremely complex operations, it essentially operates by carrying out a sequence of simple arithmetic (add, subtract) and/or logical (if, then, or) steps, according to a sequence of instructions specified by the user. The series of related instructions required to deal with a particular problem or activity (like sorting data into tables, or calculating and comparing the means of two samples) form a *program*, which provides a step-by-step routine for the computer to follow. (Such programs are described as computer *software*; the pieces of physical equipment are the *hardware*.) Of course, if a problem cannot be defined and formulated in a detailed and logical way, then it is not possible to program it for solution by the computer. Quite often, it is the definition of the problem that creates the most difficulty. Special programs are required to control the activities of the computer system itself, and these are given the general name of 'system software'.

Non-specialized computers are often categorized into three groups — microcomputers, minicomputers and mainframes — according to size, power and cost, although the distinction between these groups is somewhat imprecise (for example, a large minicomputer may be much more powerful than a small mainframe) and it is quite likely that these categories will soon become obsolete in the light of rapid technological developments. Best-known to the general public are the so-called *microcomputers*, which range from the very small 'personal' or 'home' computer to the compact desk-top type computer suitable for business, academic and similar applications. Microcomputer hardware and software is now the fastest growing section of the computer market and technical developments in microprocessor technology have meant a continuous expansion in the power, scope and sophistication of microcomputers (as well as in the number of makes available).

Minicomputers are the intermediate-size category and are designed for use in larger commercial or research organizations in which there are a number of users, who may well be located in different offices and/or laboratories, and linked to the computer by a terminal (e.g. a visual display unit [VDU] with keyboard).

The largest computer is the so-called *mainframe* which may occupy a whole floor of a building and conforms most closely to the traditional concept of a computer. It is designed for use by a very large number of users, many of whom may be quite distant and linked by landline or telephone line to the computer. In effect, although memory size is a major consideration, the important distinguishing feature of different types of computer is their operating system, especially input–output devices.

The actual physical pieces of equipment making up the computer form the 'hardware'. For a typical general purpose computer, the principal units comprise (see Fig. 12.1):

(1) The *central processing* unit (CPU) which provides central control over the functioning of the entire system and interprets the instructions of any program. Principal components of the CPU are:

(a) The *arithmetic unit* which performs all the arithmetic and logical functions of the computer, and works on the data which are held in the memory unit,

(b) The *control unit* which accepts an instruction, decodes it, and as a result, organizes the actions in and around the CPU,

(c) The *memory storage unit* which holds the programs which are being used and the actual data, in such a manner that these can be made available to the central processor during the execution of the program,

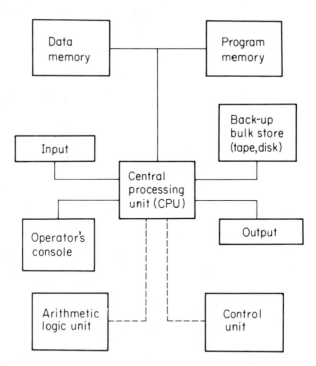

FIG. 12.1. Components of a typical computer system. Note that while separately identified in the diagram, many of these components will be contained within a single unit of physical equipment.

(d) The *input/ouput (control unit)* which provides the means by which programs and data can enter the system, and results leave it.

(2) Connected to the CPU are one or more of a number of devices or 'peripherals' including card readers, tape drives, disk drives, line printers and VDUs for actually entering programs and data, and for extracting results. The most direct way of entering data or instructions, familiar to readers with a personal computer, is by means of a keyboard, similar to that of a typewriter. Associated with this is usually a VDU (for home users, a television set) which displays what is being entered, and also acts as an output device for displaying results.

More generally, however, programs and data are recorded on auxiliary storage devices, such as punched cards, magnetic tape, magnetic disks or drums, and transmitted to the core memory of the computer as and when they are needed via such input devices as card readers, tape readers and disk drives. For many years, punched cards were the most widely used form of storage, but these have been superseded by magnetic tape and magnetic disk. Cassette tapes and paper tape systems are also used. Less familiar but increasingly used means of inputting data are bar codes, by which a pattern of bars is 'read' by a light-sensitive pen attached to the computer (often seen in retail shops), and optical character readers (OCRs), by which the computer scans a record sheet and interprets marks recorded on it (an application is in the correcting of multiple choice examination papers).

Computer output is often displayed in user-readable form on a VDU, but for permanent record it is normal to record results on paper via a printer, of which various types are available. If the results are to be used for further processing, or kept as permanent records, or sent to other users or customers, they may be recorded on tape, disk, punched cards or paper tape.

The list of instructions or program, which tells the computer what to do, has to be written in a particular form or 'language'. The computer itself operates according to a so-called machine code language which is specified by the manufacturer (and which varies with each type of machine), but to make things easier for the user, programs are usually written in a so-called 'high-level' language which can then be 'translated' by the computer into its own machine code. Programming languages in common use include FORTRAN, PASCAL, COBOL and BASIC, all of which are written in a form designed for ease of use (and learning) by the user. The computer then translates the user-languages into machine code by means of a *compiler* (roughly analogous to a dictionary); a separate compiler is needed for each high-level language, and some machines will only operate on one user-language.

One of the most rapidly growing microprocessor applications at the present time is the *word processor*, which is a specialized machine designed for the production of documents, texts, drawings and similar material. A word processor system is, essentially, a microcomputer with a keyboard, a VDU, an auxiliary storage system (usually floppy disks) and a printer. The user types the text, which is simultaneously displayed on the VDU, into the computer and a draft copy of the text is printed; the draft text will also be stored on a floppy disk. Subsequently, using the floppy disk and the VDU screen, the user can edit, amend or correct the draft text without the need to retype the whole text. The final text can then be produced on a printer and also stored on disk. (For example, this book was produced on a word processor system.)

Software packages associated with word processing systems include a wide range of editorial-type routines, including automatic pagination, alignment of left-hand and right-hand margins (justification), standardized spelling, automatic indexing, and so on. The word processor is the biggest development in office technology since the typewriter, and greatly enhances the productivity of secretarial and clerical staff. Word processors may be purchased and installed as independent specialist devices, or a word processing package may be purchased and run on a general purpose (non-specialist) micro-, mini- or mainframe computer.

12.3   Computer applications

Apart from the rather specialized function of word processing, discussed briefly in the last section, there is a large and growing variety of applications of computers in medicine and health care, ranging from well-established and fairly routine data processing activities, such as invoicing and the preparation of payrolls, the organization of out-patient appointment systems, and so on, to quite complex mathematical models designed to 'simulate' particular physiological or environmental conditions. In this section some of the more important of these applications are briefly described.

In keeping with the main subject matter of this book, a major application of particular interest is the use of the computer for purposes of statistical analysis, including the recording and organization of data, the description of data, and their analysis using the techniques of statistical inference discussed in preceding chapters.

As indicated in the previous section, the undertaking of a statistical analysis requires the user to supply the computer with the data and with the instructions (the program) necessary to analyse the data, which may include, for example, sorting them into frequency distributions, calculating the means and standard deviations for different groups within the sample data, and carrying out tests of significance on the sample statistics. Depending on the scale of the study, or its complexity, this may involve the assistance of a statistician/computer programmer. However, for most computer systems there are now available a large range of pre-written statistical programs or 'packages' which can be used 'off the shelf' by the researcher, though statistical and/or programming advice is still needed to determine the statistical techniques appropriate to the study, the capability of a particular computer system to handle the survey data, and so on. Nevertheless, the availability of such packages, along with the development of more 'user-friendly' computers and programming languages, and wider acquaintance with programming techniques, have made it easier for researchers in all disciplines to undertake work on the computer, often by means of a remote-access terminal. Statistical packages, such as *SPSS* (*Statistical Package for the Social Sciences*, Nie *et al.* [1975]) which is widely used in medical and social research, now contain a large array of sub-routines for sorting, describing and analysing data (including means and standard deviations, regression, correlation, analysis of variance, Z, t and χ^2 tests, discriminant analysis, etc.), any combination of which may be selected as appropriate for a particular study.

In large-scale studies the preparation and inputting of data is generally the most labour-intensive and time-consuming aspect of the work. Typically, the data will be initially recorded on a questionnaire or record form and it is necessary to convert this into a form suitable for acceptance by the computer — for example, punched card, magnetic tape or magnetic disk. To do this, the researcher, in conjunction with the statistician and the programmer, will prepare a list of coding instructions which specify precisely how the data are to be converted to computer-readable form. Unless the questionnaire or record sheet has been expressly designed for subsequent computerization, an intermediate stage, by which the original data are transferred onto a coding form or sheet, may be required to facilitate conversion to cards, tape or disk.

Fig. 12.2 illustrates, in a simple way, the general procedures involved, beginning with the primary survey data. Here, the record form has been specially designed with subsequent coding in mind, and an intermediate coding sheet is not required.

Each person in the survey is given a number, for purposes of identification. If the number of persons in the survey runs into four figures, then four columns will be required on the card or tape. Thus, if the survey number is 259, the first column will be left blank or recorded as 0, while the numbers 2, 5 and 9 will be entered in columns 2, 3 and 4 respectively.

The coding instructions for sex are that 1 will be recorded for a male, and 2 for a female. Thus, if the patient is male, the number 1 will be ringed, and this will be entered in column 5 of the tape or card.

The treatment of variables such as age and weight depends on how precise this information must be. In the example, age groups have been used; if the patient is, say, 34 years of age the code number 3 is ringed and this will be entered in column 6.

However, it may be desirable for the data on weight to be expressed to the

		Code number	Columns
Survey number 259		0259	1−4
Sex (1.) Male		1	5
2. Female			
Age 1. Under 20 years			6
2. 20−29 years			
(3.) 30−39 years		3	
4. 40−49 years			
5. 50 years and over			
Weight (kg) 70		070	7−9

FIG. 12.2. Coding a computer record sheet.

nearest kg, in which case the actual weight of the patient is recorded (for instance 70 kg). Three columns will be required for this (allowing for weights of 100 kg or over).

In order that the data can be recorded in computer-readable form with minimum error and maximum efficiency, it is obviously important that the coding instructions be carefully established and that the lay-out of the record sheet should facilitate entering the data in the most efficient way. In the example shown, it is only necessary for the operator to read down the column headed 'code number'. It would be possible to enter the data from the left-hand column, where numbers are ringed or written in, but most record sheets contain a considerable amount of data, and reading through the data to find the appropriate number to enter can sometimes be confusing and lead to mistakes; it also takes far longer than reading down a single column of numbers. Usually, the data are first compiled by ringing or writing in the appropriate numbers under 'sex', 'age', and so on; it is then advisable to fill up the column headed 'code number', from which the operator will read the data. Where this has not been done, record sheets are often so confusing that they have to be 'reprocessed' on to a fresh coding form and this is time-consuming and irritating to all concerned.

As soon as the data have been entered, recorded and checked, and programs prepared, the computer can then be used for processing and analysis. In a survey, it is common to prepare a large number of tables, of frequency distributions, bivariate classifications and so on. For example, it may be necessary to classify male and female patients by age. Given the instructions, the computer will sort the data and print out the required table. The preparation of tables of this kind is a routine computer application.

Subsequently, the computer may be used for tests of significance, fitting regression equations and similar statistical and mathematical operations.

The preceding discussion referred to data processing (of which further examples are given below) and statistical analysis. Another interesting application of computers is in simulation techniques, of which there are various examples in medicine and health care. Briefly, this involves the formulation of a mathematical model of a system (which may be based on actual or hypothetical data), and the use of the model to 'simulate' the consequences of particular events or decisions which are specified by the model user. These are designed to reflect 'real life' possibilities and to indicate, with varying degrees of probability, what might happen in particular situations. Some of the best known examples of simulation models occur in the social sciences; economists, for example, construct computer-based models of the economy and use them to predict what might happen to output, employment and so on if, say, the government reduces taxes. As another example, flight simulation models are used to train airline pilots, including the simulation of emergencies (such as engine failure) which would be risky (and possibly disastrous) to replicate in actual flight training.

The use of simulation models in medicine and health care includes: analysis of the effects of epidemics under varying assumptions about population movement and rates of infection; determination of 'queueing' or waiting times at clinics, under varying assumptions about rates of referral, treatment times and patient throughput; training of health care administrators or managers in resource allocation decisions through simulation of the operation of health care systems (e.g hospitals). Simulation techniques are also being developed for training in diagnosis. A hypothetical patient with specific diagnostic characteristics is simulated on the computer, and the student asked to diagnose and prescribe treatment; it is possible to some extent to simulate response to treatment. Clearly this development offers considerable possibilities, although as a complement to, rather than a substitute for, traditional clinical training methods.

The diagnostic checks and procedures used in simulation may be also used with real patients, the computer in this case undertaking the evaluation on the basis of the patient information with which it is supplied and printing out 'its' diagnosis or, more likely, a list of possible diagnoses. For the general physician, automated diagnoses of this kind may be a particularly useful form of assistance in cases of unusual or uncommon diseases and/or symptoms since, in effect, he or she is calling upon the diagnostic skills of specialists involved in the diagnostic programming of the computer facility.

In a more comprehensive way, medical record linkage provides a continuous record of individual patients from birth to death, including illnesses, hospitalization, operations, allergies and so on. Prior to the use of computers, the linking together of different events in an individual's medical case history was extremely difficult, since individual events (treatment by family doctor, stay in hospital, etc.) were, and indeed usually still are, recorded separately at different locations with no systematic procedures for bringing together these elements of case history into a single record. With computer-based recording systems such linking becomes more feasible. Medical records can be put to better use and information stored efficiently; moreover, this information can be retrieved more rapidly than before, cumulative files for individuals can be compiled and assembled into family groups, socio-economic categories, and so on, for purposes of analysis. Longitudinal studies, which involve following up a given group or cohort over a period of time, are a well-established application of the concept of medical record linkage, and the large and comprehensive computerized data bases established through record linkage open up a wide range of potential research studies. It must be noted here, however, that the development and use of such data raise issues of confidentiality in patient records, and touch upon the much broader question of the protection of individual privacy in conditions in which many details of personal circumstances (financial status, social security history, and so on) are on computer files and may be vulnerable to unauthorized access.

A somewhat related but more specific use of computerized records and data processing arises in screening the results of routine examination of large numbers of individuals, often at regular intervals (e.g. airline pilots, military personnel, schoolchildren, or simply groups drawn from the general population). Test results can be examined and collated, results for individuals compared with standard or average results or with those of earlier tests for the same individual, and summaries printed out, including reference to potentially significant, unusual or unfavourable test results which call for priority attention. This may be seen as a special but particularly useful application of the computer for diagnostic purposes.

Substantial use of computers is now being made in clinical laboratories, in the control and monitoring of equipment and in the evaluation of results, and this has been one of the most successful and intensive areas of computer applications related to health care. Clinical data (blood pressure, temperature, respiration, etc.) can be evaluated, warning signals indicated, and printed and/or graphical output produced. For continuous monitoring of patients in intensive care, the patient may be directly linked to computer-controlled equipment which will alert staff to any significant change in conditions.

Finally, computers are extensively used on the administrative and planning side of health care, and applications here are many and varied. They range from computerized payroll and staff scheduling and stock control systems, similar to those used in industry and commerce, to more specialized applications including the monitoring of hospital waiting lists, records and analysis of bed occupancy, average length of stay in hospital, and comparisons of bed utilization rates between different units and over time. Cost data may be used to estimate the true resource cost of various forms of health care delivery, and to identify critical areas where more efficient resource allocation would improve health care productivity. On a larger scale, within national health care systems such as the British National Health Service, computer-based models of the system can be used to estimate, for example, the optimal location pattern for specific health care facilities, the areas to be served by each hospital within an administrative region, and the probable demand, and hence recommended capacity for specific facilities (surgical, obstetrical, etc.) within a newly planned hospital.

As is clear from the foregoing, the scope for the application of computers in medicine and health care is enormous. With the exception of clinical laboratories and academically based medical research programs, realization of this potential is, so far, fairly limited, although growing rapidly. Practical experience of computer applications has been mixed, with some projects abandoned and others not obviously more efficient than the 'manual' systems they replaced. As is invariably the case with new technologies, there is a 'learning-by-doing' process which requires adaptation and the acquisition of new skills and practices, and most of all an understanding on the part of the user of what a computer can and cannot do, and of what it is designed to do in the particular application for which it is installed. Too often, purchasers have ambitious but vaguely articulated expectations of what a computer can do, and are subsequently disappointed; either the computer cannot perform the tasks expected of it or the wrong system has been purchased.

12.4 Summary

This chapter has provided a simple introduction to computers, including a description of different types of computer, of what they can do, and of the configuration of a typical computer system. In medicine, as in other fields, the development of microprocessors is revolutionizing traditional practices and Section 12.3 contains a brief review of the application of computers in medicine. Such is the pace of development, however, that it may be safely asserted that this chapter will be the first in this book to merit revision!

CHAPTER 13
Bias in Medical Research

DESIGN
EXECUTION
ANALYSIS

13.1 Introduction

Bias may be defined as any factor or process which tends to produce results or conclusions that differ systematically from the truth.* Any research study in a medical field is open to bias from many sources, and it is important that the researcher be aware of these biases, and in designing, executing and analysing a study avoid them where possible. Many of the biases that can arise in the planning and execution of the study are avoidable, but a badly run study cannot be rescued by clever statistical manipulation of figures. For this reason, study design is a far more important aspect of research than pure statistical analysis.

In the body of this book, it has been indicated at various stages how bias may interfere with the eventual outcome of a study, and this chapter brings together some of these ideas and introduces some new ones. Particular forms of bias are more likely with some study designs than others, and the discussion below indicates which pitfalls are more likely in which studies.

Sackett (1979) has identified 56 sources of bias in medical research, and although all these biases are not considered individually here, the article makes for fascinating reading. This chapter considers the different biases that can arise in the context of the different stages of a study execution — the design stage, patient selection, data collection, data analysis and interpretation of results. Many of the biases, of course, fit into more than one of these categories.

13.2 Study design

The previous chapters outlined the four main study designs often used in medical research — the cross-sectional, the prospective (cohort) and retrospective (case-control) observational studies and the experimental trial. Chapter 10 considered, in some detail, the avoidance of bias in the experimental

---

* This broad definition of bias thus includes errors in analytical methodology and errors of interpretation.

trial by the use of randomization and double blind procedures. These arguments are not repeated here, but, instead, points relating to the design of studies in general are considered.

Perhaps the first question to ask about any study is whether a comparison or control group is required. In most cases, the answer will be yes, and indeed many research studies are uninterpretable without a comparison group. The fact that, for example, 80% of a group of lung cancer patients smoke does not in itself suggest a relationship between smoking and lung cancer. It is necessary to know what the percentage of smokers is in the general population (the comparison group). This fact is often overlooked. Similarly, in evaluating a preventive or therapeutic measure, there must be a comparison group against which to evaluate the results. Some studies, of course, will not require a specific comparison group. In a prospective study, for example, the comparison groups are usually defined by the variables measured at the start of the study, and an explicit comparison group need not always be built into the study design. A sample survey to estimate some parameters may also fit into this category. For instance, a study to determine the factors relating to birth weight would not require a control group.

Given, however, that many studies will require an explicit control group, it is necessary to ask if, at the end of the day, like is being compared with like. If this can be achieved by designing a study in a particular way, it is far better than adjusting for extraneous differences between groups at the analysis stage. Thus in a case-control study, some form of matching may be employed or, in an experimental trial, randomization (stratified or simple) may be used.

An important source of bias in many situations relates to the number of individuals studied. This is discussed in the context of interpreting the results in Section 13.6, but in general, professional advice should be sought in determining the appropriate sample size for any investigation (see also Appendix D). Obviously, the design of a given investigation depends critically on the question to be answered and it must be ascertained whether the study as designed will answer that question.

13.3 Selecting the sample

The selection of individuals or items to be included in a study is the area with the greatest potential for bias and relates to a large extent, but not exclusively, to whether the results of a study are generalizable. As already mentioned, for example, studies based on volunteers can cause great difficulties in this area. If, however, those studied form a random sample (in the strict sense of that term) from the population of interest, then selection bias should not be a problem, as long as results are generalized only to the actual population from which the sample was taken. Studies based on hospital admissions are not generalizable to all patients with a particular condition. Comparisons between admissions to different hospitals are also often biased for the same reason. The type of patient admitted to a particular hospital will depend on, among other things, the catchment population for the hospital, admission criteria, the fame of the doctors and surgeons, the facilities and diagnostic procedures available, and the intensity of the diagnostic process. These, and other factors which determine admission to a particular institution or hospital, are even more important when it is remembered that many studies are based on a presenting sample of patients. Admissions to a hospital will of necessity exclude, for example, patients managed in the community and patients who do not survive long enough to be admitted to hospital in the first place. A further bias (Berkson's bias) can result in spurious associations between an exposure and disease in a case-control study if the admission rates to hospital differ in different disease/exposure categories. The mechanism of this bias, which is complex, is explained by Sackett (1979).

A general rule relating to studies of any particular disease is to commence the study in all patients at some fixed point in the natural history of the disease. Failure to do this properly can be a further source of bias. This is why it is suggested in a case-control study, for instance, to include newly diagnosed (incident) cases only — diagnosis being usually a fixed point in a disease's history. Evidence of exposure to a particular factor may be masked if the disease is present for some time. A problem does arise however if some patients are diagnosed earlier than others, and the bias is often called *lead time bias.* Suppose a group of breast cancer patients, diagnosed when they presented with a definite lump in the breast, had been studied and that it is wished to compare their subsequent survival with a group of cases diagnosed by mammography (X-ray) at a screening clinic. This latter group would enter the study at an earlier stage in the natural history of the disease (before an actual lump was detectable) than the former group and thus would be likely to have a longer survival anyway, due to this earlier diagnosis. Some correction for this lead time bias would have to be made when analysing or interpreting the results.

Selecting patients at a fixed point in the natural history of a disease in a survival study is not achieved, however, by retrospectively determining the date of disease onset. Apart from problems in patient recall and adequacy of available records, such a process would result in a biased group with a spuriously long survival. A researcher who determined the survival of a group of cancer cases attending a clinic by measuring the time from their diagnosis (in the past) to the present would necessarily exclude patients who had died earlier, and would thus load the group with those who survived the longest. Such an investigation can only be performed if the survival of *all* patients is determined from diagnosis, and is best done by means of a prospective study.

For any study of disease, the diagnostic criteria must be clear and explicit. Different centres may label different conditions with the same name, and it is important (as discussed in Chapter 10) to know precisely what patients were studied, and thus to which population results can be applied. The exclusion of cases because of concomitant disease or other factors may affect the general applicability of findings, although it is usually necessary to avoid contamination of the study groups. In addition to these selection biases, the problems raised by a large number of patients refusing to participate in a study must not be forgotten. This question of non-response bias has been discussed before, and it is best reduced by making the study as simple as possible, and not in any way daunting to potential participants.

13.4   Data collection — accuracy (bias and precision)

Every study in medicine must involve some data collection or measurement, and an interaction between the observer and the patient or object being observed. Measurement bias, or measurement error as it can be called, is a factor that every researcher must be wary of. All studies should employ a predesigned data collection form with the information required, whether it be based on interview, case records, or direct measurement, laid out neatly and comprehensively. If data are to be processed by computer, the form should be laid out in a manner suitable for easy transferral of the data to machine-readable form, and a computer programmer should be consulted (see Chapter 12). The specific problems of questionnaire design are not considered here, except to note that it is much more that just writing down a list of questions which require an answer. Bennett and Richie (1975) give a detailed account of the use of questionnaires in medical research.

Some of the biases of data collection, in the context of the case-control study and the experimental trial, have been discussed, emphasizing the necessity, where possible, of blinding the observer to the particular group (case/control, treatment/control) from which information is being collected. This is to avoid biases in the observer's elicitation and interpretation of a response. Measurement bias can also, of course, be due to non-response and lack of complete follow-up, when missing items of information can cause very definite problems.

The problems of measurement go deeper than this, however, but unfortunately there is no standardized terminology in this area. The definitions given are widely, but not universally, accepted and represent an attempt to put the subject into a realistic framework. In this text an *accurate* measurement will be defined as one which is *precise* and *unbiased*. Perhaps the best way to illustrate these two terms is by reference to Fig. 13.1. This shows the hits obtained on four targets by four individuals using different air guns. Mr. A's

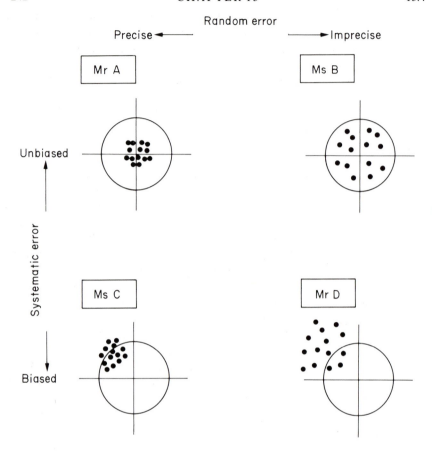

FIG. 13.1. Precision and bias. Target practice in a fairground.

shots are closely grouped around the centre of the target. From this, it might be assumed that the sight of the gun was properly aligned, so that the shots went where they were aimed, and also that he was a 'good shot', and had a steady hand, because of the close grouping around the bull's eye. Ms B did not however achieve a close bunching of her shots, although obviously, 'on average', she was hitting where she was aiming for. It might be assumed that the sight of her rifle was well-adjusted, but that her hand was not too steady, resulting in a wide spread of shots. Ms C, on the other hand, obviously had a steady hand, since her shots were grouped closely together, but she was consistently off target; either the sight of her gun was badly adjusted or there was, perhaps, a strong wind. Mr D is most unfortunate; not only is his hand a bit shaky, but by looking at where his shots are grouped, it would appear also that his sight was out of alignment.

Precision relates to the scatter of shots caused by, for instance, the random shake in an individual's hand, while bias refers to whether or not the shots are hitting the target on average. A faulty sight, or cross wind, causes a *systematic error* in one particular direction away from the bull's eye. In terms of a measurement, bias is a result of a systematic error which tends to make the actual recording of a measurement consistently above (or below) the true value. The term error in this context should only be used if the true value of the measurement is known and, in general, the term variation will be used instead. The precision of a measurement relates to the amount of *random variation* about a fixed point (be it the true value or not). An imprecise measurement will sometimes be above this fixed point, sometimes below it, and will vary randomly about it.* If the error is defined as the observed reading minus the true value, then random errors have a zero mean but any standard deviation and can be assumed to have a normal distribution. Random errors can also be considered independent of each other.

An accurate measurement, then, is one which can vary very little (precise) around the true value (unbiased) of what is being measured. For the correct classification of an individual into one group or another, on the basis of a single measurement, it is necessary that it be accurate. If a measurement is biased, the only way to solve the problem is to correct for this bias by adjusting the observed value. Thus, if an investigator were to classify individuals on the basis of a random blood glucose level, and used a small finger-prick drop of capillary blood for assay purposes, the measured values would have to be adjusted upwards by about 10% to enable estimation of the level of glucose in the venous blood.

If a measurement lacks precision, repeated measurements of the same characteristic, finally using an average of all these readings, will reduce the problem. Repeated measurements will not of course correct for bias.

What then can affect the accuracy of a given measurement? Different factors affect both precision and bias, and Fig. 13.2 displays some of these. Remember, to define bias it is necessary to know the true value of the measurement, and for the moment it will be assumed that the factor being measured is actually the factor about which information is required. (See discussion of validity below.) Thus, in evaluating measurements of blood pressure, what is being evaluated is the measurement's capability of determining the pressure exerted by the artery on the cuff of the measuring device.

Observer variation has a major impact on measurement accuracy, and can be split into two components — *within- (intra-) observer variation* and

---

* Sometimes, the term precision is used in the sense of 'a height of 2·544 metres is a more precise measurement than that of 2·5 metres'. The two usages are similar, however, in that a measurement with a large amount of random variation cannot be expressed with the same degree of exactness as one with little such variation.

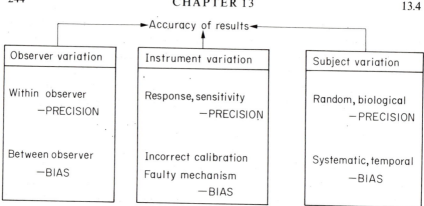

FIG. 13.2. Sources of variation in measurement results.

between- (inter-) observer variation. Within-observer variation refers to the variation between different recorded measurements by one observer, when the observations are made on different occasions. In theory, this assumes that the true value is constant, and that the differences in the measurements are due only to the observer. In practice, it is impossible to distinguish such observer variation from that of subject variation (if it exists; see below) when the same individual is tested more than once. However, if an observer is interpreting, for example, an ECG tracing or an X-ray, 'pure' within-observer variation can be detected. Within-observer variation may be caused by factors such as reading a dial, or the height of mercury in a sphygmomanometer at slightly different angles each time, or just failing to judge exactly the reading required. Slight errors in diluting a sample for assay, slightly different inflections in the voice in administering a questionnaire, or just misinterpreting a result, all contribute to within-observer variation. The important point is that within-observer variation in itself does not cause bias, but does affect precision. The variation of an observer with himself is assumed to be random.

Between-observer variation, on the other hand, can bias results and can cause great difficulty in combining measurements recorded by different individuals. Between-observer variation is the variation in a recorded measurement performed by two or more different observers. The results of between-observer variation can be severe ('doctors differ and patients die'), and in any study should be allowed for. Between-observer variation can be caused by different criteria for making a measurement (phase 4 or phase 5 in measuring diastolic blood pressure, for instance), by different techniques (blood pressure taken supine or standing), and by differing observational methods (the angle from which the level of mercury is read in a sphygmomanometer affects the observed height).

Different methods of actually recording a measurement can also lead to between-observer variation. In blood pressure again, *digit preference* is a large problem. A blood pressure of 117/89 is rarely recorded; observers tend to have a preference for certain values, or end digits, especially 5 and 10. Thus, readings of 120/85 mm Hg and similar are far more common in recorded blood pressures than would be expected on any reasonable distribution of the variable. Again, whether measurements are rounded up or down to the nearest even value or to values ending in 5 or 0, for instance, affects between-observer variation. In administering questionnaires, between-observer variability can be due to different ways of asking questions, and even the general demeanour of the interviewer. Between-observer variation due to such factors can be reduced substantially by very careful standardization of methods, and training of observers. In any study where observations are to be made by different individuals, this must be done to avoid spurious differences between groups. This is particularly so in multicentre trials for instance. Observer variation too is always a problem when clinical records or charts are being employed to gather data. Between-observer variation can also occur due to unconscious bias on the part of the observer who knows the group in which the individual has been classified. This can be avoided, as has been discussed, by blinding the observer. Between-observer variation, in essence, biases results insofar as two different observers cannot both be right. This bias is avoided, as has been said, by standardizing the methods of measurement.

A second major influence on the accuracy of observed measurements is *instrument variation*. The precision of an instrument may be low insofar as an actual reading is difficult to determine. The term instrument is used in the widest possible sense and includes physical measuring devices (weighing scales, sphygmomanometers, thermometers), questionnaires and interview schedules, and even biological assays. The precision of an instrument depends on its 'sensitivity' or response to the quantity being measured. An instrument from which a measurement is recorded by reading a pointer on a dial would be considered imprecise if the pointer hovered around but never actually stopped at a particular reading. The response or sensitivity of an instrument, however, can often not be distinguished from the effects of observer variation, or indeed (as with questionnaires for instance) from the effect of subject variation also.

Instrument variation resulting in bias is usually a result of a faulty machine or incorrect calibration. If the scale of a mercury sphygmomanometer slips down, a blood pressure reading will be higher than its true value. Careful maintenance of equipment, and testing in a situation where the true value of a measurement is known, will reduce this bias enormously.

Subject variation also affects the accuracy of test results but, of course, in one sense, it is often subject variation which is being measured — for example, a drop in blood pressure due to treatment. Random or biological subject variation relates to the fact that an individual's blood pressure, say, may vary in a random way around some fixed value. This of course affects the precision of a blood pressure's determination, and such subject variation is the main cause of the phenomenon known as regression to the mean (see Section 8.7). Random subject variation is best controlled for, of course, by repeat measurements. Systematic subject variation will cause a measurement bias. Many parameters can be affected by the subjects' mood, the conditions under which the measurements are taken, the time of day, the season and even the very fact that the subjects know that they are being observed. Such bias is of course intrinsically linked to observer variation, in that standardization of measurement technique can reduce some of the systematic variation in this area. Bias can also be due to the subjects' awareness of why they are being studied. *Recall bias*, for instance, can occur if subjects in a case-control study ruminate overmuch concerning exposure to possible causal factors, and thus remember more than if they were, in fact, controls without the disease. In a clinical trial an individual's response may be affected by his knowledge that he is in a group on a 'new wonder drug' which he knows should work (the placebo effect).

An interesting bias that can affect study results in different ways is *compliance bias*. For convenience, it is mentioned under the general heading of subject variation. If, in a controlled trial, participants in a treatment group fail to comply fully with their therapy, the apparent effect of that therapy in the full group is diluted. Also, it has been noted in some clinical trials that compliers with the placebo therapy can fare better than non-compliers with this therapy — even although there is no direct effect of the placebo. This is an interesting variation of the placebo effect. If the proportion of the compliers in the treatment and control groups differs, a biased comparison may result.

In the final analysis, however, whether variation in a measurement is random or systematic is far more important than its source. Systematic variation in any measurement is a problem; individuals will be wrongly classified on the basis of such measurements, which is serious in screening programmes or actual clinical practice. Sometimes, however, a measurement which is systematically biased (in the same direction and by the same magnitude) in each of two groups can be useful for comparative purposes. However, the size and direction of a bias is not often known, and between-group comparisons can be highly distorted if the biases occurring in each group are different.

Random variation, on the other hand, causes less of a problem. For the individual, of course, random variation can cause misclassification, but it can be controlled by taking repeat measurements on the same individual. In statistical-type investigations, analysis is performed on groups, and random variation will tend to cancel out. Thus the mean blood pressure of a group of

100 individuals may represent the true situation of the group very well, while lacking precision for any one individual. Random variation in a measurement increases its standard error, but increase of sample size can allow for this, once the amount of random variation is known. Random variation, in general, will tend to obscure group differences and reduce the magnitude of correlations between groups.

The *repeatability (reliability, reproducibility,* or *consistency)* of a measurement can be specifically determined by making replicate observations. A measure is repeatable if the same (or very nearly the same) result is obtained each time. If the same observer makes all the measurements, the repeatability of a test is directly related to its precision (amount of random variation involved) and the standard deviation of all the readings about their mean is a good measure of this random variation. Quantification and identification of the source of random variation (within-observer, instrument, or subject) is sometimes possible, depending on whether the measurements are repeated on the same individual (e.g. blood pressure) or repeated on the same test material (e.g. an ECG tracing or blood sample). When repeatability is being determined by repeated tests on the same individual or test material, by different observers, it is essentially a measure of between-observer variation. As has been said, it is important to identify, quantify and rectify this, if biased comparisons are not to result.

13.5   Data collection — validity

The last section discussed, in terms of precision and bias, problems with measurement relating to the question, 'Is the observed result the same as the true result of the measurement?' This section considers the other important question, 'Are we actually measuring what we are trying to measure?', which relates to the *validity* of a procedure. For instance, what is really required to be measured in using a sphygmomanometer, is the intra-arterial pressure exerted by the blood. This can be measured directly, and the question is whether or not the indirect measurement obtained by deflating a cuff placed on the right arm, and noting the height of a column of mercury at the appearance and disappearance of sounds is a valid method of doing this. The validity of any procedure is, thus, only determinable if some 'gold standard' of absolute truth exists, and the results of the measurement are gauged against this. Sometimes, such a gold standard may not exist and the operational definitions of the variable being measured themselves become a standard. If intelligence is defined as what is measured by an IQ test, then an IQ test is a valid measure of intelligence. The validity of a test or measurement can only, in a sense, be considered in the context of an accurate test because, obviously, problems with bias and precision will reduce a test's validity. An accurate test, however, is not necessarily a valid one. An especially important area in which validity merits attention is in the process of making a diagnosis. The 'true' diagnosis is usually made on the basis of a history, clinical examination, signs, symptoms and the results of one or more biochemical, electrical or other measurement processes. Although it may be difficult to lay down exactly what the criteria are for the diagnosis of a given condition unless autopsy reports are available and relevant, a clinical diagnosis based on all available information is, perhaps, the best available 'gold standard' for diagnosis.

Obviously, validity has important consequences in categorizing individuals. A single diagnostic test will misclassify some individuals, and this is extremely important in screening studies and in clinical practice. A *false-positive* result is a result which suggests an individual has a disease, whereas, in terms of some 'gold standard', he/she does not. A *false-negative* result categorizes an individual as disease-free, whereas, in reality, he/she has the disease. Table 13.1 shows the classification of 1000 individuals by whether or not a particular diagnostic test gave a positive result, and by their actual disease status. In general, the entries in the cells of the table are labelled *a*, *b*, *c*, and *d* as noted. In the example, there are 180 false-positives and 10 false-negatives.

The *sensitivity* of a test measures its ability to detect true cases, and is defined by the number of true-positives as a percentage of the total with the disease, or in this case, $90/100 = 90\%$. The *specificity* of a test, on the other hand, measures its ability to detect disease-free individuals, and is defined as the number of true-negatives divided by the total without the disease, or $720/900 = 80\%$. Ideally, a test should have high sensitivity and high specificity. One without the other is useless. For example, a test which defines bowel cancer to be present in all persons with a height above 0·25 metres is 100% sensitive, in that, certainly, all cases of bowel cancer will be detected.

Table 13.1 Measures relating to the validity of test results.

		Disease	
Test result	Present	Absent	Total
Positive	90(*a*)	180(*b*)	270(*a* + *b*)
Negative	10(*c*)	720(*d*)	730(*c* + *d*)
	100(*a* + *c*)	900(*b* + *d*)	1000(*n*)

Sensitivity: $a/(a+c) = 90/100 = 90\%$
Specificity: $d/(b+d) = 720/900 = 80\%$
Predictive value: $a/(a+b) = 90/270 = 33\cdot3\%$
(False-positive rate: $b/(a+b) = 180/270 = 66\cdot7\%$)
False-negative rate: $c/(c+d) = 10/730 = 1\cdot4\%$

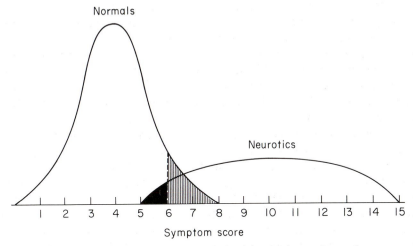

Fig. 13.3. Distribution of a symptom score in neurotic patients and normal controls.

The test which diagnosed bowel cancer as present in all persons over 2·5 metres high would be 100% specific. Unfortunately, however, sensitivity and specificity are not usually independent, and in any particular test, as one increases the other is likely to decrease. Fig. 13.3 shows the hypothetical distribution of a symptom score obtained by questionnaire in a group of psychiatric cases with a diagnosis of neurosis, compared to a normal control population. The normals have a mean score of 4 and the neurotics a mean score of 10. If a cut-off point of 6 in the symptom score was used to determine a diagnosis of neurosis, the sensitivity of the test would be fairly high, only missing neurotics with a symptom score of less than 6, as shown by the dark shaded area. The specificity of the test would not be so great, however, since it would misclassify any persons in the normal population with a score of 6 or over as denoted by the lightly shaded area in Fig. 13.3. Moving the cut-off point down to a score of 5 would give a test with a 100% sensitivity, while a test based on a score of 8 would achieve 100% specificity. Any intermediate point would result in the sensitivity and specificity indices increasing and decreasing in tandem. In a situation such as this, the best cut-off point to use can be determined only by the relative costs (to the investigator and to the patient) of the two types of misclassification. This is, obviously, a subjective judgement.

Reality is never as clear-cut as this example however. Diseased persons may just have higher values of a particular quantitative variable in a unimodal distribution and it could be questioned whether the presence of some diseases can ever be determined as definite. The grey area of uncertain diagnoses should always be allowed for. The sensitivity and specificity of a diagnostic procedure can be altered by the inclusion of more than one test to determine disease status. A diagnosis may be made only if the results of two different tests are both positive. This is called *testing in series*, and tends to increase specificity at the expense of sensitivity. Alternatively, a diagnosis might be made if either of two tests showed a positive result. Such testing *in parallel* would increase the sensitivity of the diagnostic procedure.

A word of caution should be inserted here on the question of *normal ranges*, particularly for biochemical tests. It is usually not very clear what these normal ranges represent. The first and common definition of a normal range (and for simplicity a test will be discussed in terms of abnormal values being above a specific cut-off point) is that in a general population only a certain proportion (usually 5%) of persons will have higher values than this upper limit of normal. This is a statistical definition of normality and has no relationship whatsoever to disease status. Conclusions based on such a definition will give a disease prevalence of 5% for any condition. An upper limit of a normal range could also be defined as that level above which some pathology may be present in an individual. Normal ranges based on this approach, which might be described as clinical, can be difficult to determine. A prognostic normal range, on the other hand, might define a test level above which an individual's prognosis is poor and an operational or therapeutic normal range might define that point above which medical intervention is likely to be of benefit. Prognostic or therapeutic normal ranges can only be determined on the basis of prospective studies. These four possible definitions of normal are however totally distinct and may bear no relationship to each other.

In general, individual tests not having 100% specificity and sensitivity will distort any estimates of disease prevalence. For example, in Table 13.1 the true prevalence of the disease is 10% (100 per 1000) while, on the basis of the test results, the prevalence is 27% (270 per 1000). If the validity of a test is different in two population groups being compared, spurious differences between the groups may occur. A real difference may be magnified, or it may be masked. If the validity of a test is consistent across comparison groups, the effect is always to dilute or weaken any association which may be observed between the disease and a factor.

A common error, which can lead to serious bias, can arise in studies where the validity of a test is incorrectly adjusted for. In many studies, the often small number of individuals with a positive test result are examined further to try to reduce the number of false-positives. Unfortunately, no corresponding effort is made in those with a negative test result to reduce the number of false-negatives; this will tend to result in a spuriously low prevalence estimate.

Although sensitivity and specificity may seem adequate in determining the validity of a diagnostic test, there are two further measures which are perhaps even more important in describing the effect of misclassification errors. Sensitivity and specificity can be determined independently by studying separate groups of diseased and non-diseased individuals. However, the usefulness of a diagnostic test also depends on the true prevalence of the condition in the population being studied. For the practising clinician or organizer of a screening programme, the *predictive value (diagnostic value)* of a test is a most important parameter. The predictive value of a test is the proportion of true cases among all those with a positive test result; in other words, it relates to what a clinician sees — those individuals with positive tests. In Table 13.1, the predictive value of the test is 90/270 or only 33·3%. Thus although the sensitivity and specificity of the test are 90 and 80% respectively, only one-third of the persons for whom the test results were positive actually had the disease. The usefulness of the test would be quite questionable.

The predictive value of the test can be calculated if, in addition to the test's sensitivity and specificity, the true prevalence of the disease is known, or if, as in the example, the test is performed on a sample from the population in which it is to be applied. The predictive value of a test of given sensitivity and specificity increases (decreases) as the true prevalence of the condition increases (decreases). Thus a test with a high predictive value developed in a hospital setting (where a high prevalence of any condition is to be expected) may be quite inapplicable when applied to a general population.

The *false-positive rate* for a test is calculated as the number of false-positives as a percentage of all positive test results, and is 66·7% in the example. It is, of course, 100% minus the predictive value, and is another way of looking at that parameter. The *false-negative rate* for a test is the false-negatives as a percentage of the total negative test results, and has, in the example, the low value of 1·4%. Note that the false-positive and false-negative rates are calculated with, respectively, the number of positive and negative test results as denominator, *not* the total number with or without the disease.*

Although the sensitivity and specificity of a test are measures of its validity, high values for these parameters do not in themselves make for a usable test in clinical practice. The usefulness of a test depends also on the prevalence of the condition being studied and in any evaluation of a diagnostic test predictive values and false-negative rates should be calculated if it is to be judged adequately. If the true prevalence of the condition is unknown, these calculations could be done for a series of prevalences that might be observed in practice.

---

* Some sources define the false-positive and false-negative rates with denominators of all diseased and non-diseased persons respectively. The definition given here is more generally used.

13.6   Statistical analysis and interpretation

If a study has been well-designed and well-executed, the main hurdles have been overcome. Errors in the statistical analysis and interpretation of results can of course still occur, but can be corrected. That such errors do occur is highlighted by, among others, Gore *et al.* (1977) who, in reviewing 62 reports in the *British Medical Journal* which included statistical analysis, showed that over half had statistical errors of one kind or another, that just under 30% had serious errors, and that 5 articles (8·1%) made claims that were not supportable when the data were examined carefully. Errors of interpretation can of course be on the part of the investigator, or the reader of a published paper. Errors related to the statistical analysis can arise in various ways, and most relate to failure to use appropriate statistical techniques. Errors of omission mean that a technique that should have been used on the data was not; errors of commission mean that a technique was applied incorrectly. Some of the more common errors are detailed below.

Failure to distinguish between independent and dependent observations causes many problems. If measurements are repeated on the same individual, they are not independent, and it is totally invalid to analyse them as if they were. For instance, if 20 diabetic patients were studied to determine pancreatic activity, and 5 observations were made on each patient, the data cannot be analysed for a sample size of $20 \times 5 = 100$ observations. The most important factor is the number of different individuals, and in such a case, the analysis could be performed on the 20 mean levels calculated on each individual. Analysis of variance also provides a very useful technique that can handle replicate observations in comparative studies. Failure to distinguish between independent and dependent data often arises also in clinical trials or case-control studies, where the two groups are paired or matched. The use of the independent t test or χ^2 test, instead of the paired t test or McNemar's χ^2 test, is a common error in paired comparisons.

Many errors relate to ignoring the assumptions underlying the parametric significance tests. The assumptions of approximate normality and equality of variances in group comparisons (homoscedasticity) are important in many cases, and although some tests are fairly robust (departures from some of the assumptions do not seem to matter a great deal), biased analyses can result from misapplication of tests to highly skewed data for instance. Transformation of the data may iron out such problems. With small sample sizes in particular however, assumptions can often not be checked and the non-parametric tests should perhaps be used more frequently.

Problems also arise with repeated use of significance tests. If a set of data is dredged for any significant relationships without reference to the purpose for which the study was set up, some relationships will appear statistically significant purely due to chance. A similar problem arises in a fixed sample size experimental trial, where interim analysis of results takes place before the requisite number of patients have entered. In such situations, spurious differences may appear by chance, and the p value required to declare a significant result should be decreased to allow for multiple testing. This of course will usually require an increase of sample size if the conventional levels of statistical significance are to be claimed.

Lack of understanding of the significance tests available and the type of data they can be applied to can result in biased analysis. This is particularly true in prospective studies of survival, where the problems of variable follow-up and losses to follow-up cause much difficulty. Clinical life table methods or, less preferably, the person-years at risk concept can be used to great advantage in such situations (see Sections 9.7 and 9.8).

In many studies, failure to adjust for confounding variables can result in a totally biased analysis. As has been said, however, controlling for the confounders at the design stage through randomization or matching is preferable to statistical adjustment, although the latter is often necessary.

Over-interpretation of the data is a problem that can also arise. The erroneous assumption that sensitivity and specificity, on their own, are good indicators of the usefulness of a particular diagnostic test has already been discussed. The problem also occurs when appropriate denominators are not available for the calculation of rates. For example, it is not possible to estimate absolute risk in a case-control study. Also, if a study of causes of death is being performed, only proportional mortality analyses can be carried out, unless the population from which the deaths arose is known. Thus it might be determined that 2% of all deaths under the age of 1 year were due to infectious diseases, while the proportion among deaths in those aged 1–2 years was 8%. This would not mean that the death rate (per 1000 of the population in these age groups) from infectious diseases was greater in the older age group. In fact, the death rate would be much higher in those under 1 year. When the number of deaths, only, is available for analysis the large number of deaths from all causes under the age of 1 year results in the proportional mortality for any single cause being considerably reduced.

Misinterpretations of the meaning of statistical significance abound. The confusion of statistical association with causation must be avoided (see Section 9.2) and the results should not be generalized to inappropriate populations. Also, a non-significant result does not mean a negative result; it means only that chance is a likely explanation of an observed association. Important results may be non-significant, due mainly to small sample sizes. On the other hand, a statistically significant result does not necessarily mean a medically important result. A trivial difference between two groups can always be made statistically significant with a large enough sample size.

13.7   Critical reading of the literature

One of the purposes of this book is to enable doctors to approach the medical literature with a critical mind. Many published studies are not all they seem to be at first reading, and it is up to the reader to judge a study's conclusions in the light of its design and analysis. Many biases can be detected if a report is approached with a logical mind, and if the important question 'What else could have produced the results obtained?' is asked. Errors in statistical analysis are often difficult to spot, but flaws in design and execution are more easily detectable. It goes without saying, of course, that a report must describe the study adequately in order for a judgement to be made, and many published reports fail to give sufficient information in this respect.

A report in the medical literature is usually given the following headings: 'Introduction'; 'Materials and Methods'; 'Statistical Techniques'; 'Results'; 'Conclusions'. In the introduction, there should be a clear statement of the objectives of the study, and the population to which the findings are to be related. Without this, it is difficult to see if the study design and analysis are appropriate to the question being asked. The materials and methods section, usually in small print, should give in some detail the design of the study, whether a cross-sectional retrospective or prospective observational study, or an experimental trial. Precise definitions of inclusion and exclusion criteria should be given, together with the description of the population from which the study group was formed. If random sampling was employed, this should be stated, as should also the procedure used for randomization. If matched groups are involved it should be clear whether frequency or paired matching was employed. From these descriptions it should be possible to detect any sources of selection or other biases, and to see if the researchers have made any attempt to allow for them.

There should be clear definitions of all the variables studied; this is particularly important for the major end-points of the study, and details of how the measurements were made, whether from case records, interview, direct measurement or official sources, should be indicated. If necessary, comments on the accuracy and validity of the data should be included. If patient follow-up is involved, the methods of tracing patients should be stated and an indication as to whether complete follow-up was achieved should be given.

The statistical techniques section of a paper, which is often included in 'Materials and Methods', should state, at least, which tests were performed, the significance level adopted, and whether one- or two-sided tests were used. If less common techniques were used, references, or a full description, should be given. It should be asked if appropriate techniques were actually employed, and if in fact the data were worthy of statistical analysis. This book has attempted to cover a fair proportion of the statistical techniques employed in medical research, but many techniques will be encountered that have not been detailed. In such cases, the adequateness or appropriateness of an analysis may be difficult for the general reader to judge. This section of a published paper should also, ideally, give an indication as to how the study sample size was arrived at — was any attempt made to use statistical methods, or was the size of the study group decided totally on the basis of convenience?

The results section of a paper is, without any doubt, the most important. Are the results presented clearly and in a comprehensible manner? A problem with many reports is that the results section is incomprehensible, with too much detail, too many large and complex tables, and a totally inadequate explanation as to how the results were actually arrived at. If a study is to be widely read and understood, simplicity of presentation is vital. This must be balanced, however, by the necessity to present sufficient detail for judging the adequacy and applicability of the results to the problem under investigation. The results of a study may have arisen from an extremely complex and comprehensive analysis; all aspects of this cannot be presented, and extensive summarizing may be necessary to present the kernel of what was found. There is a danger of swamping the reader with too much detail. The procedure adopted in some reports relegates such detailed results to an appendix, or to 'mini-print' tables. The results section should at least include a simple description of the distribution of the important variables studied in the different comparison groups, so that the reader may make a judgement about any confounding effects. Any statements made in a results section, such as 'males did better than females', should be backed up by summary statistics of the comparison. If confounders have to be adjusted for statistically, it is advisable that both adjusted and unadjusted results should be given, to enable the actual effect of the confounding to be seen.

The statistical significance of all comparisons should be stated, but not at the expense of failing to give the results on which the tests were based. If a study is reporting statistically non-significant results, then calculations should be presented as to whether the study was powerful enough (in terms of sample size) to detect medically important findings.

It is surprising sometimes how often numerical inconsistencies appear in published reports. Often there are discrepancies between figures given in tables and figures given in the text, or numbers in tables or percentages do not add up to the required totals. These should be checked by the reader, because although such errors are easy to make (with retyping of drafts, bad proof-reading, etc.) they may indicate more serious deficiencies in the study.* Do the numbers in the tables and text differ because some patients with missing observations were omitted from the final report but were included originally?

---

* The astute reader may discover some inconsistencies in this text!

Inconsistency may often be due to mising data (refusals, lost records, losses to follow-up), and the paper should state clearly how these problems were dealt with.

The discussion section of a paper should highlight the main results, show how they throw light on the research question being studied, and put the results in context by referring to the relevant literature.

In any study, bias may not be actually present, but the possibility of bias may put a question mark on the acceptance of final conclusions. No study can be perfect however. The important factor is whether the results do give new information which, of course, may be examined in a different way in a further investigation. If the authors of a paper identify possible sources of bias and discuss their potential influence on the results, any conclusions are all the more worthwhile. Finally, if you do discover inadequacies in a published study, ask yourself 'Could I have done it better?'. In many situations it will be found that there is no feasible alternative to that of the approach adopted, and it will be concluded that an excellent piece of research has indeed been performed.

13.8   A note on research procedures

For those who may become involved in setting up a research project, or for those who are involved in analysing or writing up a study, a few simple words of advice are offered below. Firstly, do not rush into any project. A good research project may take months, or even years, of planning before any individual is actually studied. Some statistical advice should be sought at a very early stage, especially as regards an appropriate sample size and the design of data collection forms if a computer analysis is even a possibility. A good literature survey is essential, to give an idea of what has already been done in the area of interest and to provide insights into the particular problems the study might face. It must then be decided whether the study is to be observational or experimental and what design features can reasonably be included.

The sections in this book on study design and bias in research provide an overview of the areas which must be considered, but further reading will most probably be necessary. A preliminary *pilot study* on a smaller number of individuals is often very helpful, to test data collection procedures and to provide preliminary estimates on the distribution of some variables as an aid to sample size calculations.

It is often difficult in a study to decide what variables should be measured. Do not be tempted to measure everything. The literature review and knowledge of what is being studied should be a guide to the relevant variables. A good procedure to judge what variables are really needed is to plan out in a rough way what tables would, ideally, be presented in a final report, and thus to determine the variables which are most likely to be related to the study outcome. Use only these. Avoid, too, taking measurements which will have missing information in a large number of subjects.

It is worthwhile, in the planning stages of a project, considering the type of statistical analysis that might be undertaken. This also may be a guide as to which variables to include in the data collection. It is advisable in any project to describe the complete study design, and all ancillary information in a written *protocol*. This will greatly aid in the final write-up of a study, and help ensure that the original design is strictly adhered to. Where many persons are involved in a project, and for multicentre trials, this is particularly important. This protocol can then be consulted by anyone involved in the project if there are any doubts about exactly what should be done in a particular situation. A written protocol is also necessary for submission to funding agencies (if funds are required!) and most hospitals require that research proposals be submitted to an ethics committee for approval before study commencement. A good research protocol should include a precise statement concerning the objectives of the study and its importance in the light of current medical knowledge. The actual design of the study should be given in great detail with careful attention paid to the selection of study participants (including the sample size) and potential sources of bias arising therefrom. Ethical problems must also be considered. Clear and concise definitions of the variables to be measured and the measurement techniques to be employed are essential, as are considerations of the relevance, accuracy and validity of these measurements. Data collection forms and questionnaires should be included, as should an indication of the type of statistical analysis that will be performed.

The protocol must be a practical document and should include far more than will ever appear in a published report. It should detail the manpower required for successful implementation of the study and estimate costings in terms of diagnostic tests and other procedures, stationery, printing etc., travel, computer costs and all the administrative overheads that will accrue. The likely duration of the study must be indicated and a timetable for completion of the various stages (e.g. study group selection, data collection and follow-up, analysis) should be given. How the study is to be implemented in practice, together with an outline of the responsibilities of those involved, should also be presented. Much thought should go into this area.

The execution of a study design demands careful adherence to the written protocol. All individuals involved with any of the subjects being studied should know that a special investigation is being carried out and should have read the protocol. Often, departures from the protocol may be necessary for ethical or other reasons, and careful note should be taken of such departures. Often, as a study progresses certain decisions, especially as regards exclusion or admission criteria, may have to be made in situations not considered in the original design. These too should be noted.

Once the study data have been gathered, a statistical analysis will have to be undertaken. For a large study, this may require the use of a computer and professional advice may be required. Many analyses can be undertaken by computer that would be impractical by hand, but pencil and paper methods are no more outmoded than the wheel. The statistical methods detailed in this book should be sufficient to enable a fair proportion of the data in any reasonably sized study to be analysed with the use of nothing more than a pocket calculator. This book, however, does not give computational details for any of the techniques* used to adjust for the presence of confounding variables, and if confounders are likely to be present, more advanced texts will have to be consulted.

At the end of the study, the results must be written up for publication. Choose a journal appropriate to the subject matter of the study, and read a good few articles in that journal to gauge the requirements in presentation. Also, pay careful attention to the 'instructions for authors' which are usually published in each journal on a regular basis. It is not easy to write up a research report, and a fair amount of time and effort is required. The previous section in this chapter, on the critical reading of the literature, should provide some guidelines as to what should be included in an article. Apart from that, it is all up to you.

13.9   Summary

The purpose of this chapter has been to bring together and expand on the subject of bias in medical research. Bias can arise in every stage of a research project, from design, subject selection and data collection to statistical analysis and interpretation. The chapter highlighted some, but not all, of the problems which can arise and it is hoped that it may prove useful to the reader of the medical literature and to the individual involved, for the first time, in the setting up, execution or analysis of a project.

---

* Apart from standardization in vital statistics, which can be applied to analytical study data also.

APPENDIX A
Computational Methods

A.1 Introduction

It is essential to own or have access to an electronic calculator to perform statistical computations. A simple calculator will cost very little, and as long as it has a square root function it will be sufficient for all the computations described in this book. More expensive calculators are available, which will automatically calculate means and standard deviations,* but these are not essential.

This appendix outlines some short-cut computational formulae that will simplify some of the calculations discussed in the text. In particular, simple formulae for the standard deviation, for the χ^2 test, for 2×2 tables and for regression and correlation coefficients are presented.

A.2 The standard deviation

The calculation of the standard deviation using Eqn. 2.3

$$S = \sqrt{\frac{\Sigma(X - \bar{X})^2}{n-1}}$$

is fairly cumbersome and an easier computational formula can be derived, which gives the same numerical answer. The sum of squared deviations in the numerator can be expressed

$$\Sigma(X - \bar{X})^2 = \Sigma X^2 - \frac{(\Sigma X)^2}{n} \tag{A.1}$$

so that

$$S = \sqrt{\frac{\Sigma X^2 - (\Sigma X)^2/n}{n-1}} \tag{A.2}$$

This involves squaring each observation, taking their sum (ΣX^2), and subtracting from this the square of the sum of all the observations ($\Sigma X)^2$

---

* Usually two different standard deviation functions are provided, one dividing the sum of the squared deviations by $n-1$ and the other by n. The former should always be employed.

divided by the total sample size (n). This is then divided by $n-1$ and the square root taken.

Table A.1 illustrates the layout for this calculation. Column 1 gives 6 observations (X) for which the standard deviation is to be calculated. The sum of the observations (ΣX) is given at the foot of the column. Column 2 is the square of each value (X^2) with the sum of these squares (ΣX^2) at the foot of the column. These values are then substituted into Eqn. A.1 to give the standard deviation.

It is advisable to keep as many digits in the intermediate steps as are displayed on the calculator. The final computed standard deviation need however only be expressed to two decimal places more than the original observations, unless it is to be used in further calculations. Most calculators display only eight digits and sometimes an intermediate computed quantity may exceed the display capacity. In such cases, the original observations can be rescaled to a size more manageable on the calculator. If the original units are too large, either a constant should be subtracted from each observation, or each observation should be divided by some constant. If the units are too small then each observation should be multiplied by a constant. The

Table A.1 Calculation of the standard deviation.

1 X	2 X^2
530	280 900
518	268 324
572	327 184
595	354 025
527	277 729
548	300 304
3290	1 808 466

$$n = 6$$

$$\Sigma X = 3290$$

$$(\Sigma X)^2 = 10\,824\,100$$

$$(\Sigma X)^2/n = 1\,804\,016 \cdot 7$$

$$\Sigma X^2 = 1\,808\,466$$

$$\Sigma X^2 - (\Sigma X)^2/n = 4449 \cdot 334$$

$$\frac{\Sigma X^2 - (\Sigma X)^2/n}{n-1} = 889 \cdot 8668$$

$$S = \sqrt{889 \cdot 8668} = 29 \cdot 83$$

calculations as described are carried out on the rescaled observations. If subtraction of a constant was employed in the rescaling then the computed standard deviation needs no adjustment and is the same as would have been obtained on the original data. If multiplication (or division) was employed, the computed standard deviation must be divided by (multiplied by) the chosen constant to obtain the correct result. The example in Table A.1 is recomputed in Table A.2 using rescaled values obtained by subtracting 500 from each observation and then in a separate calculation by dividing each observation by 100. The same final standard deviations are obtained. Although rescaling was not necessary in this example, the advantages of the smaller numerical quantities at each step are clear.

If a series of observations has many repeat values, or if the standard deviation of grouped data is being calculated, again there are some short-cut computational methods. In grouped data, remember that all the observations in an interval are assumed to have a value equal to the midpoint of the interval. If there are f occurrences of the value X then the standard deviation is defined

$$S = \sqrt{\frac{\Sigma f(X - \bar{X})^2}{\Sigma f - 1}} \qquad (A.3)$$

where the sample size is given by the sum of the frequencies in each class (Σf).

Table A.2 Example of rescaling in calculating standard deviations.

	Original units	-500	$\div 100$
	530	30	5·3
	518	18	5·18
	572	72	5·72
	595	95	5·95
	527	27	5·27
	548	48	5·48
ΣX	3290	290	32·90
$(\Sigma X)^2$	10 824 100	84 100	1082·41
ΣX^2	1 808 466	18 466	180·8466
$\Sigma X^2 - (\Sigma X)^2/n$	4449·334	4449·333	0·4449334
$\sqrt{\dfrac{\Sigma X^2 - (\Sigma X)^2/n}{n-1}}$	29·8306	29·8306	0·298306
S	29·83	29·83	29·83

A computationally easier formula is given by

$$S = \sqrt{\frac{\Sigma f X^2 - (\Sigma f X)^2 / \Sigma f}{\Sigma f - 1}} \qquad (A.4)$$

The application of this to calculate the standard deviation of the birth weight data discussed in Chapter 2 is illustrated in Table A.3. Column 1 gives the midpoints of each class interval which correspond to the observations X. Column 2 gives the frequencies (f) observed in each class, and the sum of their values (Σf) is the total sample size. Column 3 contains the square of each X value and column 4 gives each of these X^2 values multiplied by its frequency f. The sum of this column is $\Sigma f X^2$. Column 5 gives each observed value multiplied by its frequency giving the sum $\Sigma f X$. Σf, $\Sigma f X$ and $\Sigma f X^2$ are then substituted into Eqn. A.4 to give the standard deviation. Again the original values, X, can if necessary be rescaled to make the calculations more manageable on a pocket calculator.

Table A.3 Standard deviation for grouped data. (Birth weight data of Table 1.3.)

1 Class midpoints X	2 No. of observations f	3 X^2	4 $f X^2$	5 $f X$
1·88	4	3·5344	14·1376	7·52
2·13	3	4·5369	13·6107	6·39
2·38	12	5·6644	67·9728	28·56
2·63	34	6·9169	235·1746	89·42
2·88	115	8·2944	953·8560	331·20
3·13	175	9·7969	1714·4575	547·75
3·38	281	11·4244	3210·2564	949·78
3·63	261	13·1769	3439·1709	947·43
3·88	212	15·0544	3191·5328	822·56
4·13	94	17·0569	1603·3486	388·22
4·38	47	19·1844	901·6668	205·86
4·63	14	21·4369	300·1166	64·82
4·88	6	23·8144	142·8864	29·28
5·13	2	26·3169	52·6338	10·26
	1260 (Σf)		15 840·822* $(\Sigma f X^2)$	4429·05 $(\Sigma f X)$

* 8 digits accuracy.

$$S = \sqrt{\frac{\Sigma f X^2 - (\Sigma f X)^2 / \Sigma f}{\Sigma f - 1}}$$

$$= \sqrt{\frac{15\,840 \cdot 822 - (4429 \cdot 05)^2 / 1260}{1259}}$$

$$= 0 \cdot 4650$$

A.3   The χ^2 test for independent 2×2 tables

An alternative to the usual χ^2 formula in 2×2 tables (Eqn. 7.16)

$$\chi^2 = \Sigma \frac{(O - E)^2}{E}$$

which is computationally simpler, is often used. It has the disadvantage, however, that the expected values (E) are not computed so that there is no direct check on whether all of these are greater than 5, as required in the assumptions for the use of the test.

Table A.4 shows the layout of a general 2×2 contingency table. a, b, c and d are the four observed quantities, r_1 and r_2 are the row totals and s_1 and s_2 are the column totals, n is the sample size. With this notation

$$\chi^2 = \frac{(ad - bc)^2 n}{r_1 r_2 s_1 s_2} \tag{A.5}$$

When using a pocket calculator, the numerator of this expression may exceed the capacity of the display. This can be avoided by first calculating $(ad - bc)^2$, then dividing by r_1 and r_2, multiplying by n and finally dividing by s_1 and s_2.

Table A.4   Short-cut χ^2 formula for independent 2×2 tables.

a	b	r_1	$\chi^2 = \dfrac{(ad - bc)^2 n}{r_1 r_2 s_1 s_2}$ on 1 degree of freedom
c	d	r_2	
s_1	s_2	n	

A.4   Regression and correlation

The formulae for both the regression and correlation coefficients (Eqns. 8.4 and 8.7) involve the expression

$$\Sigma (X - \bar{X})(Y - \bar{Y})$$

while the formula for the standard error of the estimate (Eqn. 8.12) requires the calculation of

$$\Sigma (Y - \hat{Y})^2$$

where the Ys are the observed values of the dependent variable and the $\hat{Y}$s are the predicted or expected values on the basis of the regression equation. As they stand, both these expressions are computationally awkward and alternatives are available. Firstly

$$\Sigma(X - \bar{X})(Y - \bar{Y}) = \Sigma XY - \frac{(\Sigma X)(\Sigma Y)}{n} \tag{A.5}$$

where n is the number of pairs on which the regression equation or correlation coefficient is being calculated. This expression involves calculating the product of each pair of X and Y variables and summing to obtain ΣXY. The ΣX and ΣY terms are the sums of the X and Y variables separately.

Table A.5 Computation of basic quantities required for simple regression calculations. (Data from Fig. 8.6.)

1 QRS score X	2 LVEF Y	3 XY	4 X^2	5 Y^2
0	51	0	0	2601
0	57	0	0	3249
0	58	0	0	3364
0	60	0	0	3600
0	66	0	0	4356
0	71	0	0	5041
1	58	58	1	3364
1	60	60	1	3600
1	65	65	1	4225
2	57	114	4	3249
3	52	156	9	2704
4	51	204	16	2601
5	44	220	25	1936
5	46	230	25	2116
6	32	192	36	1024
6	40	240	36	1600
6	42	252	36	1764
6	48	288	36	2304
7	37	259	49	1369
8	28	224	64	784
8	38	304	64	1444
9	28	252	81	784
9	31	279	81	961
9	43	387	81	1849
11	21	231	121	441
11	22	242	121	484
11	24	264	121	576
13	18	234	169	324
142 (ΣX)	1248 (ΣY)	4755 (ΣXY)	1178 (ΣX^2)	61714 (ΣY^2)

Table A.6 Regression calculations for LVEF/QRS data.

Quantity	Computational formula	Value	
$\Sigma(X-\bar{X})(Y-\bar{Y})$	$\Sigma XY-(\Sigma X)(\Sigma Y)/n$	$4755-(142)(1248)/28$	$-1574\cdot1429$
$\Sigma(X-\bar{X})^2$	$\Sigma X^2-(\Sigma X)^2/n$	$1178-(142)^2/28$	$457\cdot85714$
$\Sigma(Y-\bar{Y})^2$	$\Sigma Y^2-(\Sigma Y)^2/n$	$61714-(1248)^2/28$	$6088\cdot8572$
$\bar{X}$	$\Sigma X/n$	$142/28$	$5\cdot0714$
$\bar{Y}$	$\Sigma Y/n$	$1248/28$	$44\cdot5714$
Regression coefficient b (Eqn. 8.4)	$\Sigma(X-\bar{X})(Y-\bar{Y})/\Sigma(X-\bar{X})^2$	$-1574\cdot1429/457\cdot85714$	$-3\cdot4381$
Regression coefficient a (Eqn. 8.6)	$\bar{Y}-b\bar{X}$	$44\cdot5714+3\cdot4381(5\cdot0714)$	$62\cdot0074$
Correlation coefficient r (Eqn. 8.7)	$\dfrac{\Sigma(X-\bar{X})(Y-\bar{Y})}{\sqrt{\Sigma(X-\bar{X})^2\,\Sigma(Y-\bar{Y})^2}}$	$\dfrac{-1574\cdot1429}{\sqrt{457\cdot85714\times6088\cdot8572}}$	$-0\cdot9428$

Table A.5 shows the original data for the regression of left ventricular ejection fraction (LVEF) on the QRS score discussed in Chapter 8.* Columns 1 and 2 give the QRS values (X), and the corresponding LVEF values (Y), which summed give ΣX and ΣY. Column 3 gives the XY values obtained by multiplying each X value by its Y value, and the sum of these is ΣXY. Columns 4 and 5 give the squares of the X and Y values and their sums. These are the basic quantities required for regression and correlation calculations. The number of pairs, n, is 28. Table A.6 shows, explicitly, the calculations for the regression coefficients (Eqns. 8.4 and 8.6) and the correlation coefficient (Eqn. 8.7) for the LVEF data.

The computational expression for $\Sigma(Y-\hat{Y})^2$ is given by

$$\Sigma(Y-\bar{Y})^2 - \frac{[\Sigma(X-\bar{X})(Y-\bar{Y})]^2}{\Sigma(X-\bar{X})^2} \tag{A.6}$$

All these quantities have already been calculated and Table A.7 shows the final computations for $S_{Y.X}$ using Eqn. 8.12.

---

* These data are based on the published diagram (Palmeri *et al.*, 1982) and the resulting calculations differ slightly from those appearing in the publication.

Table A.7 Calculation of $S_{Y.X}$ for the LVEF/QRS data.

$$\Sigma(Y-\hat{Y})^2 = \Sigma(Y-\bar{Y})^2 - \frac{[\Sigma(X-\bar{X})(Y-\bar{Y})]^2}{\Sigma(X-\bar{X})^2}$$

$$= 6088 \cdot 8572 - \frac{(-1574 \cdot 1429)^2}{457 \cdot 85714}$$

$$= 676 \cdot 8501$$

$$S_{Y.X} = \sqrt{\frac{\Sigma(Y-\hat{Y})^2}{n-2}}$$

$$= \sqrt{\frac{676 \cdot 8501}{26}}$$

$$= 5 \cdot 1022$$

APPENDIX B
Statistical Tables

B.1 Introduction

This appendix gives the statistical (and other) tables necessary in the calculation of significance levels for the tests described in this book. For ease of use, an attempt has been made to employ a uniform layout for these tables and the upper and lower critical values for a range of one- and two-sided significance levels are presented. Consequently, some of the tables may have a different appearance to those which are more customary but hopefully they will prove easier to employ in practice. Note also that the tables relate to the critical values of the test statistic as described in this text, which may have a slightly different formulation (especially for the non-parametric tests) than that given in other sources. Without exception, all the tables have been reproduced or adapted from the *Geigy Scientific Tables* (Lentner, 1982) which is a very useful reference work.

Sometimes the sample size may be too large for use of the statistical tables for the non-parametric tests. In such cases, if a non-parametric test must be used, the reference cited above gives formulae for approximate large sample size significance levels. The non-parametric tests, however, tend to be used more often with small sample sizes, so this should not be a major problem in most practical applications. Note, too, that in many of the non-parametric tests, the significance levels given in the tables are not exact, due to the discrete nature of the particular distributions. The actual probability or p value associated with a given critical value may, in fact, be slightly less than that presented. The tables included in the appendix are:

B.2 Tables

Table B.1 Table of random numbers. Abbreviated from *Geigy Scientific Tables* Vol. **2**, 8th Edn. with permission.

20557	43375	50914	83628	73935	72502	48174	62551	96122	22375	96488
83936	45842	78222	88481	44933	12839	20750	47116	58973	99018	22769
36077	82577	16210	76092	87730	90049	02115	37096	20505	91937	69776
78267	31568	58297	88922	50436	86135	42726	54307	29170	13045	65527
00232	98059	07255	90786	95246	15280	61692	45137	17539	31799	64780
65869	64355	91271	49295	98354	28005	69792	01480	51557	70726	35862
35454	51623	98381	11055	32951	28363	16451	67912	66404	76254	75495
99542	44247	12762	54488	74321	36224	95619	16238	25374	13653	25345
36087	32326	52225	72447	77804	57045	27552	72387	34001	83792	66764
64899	62390	68375	42921	28545	33167	85710	11035	40171	04840	69848
11994	97820	06653	27477	61364	22681	02280	53815	47479	44017	37563
02915	81553	92012	50435	73814	96290	86827	81430	45597	82296	28947
62895	09202	48494	95974	33534	94657	71126	71770	16092	03942	90111
39202	82110	82254	03669	03281	11613	36336	98297	48100	71594	52667
53252	18175	09457	83810	46392	02705	85591	33192	65127	80852	42030
17820	50756	80608	35695	72641	26306	76298	32532	22644	96853	18610
85245	12710	60264	74650	92126	08152	32147	17457	56298	48964	64733
85822	44424	88508	66190	74060	93206	92840	44833	81146	64060	62975
24804	24720	66501	74157	42246	41688	72835	87258	89384	11251	34329
31942	85419	93017	28087	78323	77109	56832	78400	24190	37978	85863
72838	10933	99964	13468	17211	48046	51122	92668	96750	11139	06275
38546	49559	71671	53603	24491	57570	90789	32932	67449	05115	45941
38051	39391	92039	71664	40219	97707	93975	66981	19556	24605	52169
28101	38543	54214	48928	32818	51963	87353	15094	29529	87305	01361
70476	44242	54227	28598	64422	29361	20359	48577	05971	92373	22765
64999	11468	74149	81386	94127	67342	38010	92522	57728	39432	27914
73641	52165	54336	89196	40042	37889	06003	58033	59082	94988	62152
67421	83093	77038	55399	67893	89597	85630	08059	35757	49479	63531
30976	66455	90708	08450	50120	17795	55604	51222	17900	55553	02980
29660	30790	65154	19582	20942	81439	83917	90452	64753	99645	19799
82747	97297	74420	18783	93471	89055	56413	77817	10655	52915	68198
46978	87390	53319	90155	03154	20301	47831	86786	11284	49160	79852
19783	82215	35810	39852	43795	21530	96315	55657	76473	08217	46810
12249	35844	63265	26451	06986	08707	99251	06260	74779	96285	31998
58785	53473	06308	56778	30474	57277	23425	27092	47759	18422	56074
69373	73674	97914	77989	47280	71804	74587	70563	77813	50242	60398
95662	83923	90790	49474	11901	30322	80254	99608	17019	17892	76813
97758	08206	54199	41327	01170	21745	71318	07978	35440	26128	10545
72154	86385	39490	57482	32921	33795	43155	30432	48384	85430	51828
25583	74101	87573	01556	89183	64830	16779	35724	82103	61658	20296

Table B.2 The Z test: critical values for the standard normal distribution. Abbreviated and adapted from *Geigy Scientific Tables* Vol. **2**, 8th Edn. with permission.

	Area in two tails (two-sided significance level)	0·10	0·05	0·02	0·01
	Area in one tail (one-sided significance level)	0·05	0·025	0·01	0·005
Critical value Z_c		1·645	1·960	2·326	2·576

Significant result if $Z \geqslant Z_c$ or $Z \leqslant -Z_c$

Table B.3   The *t* test: critical values for the Student's *t* distribution. Abbreviated and adapted from *Geigy Scientific Tables*, Vol. **2**, 8th Edn. with permission.

	Area in two tails (two-sided significance level)	0·10	0·05	0·02	0·01
	Area in one tail (one-sided significance level)	0·05	0·025	0·01	0·005

d.f.	Critical value t_c			
1	6·314	12·706	31·821	63·657
2	2·920	4·303	6·965	9·925
3	2·353	3·182	4·541	5·841
4	2·132	2·776	3·747	4·604
5	2·015	2·571	3·365	4·032
6	1·943	2·447	3·143	3·707
7	1·895	2·365	2·998	3·499
8	1·860	2·306	2·896	3·355
9	1·833	2·262	2·821	3·250
10	1·812	2·228	2·764	3·169
11	1·796	2·201	2·718	3·106
12	1·782	2·179	2·681	3·055
13	1·771	2·160	2·650	3·012
14	1·761	2·145	2·624	2·977
15	1·753	2·131	2·602	2·947
16	1·746	2·120	2·583	2·921
17	1·740	2·110	2·567	2·898
18	1·734	2·101	2·552	2·878
19	1·729	2·093	2·539	2·861
20	1·725	2·086	2·528	2·845
21	1·721	2·080	2·518	2·831
22	1·717	2·074	2·508	2·819
23	1·714	2·069	2·500	2·807
24	1·711	2·064	2·492	2·797
25	1·708	2·060	2·485	2·787
30	1·697	2·042	2·457	2·750
40	1·684	2·021	2·423	2·704
60	1·671	2·000	2·390	2·660
80	1·664	1·990	2·374	2·639
100	1·660	1·984	2·364	2·626
∞	1·645	1·960	2·326	2·576

Significant result if $t \geqslant t_c$ or $t \leqslant -t_c$

Table B.4   The χ^2 test. Critical values for the chi-square distribution. Abbreviated and adapted from *Geigy Scientific Tables* Vol. **2**, 8th Edn. with permission.

Two-sided significance level	0·10	0·05	0·02	0·01
One-sided significance level	0·05	0·025	0·01	0·005
d.f.		Critical value χ^2_c		
1	2·706	3·841	5·412	6·635
2	4·605	5·991	7·824	9·210
3	6·251	7·815	9·837	11·345
4	7·779	9·488	11·668	13·277
5	9·236	11·070	13·388	15·086
6	10·645	12·592	15·033	16·812
7	12·017	14·067	16·622	18·475
8	13·362	15·507	18·168	20·090
9	14·684	16·919	19·679	21·666
10	15·987	18·307	21·161	23·209
11	17·275	19·675	22·618	24·725
12	18·549	21·026	24·054	26·217
13	19·812	22·362	25·472	27·688
14	21·064	23·685	26·873	29·141
15	22·307	24·996	28·259	30·578
16	23·542	26·296	29·633	32·000
17	24·769	27·587	30·995	33·409
18	25·989	28·869	32·346	34·805
19	27·204	30·144	33·687	36·191
20	28·412	31·410	35·020	37·566
21	29·615	32·671	36·343	38·932
22	30·813	33·924	37·659	40·289
23	32·007	35·172	38·968	41·638
24	33·196	36·415	40·270	42·980
25	34·382	37·652	41·566	44·314
26	35·563	38·885	42·856	45·642
27	36·741	40·113	44·140	46·963
28	37·916	41·337	45·419	48·278
29	39·087	42·557	46·693	49·588
30	40·256	43·773	47·962	50·892

Significant result if $\chi^2 \geqslant \chi^2_c$

Table B.5(a)   The Wilcoxon two-sample rank sum test for sample sizes $n_1 = 1$ to 9, $n_2 = 1$ to 35. Critical lower (T_l) and upper (T_u) values for the sum of ranks T_1 from sample sized n_1. Abbreviated and adapted from *Geigy Scientific Tables* Vol. **2**, 8th Edn. with permission.

Two-sided significance level: 0·10
One-sided significance level: 0·05

n_1	1	2	3	4	5	6	7	8	9
n_2	$T_l\ T_u$	$T_l\ T_u$	$T_l\ T_u$	$T_l\ T_u$	$T_l\ T_u$	$T_l\ T_u$	$T_l\ T_u$	$T_l\ T_u$	$T_l\ T_u$
1	—	—	—	—	—	—	—	—	—
2	—	—	—	—	15– 25	21– 33	28– 42	37– 51	46– 62
3	—	—	6–15	10– 22	16– 29	23– 37	30– 47	39– 57	49– 68
4	—	—	6–18	11– 25	17– 33	24– 42	32– 52	41– 63	51– 75
5	—	3–13	7–20	12– 28	19– 36	26– 46	34– 57	44– 68	54– 81
6	—	3–15	8–22	13– 31	20– 40	28– 50	36– 62	46– 74	57– 87
7	—	3–17	8–25	14– 34	21– 44	29– 55	39– 66	49– 79	60– 93
8	—	4–18	9–27	15– 37	23– 47	31– 59	41– 71	51– 85	63– 99
9	—	4–20	10–29	16– 40	24– 51	33– 63	43– 76	54– 90	66–105
10	—	4–22	10–32	17– 43	26– 54	35– 67	45– 81	56– 96	69–111
11	—	4–24	11–34	18– 46	27– 58	37– 71	47– 86	59–101	72–117
12	—	5–25	11–37	19– 49	28– 62	38– 76	49– 91	62–106	75–123
13	—	5–27	12–39	20– 52	30– 65	40– 80	52– 95	64–112	78–129
14	—	6–28	13–41	21– 55	31– 69	42– 84	54–100	67–117	81–135
15	—	6–30	13–44	22– 58	33– 72	44– 88	56–105	69–123	84–141
16	—	6–32	14–46	24– 60	34– 76	46– 92	58–110	72–128	87–147
17	—	6–34	15–48	25– 63	35– 80	47– 97	61–114	75–133	90–153
18	—	7–35	15–51	26– 66	37– 83	49–101	63–119	77–139	93–159
19	1–20	7–37	16–53	27– 69	38– 87	51–105	65–124	80–144	96–165
20	1–21	7–39	17–55	28– 72	40– 90	53–109	67–129	83–149	99–171
21	1–22	8–40	17–58	29– 75	41– 94	55–113	69–134	85–155	102–177
22	1–23	8–42	18–60	30– 78	43– 97	57–117	72–138	88–160	105–183
23	1–24	8–44	19–62	31– 81	44–101	58–122	74–143	90–166	108–189
24	1–25	9–45	19–62	32– 84	45–105	60–126	76–148	93–171	111–195
25	1–26	9–47	20–67	33– 87	47–108	62–130	78–153	96–176	114–201
26	1–27	9–49	21–69	34– 90	48–112	64–134	81–157	98–182	117–207
27	1–28'	10–50	21–72	35– 93	50–115	66–138	83–162	101–187	120–213
28	1–29	10–52	22–74	36– 96	51–119	67–143	85–167	104–192	123–219
29	1–30	10–54	23–76	37– 99	53–122	69–147	87–172	106–198	127–224
30	1–31	10–56	23–79	38–102	54–126	71–151	89–177	109–203	130–230
31	1–32	11–57	24–81	39–105	55–130	73–155	92–181	112–208	133–236
32	1–33	11–59	25–83	40–108	57–133	75–159	94–186	114–214	136–242
33	1–34	11–61	25–86	41–111	58–137	77–163	96–191	117–219	139–248
34	1–35	12–62	26–88	42–114	60–140	78–168	98–196	120– 224	142–254
35	1–36	12–64	27–90	43–117	61–144	80–172	101–200	122–230	145–260

Significant result if $T_1 \geqslant T_u$ or $T_1 \leqslant T_l$

Table B.5(a)   (*Continued*)

Two-sided significance level: 0·05
One-sided significance level: 0·025

n_1	1	2	3	4	5	6	7	8	9
n_2	$T_l \ T_u$	$T_l \ T_u$	$T_l \ T_u$	$T_l \ T_u$	$T_l \ T_u$	$T_l \ T_u$	$T_l \ T_u$	$T_l \ T_u$	$T_l \ T_u$
1	—	—	—	—	—	—	—	—	—
2	—	—	—	—	—	—	—	36– 52	45– 63
3	—	—	—	—	15– 30	22– 38	29– 48	38– 58	47– 70
4	—	—	—	10– 26	16– 34	23– 43	31– 53	40– 64	49– 77
5	—	—	6–21	11– 29	17– 38	24– 48	33– 58	42– 70	52– 83
6	—	—	7–23	12– 32	18– 42	26– 52	34– 64	44– 76	55– 89
7	—	—	7–26	13– 35	20– 45	27– 57	36– 69	46– 82	57– 96
8	—	3–19	8–28	14– 38	21– 49	29– 61	38– 74	49– 87	60–102
9	—	3–21	8–31	14– 42	22– 53	31– 65	40– 79	51– 93	62–109
10	—	3–23	9–33	15– 45	23– 57	32– 70	42– 84	53– 99	65–115
11	—	3–25	9–36	16– 48	24– 61	34– 74	44– 89	55–105	68–121
12	—	4–26	10–38	17– 51	26– 64	35– 79	46– 94	58–110	71–127
13	—	4–28	10–41	18– 54	27– 68	37– 83	48– 99	60–116	73–134
14	—	4–30	11–43	19– 57	28– 72	38– 88	50–104	62–122	76–140
15	—	4–32	11–46	20– 60	29– 76	40– 92	52–109	65–127	79–146
16	—	4–34	12–48	21– 63	30– 80	42– 96	54–114	67–133	82–152
17	—	5–35	12–51	21– 67	32– 83	43–101	56–119	70–138	84–159
18	—	5–37	13–53	22– 70	33– 87	45–105	58–124	72–144	87–165
19	—	5–39	13–56	23– 73	34– 91	46–110	60–129	74–150	90–171
20	—	5–41	14–58	24– 76	35– 95	48–114	62–134	77–155	93–177
21	—	6–42	14–61	25– 79	37– 98	50–118	64–139	79–161	95–184
22	—	6–44	15–63	26– 82	38–102	51–123	66–144	81–167	98–190
23	—	6–46	15–66	27– 85	39–106	53–127	68–149	84–172	101–196
24	—	6–48	16–68	27– 89	40–110	54–132	70–154	86–178	104–202
25	—	6–50	16–71	28– 92	42–113	56–136	72–159	89–183	107–208
26	—	7–51	17–73	29– 95	43–117	58–140	74–164	91–189	109–215
27	—	7–53	17–76	30– 98	44–121	59–145	76–169	93–195	112–221
28	—	7–55	18–78	31–101	45–125	61–149	78–174	96–200	115–227
29	—	7–57	19–80	32–104	47–128	63–153	80–179	98–206	118–233
30	—	8–58	19–83	33–107	48–132	64–158	82–184	101–211	121–239
31	—	8–60	20–85	34–110	49–136	66–162	84–189	103–217	123–246
32	—	8–62	20–88	34–114	50–140	67–167	86–194	105–223	126–252
33	—	8–64	21–90	35–117	52–143	69–171	88–199	108–228	129–258
34	—	8–66	21–93	36–120	53–147	71–175	90–204	110–234	132–264
35	—	9–67	22–95	37–123	54–151	72–180	92–209	113–239	134–271

Significant result if $T_1 \geqslant T_u$ or $T_1 \leqslant T_l$

Table B.5(a) *(Continued)* The Wilcoxon two-sample rank sum test for sample sizes $n_1 = 1$ to 9, $n_2 = 1$ to 35. Critical lower (T_l) and upper (T_u) values for the sum of ranks T_1 from sample sized n_1.

Two-sided significance level: 0·02
One-sided significance level: 0·01

n_1	1	2	3	4	5	6	7	8	9
n_2	$T_l\ T_u$	$T_l\ T_u$	$T_l\ T_u$	$T_l\ T_u$	$T_l\ T_u$	$T_l\ T_u$	$T_l\ T_u$	$T_l\ T_u$	$T_l\ T_u$
1	—	—	—	—	—	—	—	—	—
2	—	—	—	—	—	—	—	—	—
3	—	—	—	—	—	—	28– 49	36– 60	46– 71
4	—	—	—	—	15– 35	22– 44	29– 55	38– 66	48– 78
5	—	—	—	10– 30	16– 39	23– 49	31– 60	40– 72	50– 85
6	—	—	—	11– 33	17– 43	24– 54	32– 66	42– 78	52– 92
7	—	—	6– 27	11– 37	18– 47	25– 59	34– 71	43– 85	54– 99
8	—	—	6– 30	12– 40	19– 51	27– 63	35– 77	45– 91	56–106
9	—	—	7– 32	13– 43	20– 55	28– 68	37– 82	47– 97	59–112
10	—	—	7– 35	13– 47	21– 59	29– 73	39– 87	49–103	61–119
11	—	—	7– 38	14– 50	22– 63	30– 78	40– 93	51–109	63–126
12	—	—	8– 40	15– 53	23– 67	32– 82	42– 98	53–115	66–132
13	—	3–29	8– 43	15– 57	24– 71	33– 87	44–103	56–120	68–139
14	—	3–31	8– 46	16– 60	25– 75	34– 92	45–109	58–126	71–145
15	—	3–33	9– 48	17– 63	26– 79	36– 96	47–114	60–132	73–152
16	—	3–35	9– 51	17– 67	27– 83	37–101	49–119	62–138	76–158
17	—	3–37	10– 53	18– 70	28– 87	39–105	51–124	64–144	78–165
18	—	3–39	10– 56	19– 73	29– 91	40–110	52–130	66–150	81–171
19	—	4–40	10– 59	19– 77	30– 95	41–115	54–135	68–156	83–178
20	—	4–42	11– 61	20– 80	31– 99	43–119	56–140	70–162	85–185
21	—	4–44	11– 64	21– 83	32–103	44–124	58–145	72–168	88–191
22	—	4–46	12– 66	21– 87	33–107	45–129	59–151	74–174	90–198
23	—	4–48	12– 69	22– 90	34–111	47–133	61–156	76–180	93–204
24	—	4–50	12– 72	23– 93	35–115	48–138	63–161	78–186	95–211
25	—	4–52	13– 74	23– 97	36–119	50–142	64–167	81–191	98–217
26	—	4–54	13– 77	24–100	37–123	51–147	66–172	83–197	100–224
27	—	5–55	13– 80	25–103	38–127	52–152	68–177	85–203	103–230
28	—	5–57	14– 82	26–106	39–131	54–156	70–182	87–209	105–237
29	—	5–59	14– 85	26–110	40–135	55–161	71–188	89–215	108–243
30	—	5–61	15– 87	27–113	41–139	56–166	73–193	91–221	110–250
31	—	5–63	15– 90	28–116	42–143	58–170	75–198	93–227	113–256
32	—	5–65	15– 93	28–120	43–147	59–175	77–203	95–233	115–263
33	—	5–67	16– 95	29–123	44–151	61–179	78–209	97–239	118–269
34	—	6–68	16– 98	30–126	45–155	62–184	80–214	100–244	120–276
35	—	6–70	17–100	30–130	46–159	63–189	82–219	102–250	123–282

Significant result if $T_1 \geqslant T_u$ or $T_1 \leqslant T_l$

Table B.5(a)   (*Continued*)

Two-sided significance level: 0·01
One-sided significance level: 0·005

n_1	1	2	3	4	5	6	7	8	9
n_2	$T_l\ T_u$	$T_l\ T_u$	$T_l\ T_u$	$T_l\ T_u$	$T_l\ T_u$	$T_l\ T_u$	$T_l\ T_u$	$T_l\ T_u$	$T_l\ T_u$
1	—	—	—	—	—	—	—	—	—
2	—	—	—	—	—	—	—	—	—
3	—	—	—	—	—	—	—	—	45– 72
4	—	—	—	—	—	21– 45	28– 56	37– 67	46– 80
5	—	—	—	—	15– 40	22– 50	29– 62	38– 74	48– 87
6	—	—	—	10– 34	16– 44	23– 55	31– 67	40– 80	50– 94
7	—	—	—	10– 38	16– 49	24– 60	32– 73	42– 86	52–101
8	—	—	—	11– 41	17– 53	25– 65	34– 78	43– 93	54–108
9	—	—	6– 33	11– 45	18– 57	26– 70	35– 84	45– 99	56–115
10	—	—	6– 36	12– 48	19– 61	27– 75	37– 89	47–105	58–122
11	—	—	6– 39	12– 52	20– 65	28– 80	38– 95	49–111	61–128
12	—	—	7– 41	13– 55	21– 69	30– 84	40–100	51–117	63–135
13	—	—	7– 44	13– 59	22– 73	31– 89	41–106	53–123	65–142
14	—	—	7– 47	14– 62	22– 78	32– 94	43–111	54–130	67–149
15	—	—	8– 49	15– 65	23– 82	33– 99	44–117	56–136	69–156
16	—	—	8– 52	15– 69	24– 86	34–104	46–122	58–142	72–162
17	—	—	8– 55	16– 72	25– 90	36–108	47–128	60–148	74–169
18	—	—	8– 58	16– 76	26– 94	37–113	49–133	62–154	76–176
19	—	3–41	9– 60	17– 79	27– 98	38–118	50–139	64–160	78–183
20	—	3–43	9– 63	18– 82	28–102	39–123	52–144	66–166	81–189
21	—	3–45	9– 66	18– 86	29–106	40–128	53–150	68–172	83–196
22	—	3–47	10– 68	19– 89	29–111	42–132	55–155	70–178	85–203
23	—	3–49	10– 71	19– 93	30–115	43–137	57–160	71–185	88–209
24	—	3–51	10– 74	20– 96	31–119	44–142	58–166	73–191	90–216
25	—	3–53	11– 76	20–100	32–123	45–147	60–171	75–197	92–223
26	—	3–55	11– 79	21–103	33–127	46–152	61–177	77–203	94–230
27	—	4–56	11– 82	22–106	34–131	48–156	63–182	79–209	97–236
28	—	4–58	11– 85	22–110	35–135	49–161	64–188	81–215	99–243
29	—	4–60	12– 87	23–113	36–139	50–166	66–193	83–221	101–250
30	—	4–62	12– 90	23–117	37–143	51–171	68–198	85–227	103–257
31	—	4–64	12– 93	24–120	37–148	53–175	69–204	87–233	106–263
32	—	4–66	13– 95	24–124	38–152	54–180	71–209	89–239	108–270
33	—	4–68	13– 98	25–127	39–156	55–185	72–215	91–245	110–277
34	—	4–70	13–101	26–130	40–160	56–190	74–220	93–251	113–283
35	—	4–72	14–103	26–134	41–164	58–194	75–226	95–257	115–290

Significant result if $T_1 \geqslant T_u$ or $T_1 \geqslant T_l$

Table B.5(b) The Wilcoxon two-sample rank sum test for sample sizes $n_1 = 10$ to 17, $n_2 = 1$ to 35. Critical lower (T_l) and upper (T_u) values for the sum of ranks T_1 from sample sized n_1. Abbreviated and adapted from *Geigy Scientific Tables* Vol. **2**, 8th Edn. with permission.

Two-sided significance level: 0·10
One-sided significance level: 0·05

n_1	10	11	12	13	14	15	16	17
n_2	T_l T_u	T_l T_u	T_l T_u	T_l T_u	T_l T_u	T_l T_u	T_l T_u	T_l T_u
1	—	—	—	—	—	—	—	—
2	56– 74	67– 87	80–100	93–115	108–130	123–147	139–165	156–184
3	59– 81	71– 94	83–109	97–124	112–140	127–158	144–176	162–195
4	62– 88	74–102	87–117	101–133	116–150	132–168	150–186	168–206
5	66– 94	78–109	91–125	106–141	121–159	138–177	155–197	173–218
6	69–101	82–116	95–133	110–150	126–168	143–187	161–207	179–229
7	72–108	85–124	99–141	115–158	131–177	148–197	166–218	186–239
8	75–115	89–131	104–148	119–167	136–186	153–207	172–228	192–250
9	79–121	93–138	108–156	124–175	141–195	159–216	178–238	198–261
10	82–128	97–145	112–164	128–184	146–204	164–226	184–248	204–272
11	86–134	100–153	116–172	133–192	151–213	170–235	190–258	210–283
12	89–141	104–160	120–180	138–200	156–222	175–245	196–268	217–293
13	92–148	108–167	125–187	142–209	161–231	181–254	201–279	223–304
14	96–154	112–174	129–195	147–217	166–240	186–264	207–289	230–314
15	99–161	116–181	133–203	152–225	171–249	192–273	213–299	236–325
16	103–167	120–188	138–210	156–234	176–258	197–283	219–309	242–336
17	106–174	123–196	142–218	161–242	182–266	203–292	225–319	249–346
18	110–180	127–203	146–226	166–250	187–275	208–302	231–329	255–357
19	113–187	131–210	150–234	171–258	192–284	214–311	237–339	262–367
20	117–193	135–217	155–241	175–267	197–293	220–320	243–349	268–378
21	120–200	139–224	159–249	180–275	202–302	225–330	249–359	274–389
22	123–207	143–231	163–257	185–283	207–311	231–339	255–369	281–399
23	127–213	147–238	168–264	189–292	212–320	236–349	261–379	287–410
24	130–220	151–245	172–272	194–300	218–328	242–358	267–389	294–420
25	134–226	155–252	176–280	199–308	223–337	248–367	273–399	300–431
26	137–233	158–260	181–287	204–316	228–346	253–377	279–409	307–441
27	141–239	162–267	185–295	208–325	233–355	259–386	285–419	313–452
28	144–246	166–274	189–303	213–333	238–364	264–396	292–428	320–462
29	148–252	170–281	194–310	218–341	243–373	270–405	298–438	326–473
30	151–259	174–288	198–318	223–349	249–381	276–414	304–448	333–483
31	155–265	178–295	202–326	227–358	254–390	281–424	310–458	339–494
32	158–272	182–302	206–334	232–366	259–399	287–433	316–468	346–504
33	162–278	186–309	211–341	237–374	264–408	292–443	322–478	352–515
34	165–285	190–316	215–349	242–382	269–417	298–452	328–488	359–525
35	169–291	194–323	219–357	247–390	275–425	304–461	334–498	365–536

Significant result if $T_1 \geqslant T_u$ or $T_1 \leqslant T_l$

Table B.5(b) *(Continued)*

Two-sided significance level: 0·05
One-sided significance level: 0·025

n_1	10	11	12	13	14	15	16	17
n_2	$T_l\ T_u$	$T_l\ T_u$	$T_l\ T_u$	$T_l\ T_u$	$T_l\ T_u$	$T_l\ T_u$	$T_l\ T_u$	$T_l\ T_u$
1	—	—	—	—	—	—	—	—
2	55– 75	66– 88	79–101	92–116	106–132	121–149	137–167	155–185
3	58– 82	69– 96	82–110	95–126	110–142	125–160	142–178	159–198
4	60– 90	72–104	85–119	99–135	114–152	130–170	147–189	164–210
5	63– 97	75–112	89–127	103–144	118–162	134–181	151–201	170–221
6	66–104	79–119	92–136	107–153	122–172	139–191	157–211	175–233
7	69–111	82–127	96–144	111–162	127–181	144–201	162–222	181–244
8	72–118	85–135	100–152	115–171	131–191	149–211	167–233	187–255
9	75–125	89–142	104–160	119–180	136–200	154–221	173–243	192–267
10	78–132	92–150	107–169	124–188	141–209	159–231	178–254	198–278
11	81–139	96–157	111–177	128–197	145–219	164–241	183–265	204–289
12	84–146	99–165	115–185	132–206	150–228	169–251	189–275	210–300
13	88–152	103–172	119–193	136–215	155–237	174–261	195–285	216–311
14	91–159	106–180	123–201	141–223	160–246	179–271	200–296	222–322
15	94–166	110–187	127–209	145–232	164–256	184–281	206–306	228–333
16	97–173	113–195	131–217	150–240	169–265	190–290	211–317	234–344
17	100–180	117–202	135–225	154–249	174–274	195–300	217–327	240–355
18	103–187	121–209	139–233	158–258	179–283	200–310	222–338	246–366
19	107–193	124–217	143–241	163–266	183–293	205–320	228–348	252–377
20	110–200	128–224	147–249	167–275	188–302	210–330	234–358	258–388
21	113–207	131–232	151–257	171–284	193–311	216–339	239–369	264–399
22	116–214	135–239	155–265	176–292	198–320	221–349	245–379	270–410
23	119–221	139–246	159–273	180–301	203–329	226–359	251–389	276–421
24	122–228	142–254	163–281	185–309	207–339	231–369	256–400	282–432
25	126–234	146–261	167–289	189–318	212–348	237–378	262–410	288–443
26	129–241	149–269	171–297	193–327	217–357	242–388	268–420	294–454
27	132–248	153–276	175–305	198–335	222–366	247–398	273–431	300–465
28	135–255	156–284	179–313	202–344	227–375	252–408	279–441	307–475
29	138–262	160–291	183–321	207–352	232–384	258–417	285–451	313–486
30	142–268	164–298	187–329	211–361	236–394	263–427	290–462	319–497
31	145–275	167–306	191–337	216–369	241–403	268–437	296–472	325–508
32	148–282	171–313	195–345	220–378	246–412	273–447	302–482	331–519
33	151–289	174–321	199–353	224–387	251–421	279–456	307–493	337–530
34	154–296	178–328	203–361	229–395	256–430	284–466	313–503	343–541
35	158–302	182–335	207–369	233–404	261–439	289–476	319–513	349–552

Significant result if $T_1 \geqslant T_u$ or $T_1 \leqslant T_l$

Table B.5(b) (*Continued*)   The Wilcoxon two-sample rank sum test for sample sizes $n_1 = 10$ to 17, $n_2 = 1$ to 35. Critical lower (T_l) and upper (T_u) values for the sum of ranks T_1 from sample sized n_1.

Two-sided significance level: 0·02
One-sided significance level: 0·01

n_1	10	11	12	13	14	15	16	17
n_2	$T_l\ T_u$	$T_l\ T_u$	$T_l\ T_u$	$T_l\ T_u$	$T_l\ T_u$	$T_l\ T_u$	$T_l\ T_u$	$T_l\ T_u$
1	—	—	—	—	—	—	—	—
2	—	—	—	91–117	105–133	120–150	136–168	153–187
3	56– 84	67– 98	80–112	93–128	107–145	123–162	139–181	157–200
4	58– 92	70–106	83–121	96–138	111–155	127–173	143–193	161–213
4	61– 99	73–114	86–130	100–147	115–165	131–184	148–204	166–225
6	63–107	75–123	89–139	103–157	118–176	135–195	152–216	171–237
7	66–114	78–131	92–148	107–166	122–186	139–206	157–227	176–249
8	68–122	81–139	95–157	111–175	127–195	144–216	162–238	181–261
9	71–129	84–147	99–165	114–185	131–205	148–227	167–249	186–273
10	74–136	88–154	102–174	118–194	135–215	153–237	172–260	191–285
11	77–143	91–162	106–182	122–203	139–225	157–248	177–271	197–296
12	79–151	94–170	109–191	126–212	143–235	162–258	182–282	202–308
13	82–158	97–178	113–199	130–221	148–244	167–268	187–293	208–319
14	85–165	100–186	116–208	134–230	152–254	171–279	192–304	213–331
15	88–172	103–194	120–216	138–239	156–264	176–289	197–315	219–342
16	91–179	107–201	124–224	142–248	161–273	181–299	202–326	224–354
17	93–187	110–209	127–233	146–257	165–283	186–309	207–337	230–365
18	96–194	113–217	131–241	150–266	170–292	190–320	212–348	235–377
19	99–201	116–225	134–250	154–275	174–302	195–330	218–358	241–388
20	102–208	119–233	138–258	158–284	178–312	200–340	223–369	246–400
21	105–215	123–240	142–266	162–293	183–321	205–350	228–380	252–411
22	108–222	126–248	145–275	166–302	187–331	210–360	233–391	258–422
23	110–230	129–256	149–283	170–311	192–340	214–371	238–402	263–434
24	113–237	132–264	153–291	174–320	196–350	219–381	244–412	269–445
25	116–244	136–271	156–300	178–329	200–360	224–391	249–423	275–456
26	119–251	139–279	160–308	182–338	205–369	229–401	254–434	280–468
27	122–258	142–287	163–317	186–347	209–379	234–411	259–445	286–479
28	125–265	145–295	167–325	190–356	214–388	239–421	265–455	292–490
29	128–272	149–302	171–333	194–365	218–398	243–432	270–466	297–502
30	131–279	152–310	174–342	198–374	223–407	248–442	275–477	303–513
31	133–287	155–318	178–350	202–383	227–417	253–452	280–488	309–524
32	136–294	158–326	182–358	206–392	232–426	258–462	286–498	314–536
33	139–301	162–333	185–367	210–401	236–436	263–472	291–509	320–547
34	142–308	165–341	189–375	214–410	240–446	268–482	296–520	326–558
35	145–315	168–349	193–383	218–419	245–455	273–492	301–531	331–570

Significant result if $T_1 \geqslant T_u$ or $T_1 \leqslant T_l$

Table B.5(b)   (*Continued*)

Two-sided significance level: 0·01
One-sided significance level: 0·005

n_1	10	11	12	13	14	15	16	17
n_2	T_l T_u	T_l T_u	T_l T_u	T_l T_u	T_l T_u	T_l T_u	T_l T_u	T_l T_u
1	—	—	—	—	—	—	—	—
2	—	—	—	—	—	—	—	—
3	55– 85	66– 99	79–113	92–129	106–146	122–163	138–182	155–202
4	57– 93	68–108	81–123	94–140	109–157	125–175	141–195	159–215
5	59–101	71–116	84–132	98–149	112–168	128–187	145–207	163–228
6	61–109	73–125	87–141	101–159	116–178	132–198	149–219	168–240
7	64–116	76–133	90–150	104–169	120–188	136–209	154–230	172–253
8	66–124	79–141	93–159	108–178	123–199	140–220	158–242	177–265
9	68–132	82–149	96–168	111–188	127–209	144–231	163–253	182–277
10	71–139	84–158	99–177	115–197	131–219	149–241	167–265	187–289
11	73–147	87–166	102–186	118–207	135–229	153–252	172–276	192–301
12	76–154	90–174	105–195	122–216	139–239	157–263	177–287	197–313
13	79–161	93–182	109–203	125–226	143–249	162–273	181–299	202–325
14	81–169	96–190	112–212	129–235	147–259	166–284	186–310	207–337
15	84–176	99–198	115–221	133–244	151–269	171–294	191–321	213–348
16	86–184	102–206	119–229	136–254	155–279	175–305	196–332	218–360
17	89–191	105–214	122–238	140–263	159–289	180–315	201–343	223–372
18	92–198	108–222	125–247	144–272	163–299	184–326	206–354	228–384
19	94–206	111–230	129–255	148–281	168–308	189–336	210–366	234–395
20	97–213	114–238	132–264	151–291	172–318	193–347	215–377	239–407
21	99–221	117–246	136–272	155–300	176–328	198–357	220–388	244–419
22	102–228	120–254	139–281	159–309	180–338	202–368	225–399	249–431
23	105–235	123–262	142–290	163–318	184–348	207–378	230–410	255–442
24	107–243	126–270	146–298	166–328	188–358	211–389	235–421	260–454
25	110–250	129–278	149–307	170–337	192–368	216–399	240–432	265–466
26	113–257	132–286	152–316	174–346	197–377	220–410	245–443	271–477
27	115–265	135–294	156–324	178–355	201–387	225–420	250–454	276–489
28	118–272	138–302	159–333	182–364	205–397	229–431	255–465	281–501
29	121–279	141–310	163–341	185–374	209–407	234–441	260–476	287–512
30	123–287	144–318	166–350	189–383	213–417	239–451	265–487	292–524
31	126–294	147–326	170–358	193–392	218–426	243–462	270–498	298–535
32	129–301	150–334	173–367	197–401	222–436	248–472	275–509	303–547
33	131–309	153–342	176–376	201–410	226–446	252–483	280–520	308–559
34	134–316	156–350	180–384	204–420	230–456	257–493	285–531	314–570
35	137–323	159–358	183–393	208–429	234–466	262–503	290–542	319–582

Significant result if $T_1 \geqslant T_u$ or $T_1 \leqslant T_l$

Table B.5(c)   The Wilcoxon two-sample rank sum test for samples sizes $n_1 = 18$ to 25, $n_2 = 1$ to 35. Critical lower (T_l) and upper (T_u) values for the sum of ranks T_1 from sample sized n_1. Abbreviated and adapted from *Geigy Scientific Tables* Vol. **2**, 8th Edn. with permission.

Two-sided significance level: 0·10
One-sided significance level: 0·05

n_1	18	19	20	21	22	23	24	25
n_2	$T_l\ T_u$	$T_l\ T_u$	$T_l\ T_u$	$T_l\ T_u$	$T_l\ T_u$	$T_l\ T_u$	$T_l\ T_u$	$T_l\ T_u$
1	—	190–209	210–230	231–252	253–275	276–299	300–324	325–350
2	175–203	194–224	214–246	236–268	258–292	281–317	306–342	331–369
3	180–216	200–237	221–259	242–283	265–307	289–332	313–359	339–386
4	187–227	207–249	228–272	250–296	273–321	297–347	322–374	348–402
4	193–239	213–262	235–285	257–310	281–335	305–362	330–390	357–418
6	199–251	220–274	242–298	265–323	289–349	313–377	339–405	366–434
7	206–262	227–286	249–311	272–337	297–363	322–391	348–420	375–450
8	212–274	234–298	257–323	280–350	305–377	330–406	357–435	385–465
9	219–285	241–310	264–336	288–363	313–391	339–420	366–450	394–481
10	226–296	248–322	272–348	296–376	321–405	348–434	375–465	404–496
11	232–308	255–334	279–361	304–389	330–418	357–448	385–479	414–511
12	239–319	262–346	287–373	312–402	338–432	366–462	394–494	423–527
13	246–330	270–357	294–386	320–415	347–445	374–477	403–509	433–542
14	253–341	277–369	302–398	328–428	355–459	383–491	413–523	443–557
15	259–353	284–381	310–410	336–441	364–472	392–505	422–538	453–572
16	266–364	291–393	317–423	344–454	372–486	401–519	431–553	462–588
17	273–375	299–404	325–435	352–467	381–499	410–533	441–567	472–603
18	280–386	306–416	333–447	361–479	389–513	419–547	450–582	482–618
19	287–397	313–428	340–460	369–492	398–526	428–561	460–596	492–633
20	294–408	320–440	348–472	377–505	407–539	437–575	469–611	502–648
21	301–419	328–451	356–484	385–518	415–553	446–589	479–625	512–663
22	307–431	335–463	364–496	393–531	424–566	455–603	488–640	522–678
23	314–442	342–475	371–509	401–544	432–580	465–616	498–654	532–693
24	321–453	350–486	379–521	410–556	441–593	474–630	507–669	542–708
25	328–464	357–498	387–533	418–569	450–606	483–644	517–683	552–723
26	335–475	364–510	395–545	426–582	458–620	492–658	526–698	562–738
27	342–486	372–521	402–558	434–595	467–633	501–672	536–712	572–753
28	349–497	379–533	410–570	443–607	476–646	510–686	545–727	582–768
29	356–508	386–545	418–582	451–620	484–660	519–700	555–741	592–783
30	363–519	394–556	426–594	459–633	493–673	528–714	564–756	602–798
31	370–530	401–568	434–606	467–646	502–686	537–728	574–770	612–813
32	377–541	408–580	441–619	475–659	510–700	547–741	584–784	622–828
33	383–553	416–591	449–631	484–671	519–713	556–755	593–799	632–843
34	390–564	423–603	457–643	492–684	528–726	565–769	603–813	642–858
35	397–575	431–614	465–655	500–697	537–739	574–783	612–828	652–873

Significant result if $T_1 \geqslant T_u$ or $T_1 \leqslant T_l$

Table B.5(c)   (*Continued*)

Two-sided significance level: 0·05
One-sided significance level: 0·025

n_1	18	19	20	21	22	23	24	25
n_2	$T_l\ T_u$	$T_l\ T_u$	$T_l\ T_u$	$T_l\ T_u$	$T_l\ T_u$	$T_l\ T_u$	$T_l\ T_u$	$T_l\ T_u$
1	—	—	—	—	—	—	—	—
2	173–205	192–226	212–248	234–270	256–294	279–319	303–345	328–372
2	178–218	197–240	218–262	239–286	262–310	285–336	310–362	335–390
4	183–231	203–235	224–276	246–300	269–325	293–351	317–379	343–407
5	189–243	209–266	230–290	253–314	276–340	300–367	325–395	352–423
6	195–255	215–279	237–303	260–328	283–355	308–382	333–411	360–440
7	201–267	222–291	244–316	267–342	291–269	316–397	342–426	369–456
8	207–279	228–304	251–329	274–356	298–384	324–412	350–442	378–472
9	213–291	235–316	258–342	281–370	306–398	332–427	359–457	387–488
10	219–303	242–328	265–355	289–383	314–412	340–442	367–473	396–504
11	226–314	248–341	272–368	296–397	322–426	349–456	376–488	405–520
12	232–326	255–353	279–381	304–410	330–440	357–471	385–503	414–536
13	238–338	262–365	286–394	311–424	338–454	365–486	394–518	423–552
14	245–349	268–378	293–407	319–437	346–468	374–500	402–534	432–568
15	251–361	275–390	300–420	7–450	354–482	382–515	411–549	442–583
16	257–373	282–402	308–432	334–464	362–496	391–529	420–564	451–599
17	264–384	289–414	315–445	342–477	370–510	399–544	429–579	460–615
18	270–396	296–426	322–458	350–490	378–524	408–558	438–594	470–630
19	277–407	303–438	329–471	357–504	386–538	416–573	447–609	479–646
20	283–419	309–451	337–483	365–517	394–552	425–587	456–624	488–662
21	290–430	316–463	344–496	373–530	4035656	433–602	465–639	498–677
22	296–442	323–475	351–509	381–543	411–579	442–616	474–654	507–693
23	303–453	330–487	359–521	388–557	419–593	451–630	483–669	517–708
24	309–465	337–499	366–534	3965707	427–607	459–645	492–684	724
25	316–476	344–511	373–547	404–583	435–621	468–659	501–699	536–739
26	322–488	351–523	381–559	412–596	444–634	476–674	510–714	545–755
27	329–499	358–535	388–572	419–610	452–648	485–688	519–729	555–770
28	335–511	365–547	396–584	427–623	460–662	494–702	528–744	564–786
29	342–522	372–559	403–597	435–636	468–676	502–717	538–758	574–801
30	348–534	379–571	410–610	443–649	476–690	511–731	547–773	583–817
31	355–545	386–583	418–622	451–662	485–703	520–745	556–788	593–832
32	361–557	393–595	425–635	458–676	493–717	528–760	565–803	602–848
33	368–568	400–607	432–648	466–689	501–731	537–774	574–818	612–863
34	374–580	407–619	440–660	474–702	509–745	546–788	583–833	622–878
35	381–591	414–631	447–673	482–715	518–758	554–803	592–848	631–894

Significant result if $T_1 \geqslant T_u$ or $T_1 \leqslant T_l$

Table B.5(c) (*Continued*) The Wilcoxon two-sample rank sum test for sample sizes $n_1 = 18$ to 25, $n_2 = 1$ to 35. Critical lower (T_l) and upper (T_u) values for the sum of ranks T_1 from sample sized n_1.

Two-sided significance level: 0·02
One-sided significance level: 0·01

n_1	18	19	20	21	22	23	24	25
n_2	$T_l\ T_u$	$T_l\ T_u$	$T_l\ T_u$	$T_l\ T_u$	$T_l\ T_u$	$T_l\ T_u$	$T_l\ T_u$	$T_l\ T_u$
1	—	—	—	—	—	—	—	—
2	171–207	191–227	211–249	232–272	254–296	277–321	301–347	326–374
3	175–221	194–243	215–265	236–289	259–313	282–339	306–366	332–393
4	180–234	199–257	220–280	242–304	264–330	288–356	313–383	338–412
5	185–247	205–270	226–294	248–319	271–345	295–372	320–400	346–429
6	190–260	210–284	232–308	254–334	277–361	302–388	327–417	354–446
7	195–273	216–297	238–322	261–348	284–376	309–404	335–433	361–464
8	201–285	222–310	244–336	267–363	291–391	316–420	342–450	370–480
9	207–297	228–323	250–350	274–377	298–406	324–435	350–466	378–497
10	212–310	234–336	257–363	281–391	306–420	331–451	358–482	386–514
11	218–322	240–349	263–377	288–405	313–435	339–466	366–498	395–530
12	224–334	246–362	270–390	295–419	320–450	347–481	375–513	403–547
13	230–346	253–374	277–403	302–433	328–464	355–496	383–529	412–563
14	236–358	259–387	283–417	309–447	335–479	363–511	391–545	420–580
15	241–371	265–400	290–430	316–461	343–493	370–527	399–561	429–596
16	247–383	272–412	297–443	323–475	350–508	378–542	408–576	438–612
17	253–395	278–425	303–457	330–489	358–522	386–557	416–592	447–628
18	259–407	284–438	310–470	337–503	365–537	394–572	424–608	455–645
19	265–419	291–450	317–483	344–517	373–551	402–587	433–623	464–661
20	271–431	297–463	324–496	352–530	380–566	410–602	441–639	473–677
21	277–443	303–476	331–509	359–544	388–580	418–617	450–654	482–693
22	283–455	310–488	337–523	366–558	396–594	426–632	458–670	491–709
23	289–467	316–501	344–536	373–572	403–609	434–647	467–685	500–725
24	295–479	323–513	351–549	381–585	411–623	443–661	475–701	509–741
25	301–491	329–526	358–562	388–599	419–637	451–676	484–716	517–758
26	307–503	336–538	365–575	395–613	426–652	459–691	492–732	526–774
27	313–515	342–551	372–588	402–627	434–666	467–706	501–747	535–790
28	320–526	349–563	379–601	410–640	442–680	475–721	509–763	544–806
29	326–538	355–576	386–614	417–654	450–694	483–736	518–778	553–822
30	332–550	362–588	392–628	424–668	457–709	491–751	526–794	562–838
31	338–562	368–601	399–641	432–681	465–723	499–766	535–809	571–854
32	344–574	375–613	406–654	439–695	473–737	508–780	543–825	580–870
33	350–586	381–626	413–667	446–709	481–751	516–795	552–840	589–886
34	356–598	388–638	420–680	454–722	488–766	524–810	561–855	598–902
35	362–610	394–651	427–693	461–736	496–780	532–825	569–871	607–918

Significant result if $T_1 \geqslant T_u$ or $T_1 \leqslant T_l$

Table B.5(c) *(Continued)*

Two-sided significance level: 0·01
One-sided significance level: 0·005

n_1	18	19	20	21	22	23	24	25
n_2	$T_l\ T_u$	$T_l\ T_u$	$T_l\ T_u$	$T_l\ T_u$	$T_l\ T_u$	$T_l\ T_u$	$T_l\ T_u$	$T_l\ T_u$
1	—	—	—	—	—	—	—	—
2	—	190–228	210–250	231–273	253–297	276–322	300–348	325–375
3	173–223	193–244	213–267	234–291	257–315	280–341	304–368	330–395
4	177–237	197–259	218–282	239–307	262–332	285–359	310–386	335–415
5	182–250	202–273	223–297	245–322	267–349	291–376	316–404	342–433
6	187–263	207–287	228–312	250–338	274–364	298–392	323–421	349–451
7	192–276	212–301	234–326	256–353	280–380	305–408	330–438	357–468
8	197–289	218–314	240–340	263–367	287–395	311–425	337–455	364–486
9	202–302	223–328	246–354	269–382	293–411	319–440	345–471	372–503
10	208–314	229–341	252–368	275–397	300–426	326–456	352–488	380–520
11	213–327	235–354	258–382	282–411	307–441	333–472	360–504	388–537
12	218–340	241–367	264–396	289–425	314–456	340–488	368–520	396–554
13	224–352	247–380	270–410	295–440	321–471	348–503	375–537	404–571
14	229–365	253–393	277–423	302–454	328–486	355–519	383–553	412–588
15	235–377	259–406	283–437	309–468	335–501	363–534	391–569	421–604
16	241–389	264–420	289–451	315–483	342–516	370–550	399–585	429–621
17	246–402	271–432	296–464	322–497	349–531	378–565	407–601	437–638
18	252–414	277–445	302–478	329–511	357–545	385–581	415–617	446–654
19	258–426	283–458	309–491	336–525	364–560	393–596	423–633	454–671
20	263–439	289–471	315–505	343–539	371–575	401–611	431–649	463–687
21	269–451	295–484	322–518	349–554	378–590	408–627	439–665	471–704
22	275–463	301–497	328–532	356–568	386–604	416–642	447–681	480–720
23	280–476	307–510	335–545	363–582	393–619	424–657	455–697	488–737
24	286–488	313–523	341–559	370–596	400–634	431–673	464–712	497–753
25	292–500	319–536	348–572	377–610	408–648	439–688	472–728	505–770
26	298–512	325–549	354–586	384–624	415–663	447–703	480–744	514–786
27	303–525	332–561	361–599	391–638	422–678	455–718	488–760	522–803
28	309–537	338–574	367–613	398–652	430–692	462–734	496–776	531–819
29	315–549	344–587	374–626	405–666	437–707	470–749	504–792	540–835
30	321–561	350–600	380–640	412–680	444–722	478–764	513–807	548–852
31	326–574	356–613	387–653	419–694	452–736	486–779	521–823	557–868
32	332–586	362–626	394–666	426–708	459–751	494–794	529–839	565–885
33	338–598	369–638	400–680	433–722	467–765	501–810	537–855	574–901
34	344–610	375–651	407–693	440–736	474–780	509–825	545–871	583–917
35	350–622	381–664	413–707	447–750	482–794	517–840	554–886	591–934

Significant result if $T_1 \geqslant T_u$ or $T_1 \leqslant T_l$

Table B.6 (a) The sign test (paired data). Critical lower (S_l) and upper (S_u) values for the number of positive differences n_+ from a sample with n non-zero differences.

(b) The exact test for correlated proportions. Critical values for the number of untied pairs 'c' in favour of one of the 'treatments' with n untied pairs altogether. Abbreviated and adapted from *Geigy Scientific Tables* Vol. **2**, 8th Edn. with permission.

Two-sided significance level	0·10	0·05	0·02	0·01
One-sided significance level	0·05	0·025	0·01	0·005
n	$S_l \; S_u$	$S_l \; S_u$	$S_l \; S_u$	$S_l \; S_u$
5	0–5	—	—	—
6	0–6	0–6	—	—
7	0–7	0–7	0–7	—
8	1–7	0–8	0–8	0–8
9	1–8	1–8	0–9	0–9
10	1–9	1–9	0–10	0–10
11	2–9	1–10	1–10	0–11
12	2–10	2–10	1–11	1–11
13	3–10	2–11	1–12	1–12
14	3–11	2–12	2–12	1–13
15	3–12	3–12	2–13	2–13
16	4–12	3–13	2–14	2–14
17	4–13	4–13	3–14	2–15
18	5–13	4–14	3–15	3–15
19	5–14	4–15	4–15	3–16
20	5–15	5–15	4–16	3–17
21	6–15	5–16	4–17	4–17
22	6–16	5–17	5–17	4–18
23	7–16	6–17	5–18	4–19
24	7–17	6–18	6–19	5–20
25	7–18	7–18	6–19	5–20
26	8–18	7–19	6–20	6–20
27	8–19	7–20	7–20	6–21
28	9–19	8–20	7–21	6–22
29	9–20	8–21	7–22	7–22
30	10–20	9–21	8–22	7–23
31	10–21	9–22	8–23	7–24
32	10–22	9–23	8–24	8–24
33	11–22	10–23	9–24	8–25
34	11–23	10–24	9–25	9–25
35	12–23	11–24	10–25	9–26

Significant result if (a) $n_+ \geqslant S_u$ or $n_+ \leqslant S_l$

(b) $c \geqslant S_u$ or $c \leqslant S_l$

Table B.6 (*Continued*)

Two-sided significance level	0·10	0·05	0·02	0·01
One-sided significance level	0·05	0·025	0·01	0·005
n	S_l S_u	S_l S_u	S_l S_u	S_l S_u
36	12–24	11–25	10–26	9–27
37	13–24	12–25	10–27	10–27
38	13–25	12–26	11–27	10–28
39	13–26	12–57	11–28	11–28
40	14–26	13–27	12–28	11–29
41	14–27	13–28	12–29	11–30
42	15–27	14–28	13–29	12–30
43	15–28	14–29	13–30	12–31
44	16–28	15–29	13–31	13–31
45	16–29	15–30	14–31	13–32
46	16–30	15–31	14–32	13–33
47	17–30	16–31	15–32	14–33
48	17–31	16–32	15–33	14–34
49	18–31	17–32	15–34	15–34
50	18–32	17–33	16–34	15–35
51	19–32	18–33	16–35	15–36
52	19–33	18–34	17–35	16–36
53	20–33	18–35	17–36	16–37
54	20–34	19–35	18–36	17–37
55	20–35	19–36	18–37	17–38
56	21–35	20–36	18–38	17–39
57	21–36	20–37	19–38	18–39
58	22–36	21–37	19–39	18–40
59	22–37	21–38	20–39	19–40
60	23–37	21–39	20–40	19–41
61	23–38	22–39	20–41	20–41
62	24–38	22–40	21–41	20–42
63	24–39	23–40	21–42	20–43
64	24–40	23–41	22–42	21–43
65	25–40	24–41	22–43	21–44
66	25–41	24–42	23–43	22–44
67	26–41	25–42	23–44	22–45
68	26–42	25–43	23–45	22–46
69	27–42	25–44	24–45	23–46
70	27–43	26–44	24–46	23–47

Significant result if (a) $n_+ \geqslant S_u$ or $n_+ \leqslant S_l$
(b) $c \geqslant S_u$ or $c \leqslant S_l$

Table B.6 (*Continued*) (a) The sign test (paired data). Critical lower (S_l) and upper (S_u) values for the number of positive differences n_+ from a sample with n non-zero differences.

                (b) The exact test for correlated proportions. Critical values for the number of untied pairs 'c' in favour of one of the 'treatments' with n untied pairs altogether.

Two-sided significance level	0·10	0·05	0·02	0·01
One-sided significance level	0·05	0·025	0·01	0·005
n	$S_l\ S_u$	$S_l\ S_u$	$S_l\ S_u$	$S_l\ S_u$
71	28–43	26–45	25–46	24–47
72	28–44	27–45	25–47	24–48
73	28–45	27–46	26–47	25–48
74	29–45	28–46	26–48	25–49
75	29–46	28–47	26–49	25–50
76	30–46	28–48	27–49	26–50
77	30–47	29–48	27–50	26–51
78	31–47	29–40	28–50	27–51
79	31–48	30–49	28–51	27–52
80	32–48	30–50	29–51	28–52
81	32–49	31–50	29–52	28–53
82	33–49	31–51	30–52	28–54
83	33–50	32–51	30–53	29–54
84	33–51	31–52	30–54	29–55
85	34–51	32–53	31–54	30–55
86	34–52	33–53	31–55	30–56
87	35–52	33–54	32–55	31–56
88	35–53	34–54	32–56	31–57
89	36–53	34–55	33–56	31–58
90	36–54	35–55	33–57	32–58
91	37–54	35–56	33–58	32–59
92	37–55	36–56	34–58	33–59
93	38–55	36–57	34–59	33–60
94	38–56	37–57	35–59	34–60
95	38–57	37–58	35–60	34–61
96	39–57	37–59	36–60	34–62
97	39–58	38–59	36–61	35–62
98	40–58	38–60	37–61	35–63
99	40–59	39–60	37–62	36–63
100	41–59	38–61	37–63	36–64

Significant result if (a) $n_+ \geqslant S_u$ or $n_+ \leqslant S_l$

(b) $c \geqslant S_u$ or $c \leqslant S_l$

Table B.7   The Wilcoxon signed rank test (paired data). Critical lower (T_l) and upper (T_u) values for the sum of the positive ranks (T_+) from a study with n non-zero differences. Abbreviated and adapted from *Geigy Scientific Tables* Vol. **2**, 8th Edn. with permission.

Two-sided significance level	0·10	0·05	0·02	0·01
One-sided significance level	0·05	0·025	0·01	0·005
n	T_l T_u	T_l T_u	T_l T_u	T_l T_u
5	0– 15	—	—	—
6	2– 19	0– 21	—	—
7	3– 25	2– 26	0– 28	—
8	5– 31	3– 33	1– 35	0– 36
9	8– 37	5– 40	3– 42	1– 44
10	10– 45	8– 47	5– 50	3– 52
11	13– 53	10– 56	7– 59	5– 61
12	17– 61	13– 65	9– 69	7– 71
13	21– 70	17– 74	12– 79	9– 82
14	25– 80	21– 84	15– 90	12– 93
15	30– 90	25– 95	19–101	15–105
16	35–101	29–107	23–113	19–117
17	41–112	34–119	28–125	23–130
18	47–124	40–131	32–139	27–144
19	53–137	46–144	37–153	32–158
20	60–150	52–158	43–167	37–173
21	67–164	58–173	49–182	42–189
22	75–178	66–187	55–198	48–205
23	83–193	73–203	62–214	54–222
24	91–209	81–219	69–231	61–239
25	100–225	89–236	76–249	68–257

Significant result if $T_+ \geqslant T_u$ or $T_+ \leqslant T_l$

Table B.8 Logs of the factorials of $n = 0$ to 99. Abbreviated from *Geigy Scientific Tables* Vol. **2**, 8th Edn. with permission.

n	0	1	2	3	4	5	6	7	8	9
0	0·00000	0·00000	0·30103	0·77815	1·38021	2·07918	2·85733	3·70243	4·60552	5·55976
10	6·55976	7·60116	8·68034	9·79428	10·94041	12·11650	13·32062	14·55107	15·80634	17·08509
20	18·38612	19·70834	21·05077	22·41249	23·79271	25·19065	26·60562	28·03698	29·48414	30·94654
30	32·42366	33·91502	35·42017	36·93869	38·47016	40·01423	41·57054	43·13874	44·71852	46·30959
40	47·91165	49·52443	51·14768	52·78115	54·42460	56·07781	57·74057	59·41267	61·09391	62·78410
50	64·48307	66·19064	67·90665	69·63092	71·36332	73·10368	74·85187	76·60774	78·37117	80·14202
60	81·92017	83·70550	85·49790	87·29724	89·10342	90·91633	92·73587	94·56195	96·39446	98·23331
70	100·07841	101·92966	103·78700	105·65032	107·51955	109·39461	111·27543	113·16192	115·05401	116·95164
80	118·85473	120·76321	122·67703	124·59610	126·52038	128·44980	130·38430	132·32382	134·26830	136·21769
90	138·17194	140·13098	142·09476	144·06325	146·03638	148·01410	149·99637	151·98314	153·97437	155·97000

Table B.9   Antilogarithm table. Reprinted from *Geigy Scientific Tables*, Vol. **2**, 8th Edn. with permission.

$\log_{10}x$	0	1	2	3	4	5	6	7	8	9		1	2	3	4	5	6	7	8	9
0·00	1000	1002	1005	1007	1009	1012	1014	1016	1019	1021		0	0	1	1	1	1	2	2	2
0·01	1023	1026	1028	1030	1033	1035	1038	1040	1042	1045		0	0	1	1	1	1	2	2	2
0·02	1047	1050	1052	1054	1057	1059	1062	1064	1067	1069		0	0	1	1	1	1	2	2	2
0·03	1072	1074	1076	1079	1081	1084	1086	1089	1091	1094		0	0	1	1	1	1	2	2	2
0·04	1096	1099	1102	1104	1107	1109	1112	1114	1117	1119		0	1	1	1	1	2	2	2	2
0·05	1122	1125	1127	1130	1132	1135	1138	1140	1143	1146		0	1	1	1	1	2	2	2	2
0·06	1148	1151	1153	1156	1159	1161	1164	1167	1169	1172		0	1	1	1	1	2	2	2	2
0·07	1175	1178	1180	1183	1186	1189	1191	1194	1197	1199		0	1	1	1	1	2	2	2	2
0·08	1202	1205	1208	1211	1213	1216	1219	1222	1225	1227		0	1	1	1	1	2	2	2	3
0·09	1230	1233	1236	1239	1242	1245	1247	1250	1253	1256		0	1	1	1	1	2	2	2	3
0·10	1259	1262	1265	1268	1271	1274	1276	1279	1282	1285		0	1	1	1	1	2	2	2	3
0·11	1288	1291	1294	1297	1300	1303	1306	1309	1312	1315		0	1	1	1	2	2	2	2	3
0·12	1318	1321	1324	1327	1330	1334	1337	1340	1343	1346		0	1	1	1	2	2	2	2	3
0·13	1349	1352	1355	1358	1361	1365	1368	1371	1374	1377		0	1	1	1	2	2	2	3	3
0·14	1380	1384	1387	1390	1393	1396	1400	1403	1406	1409		0	1	1	1	2	2	2	3	3
0·15	1413	1416	1419	1422	1426	1429	1432	1435	1439	1442		0	1	1	1	2	2	2	3	3
0·16	1445	1449	1452	1455	1459	1462	1466	1469	1472	1476		0	1	1	1	2	2	2	3	3
0·17	1479	1483	1486	1489	1493	1496	1500	1503	1507	1510		0	1	1	1	2	2	2	3	3
0·18	1514	1517	1521	1524	1528	1531	1535	1538	1542	1545		0	1	1	1	2	2	2	3	3
0·19	1549	1552	1556	1560	1563	1567	1570	1574	1578	1581		0	1	1	1	2	2	3	3	3
0·20	1585	1589	1592	1596	1600	1603	1607	1611	1614	1618		0	1	1	1	2	2	3	3	3
0·21	1622	1626	1629	1633	1637	1641	1644	1648	1652	1656		0	1	1	2	2	2	3	3	3
0·22	1660	1663	1667	1671	1675	1679	1683	1687	1690	1694		0	1	1	2	2	2	3	3	3
0·23	1698	1702	1706	1710	1714	1718	1722	1726	1730	1734		0	1	1	2	2	2	3	3	4
0·24	1738	1742	1746	1750	1754	1758	1762	1766	1770	1774		0	1	1	2	2	2	3	3	4

x   Proportional parts

Table B.9 *(Continued)* Antilogarithm table.

$\log_{10} x$	0	1	2	3	4	5	6	7	8	9	1	2	3	4	5	6	7	8	9
					x										Proportional parts				
0·25	1778	1782	1786	1791	1795	1799	1803	1807	1811	1816	0	1	1	2	2	2	3	3	4
0·26	1820	1824	1828	1832	1837	1841	1845	1849	1854	1858	0	1	1	2	2	3	3	3	4
0·27	1862	1866	1871	1875	1879	1884	1888	1892	1897	1901	0	1	1	2	2	3	3	3	4
0·28	1905	1910	1914	1919	1923	1928	1932	1936	1941	1945	0	1	1	2	2	3	3	4	4
0·29	1950	1954	1959	1963	1968	1972	1977	1982	1986	1991	0	1	1	2	2	3	3	4	4
0·30	1995	2000	2004	2009	2014	2018	2023	2028	2032	2037	0	1	1	2	2	3	3	4	4
0·31	2042	2046	2051	2056	2061	2065	2070	2075	2080	2084	0	1	1	2	2	3	3	4	4
0·32	2089	2094	2099	2104	2109	2113	2118	2123	2128	2133	0	1	1	2	2	3	3	4	4
0·33	2138	2143	2148	2153	2158	2163	2168	2173	2178	2183	0	1	1	2	2	3	3	4	4
0·34	2188	2193	2198	2203	2208	2213	2218	2223	2228	2234	1	1	2	2	3	3	4	4	5
0·35	2239	2244	2249	2254	2259	2265	2270	2275	2280	2286	1	1	2	2	3	3	4	4	5
0·36	2291	2296	2301	2307	2312	2317	2323	2328	2333	2339	1	1	2	2	3	3	4	4	5
0·37	2344	2350	2355	2360	2366	2371	2377	2382	2388	2393	1	1	2	2	3	3	4	4	5
0·38	2399	2404	2410	2415	2421	2427	2432	2438	2443	2449	1	1	2	2	3	3	4	4	5
0·39	2455	2460	2466	2472	2477	2483	2489	2495	2500	2506	1	1	2	2	3	3	4	5	5
0·40	2512	2518	2523	2529	2535	2541	2547	2553	2559	2564	1	1	2	2	3	4	4	5	5
0·41	2570	2576	2582	2588	2594	2600	2606	2612	2618	2624	1	1	2	2	3	4	4	5	5
0·42	2630	2636	2642	2649	2655	2661	2667	2673	2679	2685	1	1	2	3	3	4	4	5	6
0·43	2692	2698	2704	2710	2716	2723	2729	2735	2742	2748	1	1	2	3	3	4	4	5	6
0·44	2754	2761	2767	2773	2780	2786	2793	2799	2805	2812	1	1	2	3	3	4	4	5	6
0·45	2818	2825	2831	2838	2844	2851	2858	2864	2871	2877	1	1	2	3	3	4	5	5	6
0·46	2884	2891	2897	2904	2911	2917	2924	2931	2938	2944	1	1	2	3	3	4	5	5	6
0·47	2951	2958	2965	2972	2979	2985	2992	2999	3006	3013	1	1	2	3	3	4	5	5	6
0·48	3020	3027	3034	3041	3048	3055	3062	3069	3076	3083	1	1	2	3	4	4	5	6	6
0·49	3090	3097	3105	3112	3119	3126	3133	3141	3148	3155	1	1	2	3	4	4	5	6	6

x	0	1	2	3	4	5	6	7	8	9	1	2	3	4	5	6	7	8	9
0·50	3162	3170	3177	3184	3192	3199	3206	3214	3221	3228	1	1	2	3	4	4	5	6	7
0·51	3236	3243	3251	3258	3266	3273	3281	3289	3296	3304	1	2	2	3	4	5	5	6	7
0·52	3311	3319	3327	3334	3342	3350	3357	3365	3373	3381	1	2	2	3	4	5	5	6	7
0·53	3388	3396	3404	3412	3420	3428	3436	3443	3451	3459	1	2	2	3	4	5	6	6	7
0·54	3467	3475	3483	3491	3499	3508	3516	3524	3532	3540	1	2	2	3	4	5	6	6	7
0·55	3548	3556	3565	3573	3581	3589	3597	3606	3614	3622	1	2	2	3	4	5	6	7	7
0·56	3631	3639	3648	3656	3664	3673	3681	3690	3698	3707	1	2	3	3	4	5	6	7	8
0·57	3715	3724	3733	3741	3750	3758	3767	3776	3784	3793	1	2	3	3	4	5	6	7	8
0·58	3802	3811	3819	3828	3837	3846	3855	3864	3873	3882	1	2	3	4	4	5	6	7	8
0·59	3890	3899	3908	3917	3926	3936	3945	3954	3963	3972	1	2	3	4	5	5	6	7	8
0·60	3981	3990	3999	4009	4018	4027	4036	4046	4055	4064	1	2	3	4	5	6	6	7	8
0·61	4074	4083	4093	4102	4111	4121	4130	4140	4150	4159	1	2	3	4	5	6	7	8	9
0·62	4169	4178	4188	4198	4207	4217	4227	4236	4246	4256	1	2	3	4	5	6	7	8	9
0·63	4266	4276	4285	4295	4305	4315	4325	4335	4345	4355	1	2	3	4	5	6	7	8	9
0·64	4365	4375	4385	4395	4406	4416	4426	4436	4446	4457	1	2	3	4	5	6	7	8	9
0·65	4467	4477	4487	4498	4508	4519	4529	4539	4550	4560	1	2	3	4	5	6	7	8	9
0·66	4571	4581	4592	4603	4613	4624	4634	4645	4656	4667	1	2	3	4	5	6	7	9	10
0·67	4677	4688	4699	4710	4721	4732	4742	4753	4764	4775	1	2	3	4	5	7	8	9	10
0·68	4786	4797	4808	4819	4831	4842	4853	4864	4875	4887	1	2	3	4	6	7	8	9	10
0·69	4898	4909	4920	4932	4943	4955	4966	4977	4989	5000	1	2	3	5	6	7	8	9	10
0·70	5012	5023	5035	5047	5058	5070	5082	5093	5105	5117	1	2	4	5	6	7	8	9	11
0·71	5129	5140	5152	5164	5176	5188	5200	5212	5224	5236	1	2	4	5	6	7	8	10	11
0·72	5248	5260	5272	5284	5297	5309	5321	5333	5346	5358	1	2	4	5	6	8	9	10	11
0·73	5370	5383	5395	5408	5420	5433	5445	5458	5470	5483	1	2	4	5	6	8	9	10	11
0·74	5495	5508	5521	5534	5546	5559	5572	5585	5598	5610	1	3	4	5	6	8	9	10	12
0·75	5623	5636	5649	5662	5675	5689	5702	5715	5728	5741	1	3	4	5	7	8	9	10	12
0·76	5754	5768	5781	5794	5808	5821	5834	5848	5861	5875	1	3	4	5	7	8	9	11	12
0·77	5888	5902	5916	5929	5943	5957	5970	5984	5998	6012	1	3	4	5	7	8	10	11	12
0·78	6026	6039	6053	6067	6081	6095	6109	6124	6138	6152	1	3	4	6	7	8	10	11	13
0·79	6166	6180	6194	6209	6223	6237	6252	6266	6281	6295	1	3	4	6	7	9	10	11	13

Table B.9 (*Continued*) Antilogarithm table.

$\log_{10} x$	0	1	2	3	4	5	6	7	8	9	1	2	3	4	5	6	7	8	9
						x								Proportional parts					
0·80	6310	6324	6339	6353	6368	6383	6397	6412	6427	6442	1	3	4	6	7	9	10	12	13
0·81	6457	6471	6486	6501	6516	6531	6546	6561	6577	6592	2	3	5	6	8	9	11	12	14
0·82	6607	6622	6637	6653	6668	6683	6699	6714	6730	6745	2	3	5	6	8	9	11	12	14
0·83	6761	6776	6792	6808	6823	6839	6855	6871	6887	6902	2	3	5	6	8	9	11	13	14
0·84	6918	6934	6950	6966	6982	6998	7015	7031	7047	7063	2	3	5	6	8	10	11	13	15
0·85	7079	7096	7112	7129	7145	7161	7178	7194	7211	7228	2	3	5	7	8	10	12	13	15
0·86	7244	7261	7278	7295	7311	7328	7345	7362	7379	7396	2	3	5	7	8	10	12	13	15
0·87	7413	7430	7447	7464	7482	7499	7516	7534	7551	7568	2	3	5	7	9	10	12	14	16
0·88	7586	7603	7621	7638	7656	7674	7691	7709	7727	7745	2	4	5	7	9	11	12	14	16
0·89	7762	7780	7798	7816	7834	7852	7870	7889	7907	7925	2	4	5	7	9	11	13	14	16
0·90	7943	7962	7980	7998	8017	8035	8054	8072	8091	8110	2	4	6	7	9	11	13	15	17
0·91	8128	8147	8166	8185	8204	8222	8241	8260	8279	8299	2	4	6	8	9	11	13	15	17
0·92	8318	8337	8356	8375	8395	8414	8433	8453	8472	8492	2	4	6	8	10	12	14	15	17
0·93	8511	8531	8551	8570	8590	8610	8630	8650	8670	8690	2	4	6	8	10	12	14	16	18
0·94	8710	8730	8750	8770	8790	8810	8831	8851	8872	8892	2	4	6	8	10	12	14	16	18
0·95	8913	8933	8954	8974	8995	9016	9036	9057	9078	9099	2	4	6	8	10	12	15	17	19
0·96	9120	9141	9162	9183	9204	9226	9247	9268	9290	9311	2	4	6	8	11	13	15	17	19
0·97	9333	9354	9376	9397	9419	9441	9462	9484	9506	9528	2	4	7	9	11	13	15	17	20
0·98	9550	9572	9594	9616	9638	9661	9683	9705	9727	9750	2	4	7	9	11	13	16	18	20
0·99	9772	9795	9817	9840	9863	9886	9908	9931	9954	9977	2	5	7	9	11	14	16	18	20

Table B.10 Spearman's rank correlation coefficient: critical values for the correlation coefficient r_s calculated on n pairs of observations. Abbreviated from *Geigy Scientific Tables*, Vol. **2**, 8th Edn. with permission.

Two-sided significance level	0·10	0·05	0·02	0·01
One-sided significance level	0·05	0·025	0·01	0·005

n	Critical values r_c			
4	0·9999	—	—	—
5	0·9000	0·9999	0·9999	—
6	0·8286	0·8857	0·9429	0·9999
7	0·7143	0·7857	0·8929	0·9286
8	0·6429	0·7381	0·8333	0·8810
9	0·6000	0·6833	0·7833	0·8333
10	0·5636	0·6485	0·7333	0·7939
11	0·5364	0·6182	0·7000	0·7545
12	0·5035	0·5874	0·6783	0·7343
13	0·4835	0·5604	0·6484	0·7033
14	0·4637	0·5385	0·6264	0·6791
15	0·4464	0·5214	0·6036	0·6571
16	0·4294	0·5029	0·5853	0·6353
17	0·4142	0·4877	0·5662	0·6176
18	0·4014	0·4737	0·5501	0·5996
19	0·3912	0·4596	0·5351	0·5842
20	0·3805	0·4466	0·5218	0·5699
21	0·3701	0·4364	0·5091	0·5558
22	0·3608	0·4252	0·4975	0·5438
23	0·3528	0·4160	0·4862	0·5316
24	0·3443	0·4070	0·4757	0·5209
25	0·3369	0·3985	0·4662	0·5108
26	0·3306	0·3901	0·4571	0·5009
27	0·3242	0·3828	0·4487	0·4921
28	0·3180	0·3755	0·4406	0·4833
29	0·3118	0·3690	0·4325	0·4749
30	0·3063	0·3624	0·4256	0·4670

Significant result if $r_s \geqslant r_c$ or $r_s \leqslant -r_c$

APPENDIX C
Statistical Analyses

C.1 Introduction

The purpose of this appendix is to summarize the statistical techniques discussed in the book, by outlining their areas of applicability and by providing a step-by-step guide to their calculation.

The simplest situation encountered was the analysis of a single variable in one sample. Estimation of population parameters such as a mean or proportion via confidence intervals was described, as were the one-sample tests for means and proportions. Table C.1 summarizes these different techniques and indicates where they are discussed in the body of the book and where they are to be found in the appendix.

Many applications however concern one or more variables in one or more samples and, as discussed previously, membership of a particular sample can be considered a qualitative variable whose categories are the different samples being studied. From this point of view a statistical analysis can be viewed as an examination of the associations between two or more variables. Thus, for example, an association between blood pressure levels (a quantitative variable) and treatment group (a qualitative variable) in a clinical trial might be examined, as might the association between blood pressure and weight (two quantitative variables) in a group of schoolchildren.

Table C.1 Statistical analysis in the one-sample, one-variable situation. (Section and appendix numbers where the procedures are discussed are given in parenthesis.)

Type of data	Purpose of analysis	
	Estimation	Hypothesis testing
Quantitative	CI for means (4.4; 4.7; C.2)	One-sample Z and t tests (6.6; 6.8; C.2)
Qualitative (2 categories)	CI for proportions (4.8; C.3)	One-sample Z test (6.9; C.3)
Qualitative (>2 categories)	As above	One-sample χ^2 test (6.10; C.4)

CI = Confidence interval

In statistical terms, variables which are not associated or correlated with each other are considered as independent of each other, and statistical tests of association and statistical tests of independence are just opposite sides of the same coin, differing only in terminology.

Nearly all statistical tests follow the same general structure. A null hypothesis, usually of no association between the variables, is postulated. A test statistic (e.g. t or Z), which is known to have a particular theoretical distribution if the null hypothesis is true, is calculated on the basis of the observed results. If, on the assumption of the null hypothesis, the probability of obtaining this calculated statistic, or one even more extreme, is less than a specified level — the significance level of the test — this is considered as evidence to doubt the null hypothesis.

This probability is determined by referring the test statistic to a table which gives the critical values appropriate to the test and to the chosen one- or two-sided significance level (usually 5%). These critical values determine the acceptance and rejection regions for the test. If the test statistic lies in the acceptance region the null hypothesis is not rejected and a non-significant result obtains. If, on the other hand, the test statistic lies in the rejection region — in the tail(s) of its particular distribution — the null hypothesis can be rejected and a significant result declared at the given level of significance.

The terms independent and dependent are also used to describe the variables in an analysis rather than the relationship between them. Usually, there is only one dependent variable and one or more independent ones. If there are only two variables in an analysis and one of them is qualitative it does not matter, generally, which is referred to as independent and which as dependent; such an analysis can be seen in terms of a comparison between the groups defined by the qualitative variable and the techniques of Chapters 6 and 7 are appropriate. Table C.2 summarizes some of the different tests which can be used for comparisons between groups. The appropriate test depends on whether the groups are independently chosen or are matched, and on the measurement scale of the variable being analysed. The computational details for all the tests are not described in this text but the table notes the appropriate sections where the tests are discussed and the sections in this appendix where the tests are summarized.

If the only two variables in an analysis are quantitative then a correlation analysis may suffice. If a regression analysis is required then the determination of the independent and dependent variable is important. Chapter 8 discusses these techniques.

When there is more than one independent variable in an analysis the statistical techniques become much more complex and either analysis of variance or covariance, multiple regression or some sort of standardization technique must be used. These approaches were briefly discussed in the text without detailing the computations required.

Table C.2　Significance testing in the comparison of groups. (Section and appendix numbers where the tests are discussed are given in parenthesis.)

Type of data	Comparison of 2 groups		Comparison of >2 groups	
	Independent	Matched	Independent	Matched
Quantitative	t test (7.4; C.5)	Paired t test (7.6; C.7)	One-way analysis of variance* (7.14)	Two-way analysis of variance* (7.14)
Qualitative (ordinal or ranked)	Wilcoxon rank sum test (7.5; C.6)	Sign test (7.7; C.8) Wilcoxon signed rank test (7.8; C.9)	Kruskal–Wallis test* (7.14)	Friedman test* (7.14)
Qualitative (nominal; 2 categories)	Z test (7.9; C.10) χ^2 test (7.10; C.11) Fisher's exact test (7.11; C.12)	McNemar's test (7.13; C.13)	χ^2 test (7.12; C.11)	—
Qualitative (nominal; >2 categories)	χ^2 test (7.12; C.11)	—	χ^2 test (7.12; C.11)	—

*Computational details not given in this text.

Table C.3 outlines the various tests discussed for the general statistical analysis of two or more variables. There is some overlap with Table C.2 and the tables only give a guide to when these techniques can be used. The remainder of the appendix summarizes the computational steps for all the tests detailed in the body of this book and should provide a handy reference for practical use.

Note, however, particularly for the non-parametric tests, that the description of the test statistic to be employed may differ slightly from that given in other textbooks, and consequently, the statistical tables (Appendix B) may differ from those in other books in both layout and content. It is suggested that you become familiar with one set of tables and their appropriate test statistics to avoid unnecessary confusion.

Table C.3 An outline of some statistical tests used in the analysis of two or more variables. (Section and appendix numbers where the procedures are discussed are given in parenthesis.)

Dependent variable(s)	Independent variable	
	Quantitative	Qualitative
1 Quantitative	Simple regression; correlation (Chap. 8; C.14)	t tests; ANOVA* (see Table C.2)
1 Qualitative	t tests; ANOVA* (see Table C.2)	χ^2 test (see Table C.2)
>1 Quantitative	Multiple regression* (8.8)	Logistic regression* (8.9)
>1 Qualitative	ANOVA* (7.14; 7.15)	Standardization techniques* (7.15)
Quantitative and qualitative	Analysis of covariance* (7.15; 8.9)	Logistic regression* (8.9)

*Computational details not given in this text.

ANOVA = analysis of variance

C.2 The one-sample Z and t tests. Confidence intervals for a mean

These procedures are discussed in Sections 4.4, 4.6, 4.7, 6.6 and 6.8.

Situation
Random sample size n from a population; quantitative variable of unknown mean μ.

Assumptions/requirements
That the distribution of the variable in the population is not markedly skewed.

Null hypothesis
That the mean μ of the population is equal to μ_0 (a numerical value).

Method
(1) Calculate the mean, $\bar{X}$, and the standard deviation, S, in the sample.
(2) If the standard deviation σ in the population is known, calculate the Z statistic (equivalent to the t statistic on infinite degrees of freedom).

$$Z = \frac{\bar{X} - \mu_0}{\sigma/\sqrt{n}}$$

If the standard deviation in the population is not known, calculate the t statistic on $n-1$ degrees of freedom.

$$t = \frac{\bar{X} - \mu_0}{S/\sqrt{n}}$$

(3) Look up the critical value t_c of the t distribution for degrees of freedom $n-1$ or infinity at the required one- or two-sided significance level (Table B.3).

One-sided test
If $t \geqslant t_c$	conclude $\mu > \mu_0$
If $t \leqslant -t_c$	conclude $\mu < \mu_0$
If $-t_c < t < t_c$	conclude $\mu = \mu_0$

Two-sided test
If $t \geqslant t_c$ or $t \leqslant -t_c$	conclude $\mu \neq \mu_0$
If $-t_c < t < t_c$	conclude $\mu = \mu_0$

Confidence intervals
95% and 99% confidence intervals for μ are calculated as

$$\bar{X} \pm t_c \sigma/\sqrt{n} \quad (\sigma \text{ known})$$
$$\text{or} \quad \bar{X} \pm t_c S/\sqrt{n} \quad (\sigma \text{ unknown})$$

where t_c on $n-1$ (σ unknown) or infinite (σ known) degrees of freedom is the two-sided 5% or 1% critical value for the t distribution.

C.3 The one-sample Z test for a proportion. Confidence intervals for a proportion

These procedures are discussed in Sections 4.8 and 6.9.

Situation
Random sample size n from a population; qualitative binary variable with unknown proportion π in one category.

Assumptions/requirements
That $n\pi$ and $n(1-\pi)$ are both greater than 5.

Null hypothesis
That the proportion π in the population is equal to π_0 (a numerical value).

Method
(1) Calculate the proportion p observed in the sample.
(2) Calculate the Z statistic.

$$Z = \frac{p - \pi_0}{\sqrt{\dfrac{\pi_0(1 - \pi_0)}{n}}}$$

(3) Look up the critical value Z_c of the normal distribution at the required one- or two-sided significance level (Table B.2).

One-sided test

If $Z \geqslant Z_c$ conclude $\pi > \pi_0$

If $Z \leqslant -Z_c$ conclude $\pi < \pi_0$

If $-Z_c < Z < Z_c$ conclude $\pi = \pi_0$

Two-sided test

If $Z \geqslant Z_c$ or $Z \leqslant -Z_c$ conclude $\pi \neq \pi_0$

If $-Z_c < Z < Z_c$ conclude $\pi = \pi_0$

Confidence intervals

95% and 99% confidence intervals for π are calculated as

$$P \pm Z_c \sqrt{p(1-p)/n}$$

where Z_c is the two-sided 5% or 1% critical value for the normal distribution.

C.4   The one-sample χ^2 test for many proportions

This procedure is discussed in Section 6.10.

Situation

Random sample size n from a population; qualitative variable with two or more categories.

Assumptions/requirements

That not more than 20% of the expected numbers (see below) in the categories are less than 5, and that no expected number is less than one.

Null hypothesis

That the proportions in each category of the variable in the population have certain values defined independently of the data.

Method

(1) Calculate the expected numbers (E) in each category of the variable by multiplying the sample size n by the each of the hypothesized proportions.

(2) Calculate the χ^2 statistic on degrees of freedom one less than the number of categories.

$$\chi^2 = \sum \frac{(O - E)^2}{E}$$

where Os are the observed numbers in each category of the variable, and the summation is over all the categories.

(3) Look up the critical value χ^2_c of the chi-square distribution for the

appropriate degrees of freedom at the required two-sided significance level (Table B.4).

If $\chi^2 \geqslant \chi^2_c$　　　reject the null hypothesis
If $\chi^2 < \chi^2_c$　　　do not reject the null hypothesis

C.5　The two-sample independent t tests. Confidence intervals for a difference

These procedures are discussed in Section 7.4.

Situation
Two independent random samples size n_1 and n_2 from two populations; quantitative variable with means μ_1 and μ_2 in the two populations.

Assumptions/requirements
That the distribution of the variable is not markedly skewed in either of the populations and either (a) that the population variances σ_1^2 and σ_2^2 are equal, or (b) that these variances are unequal and the sample size in both groups combined is greater than 60 with numbers in each group roughly the same.

Null hypothesis
That the means μ_1 and μ_2 of the two populations are equal, or that the mean difference is zero.

Method
(1) Calculate the means $\bar{X}_1$ and $\bar{X}_2$ and the standard deviations S_1 and S_2 in the two samples.
(2) Assumption a: calculate the pooled variance.

$$S_p^2 = \frac{(n_1 - 1)S_1^2 + (n_2 - 1)S_2^2}{n_1 + n_2 - 2}$$

and the t statistic on $n_1 + n_2 - 2$ degrees of freedom.

$$t = \frac{\bar{X}_1 - \bar{X}_2}{\sqrt{\dfrac{S_p^2}{n_1} + \dfrac{S_p^2}{n_2}}}$$

(3) Assumption b: calculate the Z statistic (equivalent to the t statistic on infinite degrees of freedom).

$$Z = \frac{\bar{X}_1 - \bar{X}_2}{\sqrt{\dfrac{S_1^2}{n_1} + \dfrac{S_2^2}{n_2}}}$$

(4) Look up the critical value t_c of the t distribution for degrees of freedom $n_1 + n_2 - 2$ (assumption a) or infinity (assumption b) at the required one- or two-sided significance level (Table B.3).

One-sided test

If $t \geqslant t_c$	conclude $\mu_1 > \mu_2$
If $t \leqslant -t_c$	conclude $\mu_1 < \mu_2$
If $-t_c < t < t_c$	conclude $\mu_1 = \mu_2$

Two-sided test

If $t \geqslant t_c$ or $t \leqslant -t_c$	conclude $\mu_1 \neq \mu_2$
If $-t_c < t < t_c$	conclude $\mu_1 = \mu_2$

Confidence intervals
95% and 99% confidence intervals for the mean difference $\mu_1 - \mu_2$ between the two populations are calculated from

$$X_1 - X_2 \pm t_c \, \text{SE}\,(X_1 - X_2)$$

where SE $(X_1 - X_2)$ is the denominator of the test statistic above, and t_c on $n_1 + n_2 - 2$ (assumption a) or infinite (assumption b) degrees of freedom is the two-sided 5% or 1% critical value for the t distribution.

C.6   The Wilcoxon two-sample rank sum test for independent data

This procedure is discussed in Section 7.5.

Situation
Two independent random samples size n_1 and n_2 from two populations; quantitative or ordinal variable with medians m_1 and m_2 in the two populations.

Assumptions/requirements
That there is an underlying continuous distribution of the variable, even if it is only measured on an ordinal scale; that there are not too many tied observations.

Null hypothesis
That the medians m_1 and m_2 in the two populations are equal.

Method
(1) Combine the observations from the two groups and order them from lowest to highest while still noting which observation came from which group. Assign a rank to each observation giving the smallest observation rank 1. If there are tied observations assign the mean of the ranks in the position concerned.

(2) Calculate the sum of the ranks assigned to the observations in the group with sample size n_1. Call this T_1.

(3) Locate the pages of the rank sum test table (Table B.5) corresponding to the sample size in group 1 (n_1). Choose the page that corresponds to the required one- or two-sided significance level, and look in the table for the entries corresponding to the sample sizes n_1 (in the row) and n_2 (in the column). These give the lower (T_l) and upper (T_u) critical values for the sum of ranks in group 1 (T_1). Relabel the groups if necessary to use the table.

One-sided test

If $T_1 \geqslant T_u$	conclude $m_1 > m_2$
If $T_1 \leqslant T_l$	conclude $m_1 < m_2$
If $T_l < T_1 < T_u$	conclude $m_1 = m_2$

Two-sided test

If $T_1 \geqslant T_u$ or $T_1 \leqslant T_1$	conclude $m_1 \neq m_2$
If $T_l < T_1 < T_u$	conclude $m_1 = m_2$

C.7 The paired t test. Confidence intervals for a difference

This procedure is discussed in Section 7.6.

Situation
Two individually matched samples each of sample size n (n pairs of observations); quantitative variable with population means μ_1 and μ_2.

Assumptions/requirements
That the distribution of the differences between pairs in the population is not too skewed.

Null hypothesis
That the population means μ_1 and μ_2 are equal, or that the mean difference is zero.

Method
(1) Calculate the difference between each pair of values, $d = X_1 - X_2$, and compute the mean, $\bar{d}$, and standard deviation, S_d, of these n differences (include zero values of d).

(2) Compute the t statistic on $n-1$ degrees of freedom.

$$t = \frac{\bar{d}}{S_d/\sqrt{n}}$$

(3) Look up the critical value t_c of the t distribution for degrees of freedom $n-1$ at the required one- or two-sided significance level (Table B.3).

One-sided test

If $t \geqslant t_c$	conclude $\mu_1 > \mu_2$
If $t \leqslant -t_c$	conclude $\mu_1 < \mu_2$
If $-t_c < t < t_c$	conclude $\mu_1 = u_2$

Two-sided test

If $t \geqslant t_c$ or $t \leqslant -t_c$	conclude $\mu_1 \neq \mu_2$
If $-t_c < t < t_c$	conclude $\mu_1 = \mu_2$

Confidence intervals
95% and 99% confidence intervals for the mean difference between the two populations are calculated from

$$\bar{d} \pm t_c \, S_d / \sqrt{n}$$

where t_c on $n-1$ degrees of freedom is the two-sided 5% or 1% critical value for the t distribution.

C.8 The sign test

This procedure is discussed in Section 7.7.

Situation
Two individually matched samples each of sample size N (N pairs of observations); quantitative or ordinal variable (in that one can determine which individual in each pair has a higher value than the other).

Assumptions/requirements
That there is an underlying continuous distribution of the variable even if it is only measured on an ordinal scale.

Null hypothesis
That the medians m_1 and m_2 in the two populations are equal.

Method
(1) Calculate the sign ($+$ or $-$) of the differences $X_1 - X_2$ between each pair of values. If some pairs have the same value the difference is zero. Count the number of non-zero differences and call it n. If there are no ties $N = n$.
(2) Count the number of positive ($+$) differences and call it n_+.
(3) Look up the table for the sign test (Table B.6) corresponding to the chosen one- or two-sided significance level and the number of non-zero differences n. The entry gives the lower (S_l) and upper (S_u) critical values for the number of positive differences n_+.

One-sided test

If $n_+ \geqslant S_u$.	conclude $m_1 > m_2$
If $n_+ \leqslant S_l$	conclude $m_1 < m_2$
If $S_l < n_+ < S_u$	conclude $m_1 = m_2$

Two-sided test

If $n_+ \geqslant S_u$ or $n_+ \leqslant S_l$	conclude $m_1 \neq m_2$
If $S_l < n_+ < S_u$	conclude $m_1 = m_2$

C.9 The Wilcoxon matched pairs signed rank test

This procedure is discussed in Section 7.8.

Situation
Two individually matched samples each of sample size N (N pairs of observations); quantitative or ordinal variable in that the differences between each pair can be ordered.

Assumptions/requirements
That there is an underlying continuous distribution of the variable even if it is only measured on an ordinal scale; that there are not too many ties among the differences.

Null hypothesis
That the medians m_1 and m_2 in the two populations are equal.

Method
(1) Calculate the differences between each pair of values, $d = X_1 - X_2$. Let n equal the number of non-zero differences.

(2) Rank these non-zero differences from smallest to highest ignoring the sign of the difference. Assign a rank to each of these differences giving the smallest a rank of 1. If two differences have the same magnitude assign the mean of the ranks in the positions concerned. Now affix to each rank the sign (+ or −) of the difference it represents.

(3) Add up the positive (+) ranks and call the sum T_+.

(4) Look up the table for this test (Table B.7), and find the lower (T_l) and upper (T_u) critical values for T_+ corresponding to the number of non-zero differences n and the chosen one- or two-sided significance level.

One-sided test

If $T_+ \geqslant T_u$	conclude $m_1 > m_2$
If $T_+ \leqslant T_l$	conclude $m_1 < m_2$
If $T_l < T_+ < T_u$	conclude $m_1 = m_2$

Two-sided test
If $T_+ \geqslant T_u$ or $T_+ \leqslant T_l$ conclude $m_1 \neq m_2$
If $T_l < T_+ < T_u$ conclude $m_1 = m_2$

C.10   The Z test for two independent proportions. Confidence intervals for a difference

These procedures are discussed in Section 7.9.

Situation
Two independent random samples size n_1 and n_2 from two populations; qualitative binary variable with unknown population proportions, π_1 and π_2, in one category of the variable.

Assumptions/requirements
That for total sample size, $n_1 + n_2$, less than 40, the four quantities obtained by multiplying n_1 and n_2 by p and $1 - p$ are all greater than 5, where p is the pooled proportion in the two samples combined (see below). Thus this test should not be used for total sample sizes less than 20.

Null hypothesis
That the proportions π_1 and π_2 in the populations are equal.

Method
   (1) Calculate the proportions p_1 and p_2 in each of the samples. Also calculate the overall sample proportion p in the two groups combined (the pooled value).
   (2) Calculate the Z statistic

$$Z = \frac{p_1 - p_2}{\sqrt{pq\left(\dfrac{1}{n_1} + \dfrac{1}{n_2}\right)}}$$

where $q = 1 - p$.
   (3) Look up the critical value Z_c of the normal distribution at the required one- or two-sided significance level (Table B.2).

One-sided test
If $Z \geqslant Z_c$ conclude $\pi_1 > \pi_2$
If $Z \leqslant -Z_c$ conclude $\pi_1 < \pi_2$
If $-Z_c < Z < Z_c$ conclude $\pi_1 = \pi_2$

Two-sided test
If $Z \geqslant Z_c$ or $Z \leqslant -Z_c$ conclude $\pi_1 \neq \pi_2$
If $-Z_c < Z < Z_c$ conclude $\pi_1 = \pi_2$

Confidence intervals
95% and 99% confidence intervals for the difference between the population proportions $\pi_1 - \pi_2$ are calculated from

$$p_1 - p_2 \pm Z_c \sqrt{\frac{p_1 q_1}{n_1} + \frac{p_2 q_2}{n_2}}$$

where $q_1 = 1 - p_1$, $q_2 = 1 - p_2$ and Z_c is the two-sided 5% or 1% critical value for the normal distribution.

C.11   The χ^2 test for many independent proportions and two or more samples

This procedure is discussed in Sections 7.10, 7.12 and A.3.

Situation
Independent random samples from two or more populations; qualitative variable with two or more categories. The data are usually laid out in a $I \times J$ table where I is the number of rows and J is the number of columns. The number of observations in each cell of the table must be known. The situation also arises when two qualitative variables are being examined in a single sample.

Assumptions
That not more than 20% of the expected values in the cells (see below) should be less than 5 and no cell should have an expected value of less than 1.

Null hypothesis
That the distributions of the qualitative variable in the different populations are the same or, equivalently, that two qualitative variables in a single sample are not associated.

Method
   (1) Calculate the expected values (E) in each cell in the table. The expected value for the cell in the ith row and jth column is obtained by multiplying the totals of the corresponding row, r_i, and column, s_j, and dividing by the total sample size in all groups combined (n).
   (2) Calculate the χ^2 statistic on $(I-1)(J-1)$ degrees of freedom

$$\chi^2 = \sum \frac{(O - E)^2}{E}$$

where the Os are the observed numbers in each cell and summation is over all cells in the table.

(3) If the data fit into a 2×2 table as below

a	b	r_1
c	d	r_2
s_1	s_2	n

an equivalent but easier computational procedure is to calculate on 1 degree of freedom (see Section A.3)

$$\chi^2 = \frac{(ad - bc)^2 n}{r_1 r_2 s_1 s_2}$$

(4) Look up the critical value χ^2_c of the chi-square distribution for degrees of freedom $(I-1)(J-1)$ at the required two-sided significance level (Table 8.4). (A one-sided test is only legitimate for a 2×2 table.)

If $\chi^2 \geqslant \chi^2_c$ reject the null hypothesis
If $\chi^2 < \chi^2_c$ do not reject the null hypothesis

C.12   Fisher's exact test for a 2×2 table

This procedure is discussed in Section 7.11.

Situation
Independent data laid out in a 2×2 table.

Assumptions/requirements
That the row and column totals are fixed.

Null hypothesis
That the row and column variables are not associated or, equivalently, that a binary variable is not associated with group membership in a two-sample situation.

Method
(1) Rearrange the table so that the smallest cell frequency is in the top left-hand corner.
(2) Create a new table by reducing the number in the top-left cell by 1 (unless it is zero to start with) and fill in the rest of the table so that it has the same row and column totals as the original.
(3) Repeat step 2 until a table with a zero in the top left cell is obtained. There should now be a total of $V+1$ tables, including the original, where V is the smallest cell frequency in the original. Label these tables from set 0 to set V according to the number in the top left cell. The table in set i has the form

a_i	b_i	r_1
c_i	d_i	r_2
s_1	s_2	n

where, of course, r_1, r_2, s_1 and s_2 are the row and column totals which are the same for each table. $a_0 = 0$ and $a_i = i$.

(4) Calculate the probability of the table in set 0, directly or using logs (Tables B.8 and B.9).

$$P_0 = \frac{r_2! \, s_2!}{d_0! \, n!}$$

(5) Calculate the probability of the table in the next set (if there is one) using

$$P_{i+1} = P_i \times \frac{b_i \times c_i}{a_{i+1} \times d_{i+1}}$$

(6) Repeat the last step until all the probabilities from P_0 to P_V have been calculated.

(7) Sum these $V + 1$ probabilities. This is the one-sided p value for the test. Multiply this by 2 to obtain the two-sided value. If the (one- or two-sided) p value is less than 5% the null hypothesis can be rejected.

C.13   The McNemar and exact tests for correlated or paired proportions

This procedure is discussed in Section 7.13.

Situation
Two individually matched samples each of size N (N pairs of observations); qualitative binary variable with unknown population proportions π_1 and π_2 in one category of the variable. This category is denoted by a plus sign below.

Assumptions/requirements
None.

Null hypothesis
That the proportions π_1 and π_2 in the two paired populations are equal.

Method

(1) Lay out the data in a 2×2 table as

		Group 1	
		+	−
G			
r	+	a	b
o			
u			
p	−	c	d
2			

where the classification is based on the N pairs of observations, and the plus and minus refer to the categories of the binary variable.

(2) For small sample sizes refer c (number of untied pairs in favour of group 1) to Table B.6, which gives the lower (S_l) and upper (S_u) critical values for the test, entered at $n = b + c$ which is the total number of untied pairs.

One-sided test
If $c \geqslant S_u$ conclude $\pi_1 > \pi_2$
If $c \leqslant S_l$ conclude $\pi_1 < \pi_2$
If $S_l < c < S_u$ conclude $\pi_1 = \pi_2$

Two-sided test
If $c \geqslant S_u$ or $c \leqslant S_l$ conclude $\pi_1 \neq \pi_2$
If $S_l < c < S_u$ conclude $\pi_1 = \pi_2$

(3) For large sample sizes calculate

$$\chi^2 = \frac{(b-c)^2}{b+c}$$

on 1 degree of freedom.

(4) Look up the critical value χ^2_c of the chi-square distribution on 1 degree of freedom at the required one- or two-sided significance level (Table B.4).

If $\chi^2 \geqslant \chi^2_c$ conclude $\pi_1 \neq \pi_2$
If $\chi^2 < \chi^2_c$ conclude $\pi_1 = \pi_2$

C.14   Significance tests for regression and correlation

These procedures are discussed in Section 8.5.

Situation
Random samples of a Y variable at different values of an X variable; both

variables quantitative; often assumed in random sampling from a single group; n pairs of values in all.

Assumptions/requirements
That the population distribution of Y at each fixed X is normal and that the variances of these Y distributions are all equal; that the means of the Y distributions are linearly related to X.

Null hypotheses
(1) That the population regression coefficient β is equal to a fixed value β_0 or (2) that the population correlation coefficient ρ is equal to zero.

Method — null hypothesis (1)
(1) Calculate the regression coefficient b, the sum of squares $\Sigma(X - \bar{X})^2$ and the standard error of the estimate, $S_{Y.X}$, using the methods outlined in Section A.4.
(2) Calculate the t statistic on $n-2$ degrees of freedom.

$$t = \frac{b - \beta_0}{SE(b)}$$

where

$$SE(b) = \frac{S_{Y.X}}{\sqrt{\Sigma(X - \bar{X})^2}}$$

(3) Look up the critical value t_c of the t distribution on $n-2$ degrees of freedom at the required two-sided (usually) significance level (Table B.3).

If $t \geqslant t_c$ or $t \leqslant -t_c$	conclude $\beta \neq \beta_0$
If $-t_c < t < t_c$	conclude $\beta = \beta_0$

Confidence intervals
95 and 99% confidence intervals for β are calculated from

$$b \pm t_c\, SE(b)$$

where t_c is the appropriate critical value of the t distribution on $n-1$ degrees of freedom.

Method — null hypothesis (2)
(1) Calculate the correlation coefficient r (see Section A.4).
(2) Calculate the t statistic on $n-2$ degrees of freedom.

$$t = r\sqrt{\frac{n-2}{1-r^2}}$$

(3) Look up the critical value t_c of the t distribution on $n-2$ degrees of freedom at the required two-sided (usually) significance level (Table B.3).

If $t \geqslant t_c$ or $t \leqslant -t_c$ conclude $\rho \neq 0$

If $-t_c < t < t_c$ conclude $\rho = 0$

C.15   Spearman's rank order correlation coefficient

This procedure is discussed in Section 8.11.

Situation
n pairs of observations on an X and Y variable. Both variables quantitative or ordered.

Assumptions/requirements
That there are not too many ties in the ranks of the variables.

Null hypothesis
That the population correlation ρ_s between the two variables is zero.

Method
   (1) Assign ranks to the X and Y variables separately, from lowest to highest, giving the average rank to tied observations.
   (2) For each pair subtract the rank of variable Y from the rank of variable X and call the result d.
   (3) Square each d and add to obtain Σd^2.
   (4) Spearman's rank correlation coefficient is calculated as

$$r_s = \frac{6\Sigma d^2}{n(n^2 - 1)}$$

   (5) Look up the critical value r_c for Spearman's rank correlation coefficient in Table B.10 for n equal to the number of pairs at the appropriate (usually) two-sided significance level

If $r_s \geqslant r_c$ or $r_s \leqslant -r_c$ conclude $\rho_s \neq 0$

If $-r_c < r_s < r_c$ conclude $\rho_s = 0$

APPENDIX D
Sample Size Calculations

D.1 Introduction

As has been discussed, the sample size required for an investigation should be estimated at the planning stage. No study should be carried out unless it has a reasonable chance of detecting an important effect at a given level of statistical significance. If the sample size of a study is too small, important differences may be declared statistically non-significant. This appendix gives, without derivation, some sample size formulae for use in two-group comparisons with equal numbers in each group. The sample sizes calculated assume that there are no losses from the study, and thus extra allowance should be made for patient withdrawals. The formulae also assume that (in prospective studies or clinical trials) a variable follow-up is not involved, so that the end-point of interest must be known to be either present or absent at a fixed time from study commencement in all patients.

Before a sample size can be estimated, some preliminary decisions must be made. Firstly, the investigators must decide on the minimum difference between the two groups they wish to detect. Thus in a clinical trial, a standard treatment may be known to have a five-year survival of 50%, and it is wished to see if a new therapy could increase this survival to 60%. The sample size for a two-group trial would then be estimated on the basis of a minimum survival difference between the groups of 10%. It would be accepted that a smaller effect than this might not be detected. Obviously, there will often be more than one variable of interest in a two-group comparison, and sample sizes may have to be calculated for comparisons of each of these variables, and the largest sample size chosen.

If a difference in a quantitative variable is to be tested, in addition to the minimum difference to be detected, the standard deviation of the variable is also required. If this is not available from previous studies, a pilot study would have to be performed to obtain a rough estimate.

Two other parameters must also be specified. These are the significance level (p value, probability of a type I error, α error) at which the group difference is to be detected, and the required probability of making a type II (β) error in detecting this difference. Often the β probability is set at four times the α probability. Thus for a 5% level of significance, β might be set equal to

312

0·2. See Section 6.7 for a fuller discussion of type I and type II errors in significance testing.

In the next section, sample size formulae are given for the comparison of means in independent samples, proportions in independent samples, and means in paired samples. The formulae are approximate and are not accurate for small sample sizes. Professional advice should usually be sought for sample size estimation, although the formulae presented below will give some guide as to how large a particular study should be.

D.2 Sample size formulae

For the comparison of mean values in two independent samples

$$n > \frac{2K\,\sigma^2}{\Delta^2} \tag{D.1}$$

where n is the sample size required in each of the groups. K is a constant (based on tables of the standard normal curve) which depends on the desired α and β probabilities for the comparison, and whether the significance test is to be one-sided or two-sided. Table D.1 gives these constants for varying levels of α and β. σ^2 is the variance in each of the groups being compared (equal variances are assumed). Usually, only a rough estimate of this will be available. Δ is the magnitude of the difference between the populations that it is required to detect at the stated α and β values.

Suppose a clinical trial is to be carried out to compare two different treatments for blood pressure reduction. The researchers want to have a fairly large chance of detecting, as statistically significant, a real (population) difference between the mean systolic blood pressures in the two groups of 10 mm Hg or greater. A non-stratified randomization is to be employed, so that the two groups may be considered independent. The researchers decide on a two-sided significance test at a 5% level, and on a β probability of 0·2. This

Table D.1 Multiplying factor K for sample size formulae. α = significance level (probability of a type I error). β = probability of a type II error.

		One-sided test				Two-sided test	
		α				α	
		0·05	0·01			0·05	0·01
	0·05	10·8	15·8		0·05	13·0	17·8
β	0·10	8·6	13·0	β	0·10	10·5	14·9
	0·20	6·2	10·0		0·20	7·8	11·7

means that the resulting study should have an 80% $(1-\beta$; the power of the test) chance of detecting this treatment effect. A preliminary estimate of the standard deviation of the systolic blood pressure is 20 mm Hg. Thus from Table D.1, $K = 7·9$ while $\sigma^2 = 400$ and $\Delta^2 = 100$. Using Eqn. D.1, a sample size of over 63·2 is necessary in each group. This value is rounded up to the nearest integer so that a total of 128 patients will be required.

For the comparison of means in a paired situation

$$n > \frac{K \sigma_d^2}{\Delta^2} \tag{D.2}$$

n in this case is the number of pairs required in the study, σ_d^2 is the variance of the differences between the values of the two populations, Δ is the minimum difference to be detected. K is determined as before from Table D.1 on the basis of the chosen α and β values.

Suppose that in the clinical trial discussed above, a cross-over design was to be used with each patient receiving each treatment, and that the same statistical requirements were chosen. If a preliminary estimate of the standard deviation of the paired differences was obtained as $\sigma_d = 25$ mm Hg, n (the number of pairs required) turns out to be, from Eqn. D.2, 49·375 or 50 patients, since this is a self-paired experiment.

For the comparison of proportions in two independent groups

$$n > \frac{K(p_1 q_1 + p_2 q_2)}{\Delta^2} \tag{D.3}$$

Again, n is the number of individuals required in each group, p_1 and p_2 are the presumed proportions in the two groups being compared, while, as usual, $q_1 = 1 - p_1$ and $q_2 = 1 - p_2$. Δ is the minimum difference to be detected which, of course, is nothing more than $p_1 - p_2$. Note that in this case no estimate of a standard deviation is required.

Again, taking a clinical trial sample, the sample size requirements for the situation discussed in Section D.1 will be examined. The usual 5-year survival for breast cancer patients is known to be around 50% (or, expressed as a proportion, 0·5) and it is hoped to study the effectiveness of a new therapy which might increase this to at least 60% (0·6). It is desired that this effect should be detected at a two-sided 1% significance level, with only a 0·05 chance of missing it if it does exist. A non-stratified randomization is to be employed, with follow-up of each patient for a full five years. Thus K from Table D.1 is 17·8. $p_1 = 0·5$, $q_1 = 0·5$, $p_2 = 0·6$, $q_2 = 0·4$, and $\Delta = 0·6 - 0·5 = 0·1$. Substituting these values into Eqn. D.3, the required sample size in each group is 872·2 or a total requirement of 1746 patients. Large sample sizes such as this are not uncommon in many situations.

BIBLIOGRAPHY AND REFERENCES

The bibliography lists a number of books and articles for further reading. Some of these have already been referred to in the text and the selection, although by no means comprehensive, should guide the interested reader to a more advanced treatment of some of the topics covered. The reference section includes all works cited in the text from which illustrative examples were taken. Reproduction or adaptation of tables or figures from these works was by kind permission of the authors, editors and publishers concerned.

Bibliography

ABRAMSON J. H. (1979) *Survey Methods in Community Medicine*, 2nd Edition. Edinburgh: Churchill Livingstone. A comprehensive text book on the planning and performance of medical surveys and clinical trials.

ARMITAGE P. (1971) *Statistical Methods in Medical Research*. Oxford: Blackwell Scientific Publications. A standard reference work in medical statistics which includes details of many of the more complex techniques used in medical research. A good deal more advanced than this book.

ARMITAGE P. (1975) *Sequential Medical Trials*. Oxford: Blackwell Scientific Publications. An excellent and detailed description of the sequential clinical trial. The mathematical level is considerably higher than that of this book.

ASBURY A. J. (1983) *ABC of Computing*. London: British Medical Association. Reprints of articles from the British Medical Journal which explain basic computer configurations and their application to medicine. A very useful introductory guide.

BENJAMIN B. (1968) *Health and Vital Statistics*. London: Heinemann. Good introductory text covering demography, mortality, morbidity, fertility, hospital statistics and analysis of disease mortality.

BENNETT A. E. & RITCHIE K. (1975) *Questionnaires in Medicine*. Oxford: Oxford University Press. A useful book on the design and use of questionnaires in medical research.

BRESLOW N. E. & DAY N. E. (1980) *Statistical Methods in Cancer Research*, Vol. 1. Lyon: International Agency for Research on Cancer. An excellent exposition of the case-control study, including a detailed discussion of its design and implementation. Heavy emphasis is placed on the analysis of case-control studies and how to control for confounders. Appropriate multiple regression techniques are described in detail and computer programs are given in appendices. (More up-to-date programs may be available from the authors.)

CASTLE W. M. (1972) *Statistics in Small Doses*, 2nd Edition. Edinburgh: Churchill Livingstone. A programmed instruction text which leads the reader through some of the more simple aspects of data description and analysis.

COLTON T. (1974) *Statistics in Medicine*. Boston: Little, Brown and Company. A textbook at about the same level as this work with extensive examples from the medical literature and a good introduction to study design.

COX D. R. (1972) Regression models and life-tables (with discussion). *Journal of the Royal Statistical Association*, **B34**, 187–220. A difficult statistical paper which details the applications and theory of Cox's regression model for life-table analysis.

FEINSTEIN A. R. (1977) *Clinical Biostatistics*. St Louis: C. V. Mosby & Co. A collection of articles on various topics in biostatistics, which originallly appeared as essays in the *Journal of Clinical Pharmacology and Therapeutics*. This is a very readable book which discusses many of the problems and pitfalls to be encountered in epidemiological research.

GEIGY SCIENTIFIC TABLES (1982) Vol. 2, 8th Edition. C. Lentner (Ed.) Basle: Ciba-Geigy. A useful and comprehensive handbook of statistical tables with a summary section outlining a large body of statistical theory and significance tests.

GORE S. M., JONES I. G. & RYTTER E. C. (1977) Misuse of statistical methods: critical assessment of articles in BMJ from January to March 1976. *British Medical Journal* **1**, 85–7. A survey of statistical errors in the medical literature.

GORE S. M. & ALTMAN D. G. (1982) *Statistics in Practice*. London: British Medical Association. Reprints of articles from the British Medical Journal with emphasis on the methodology and execution of clinical trials. Most of the text is in a question and answer format but should be most useful for anyone involved in the design of a trial.

HILL A. B. (1963) Medical ethics and controlled trials. *British Medical Journal* **1**, 1043–9. An early but key paper on the ethics of the clinical trial.

HILL A. B. (1971) *Principles of Medical Statistics*. London: Lancet. A classic textbook of medical statistics, at about the same level as this book.

HILLS M. & ARMITAGE P. (1979) The two-period cross-over clinical trial. *British Journal of Clinical Pharmacology* **8**, 7–20. A detailed description of the design and analysis of the cross-over clinical trial.

MacMahon B. & Pugh T. F. (1970) *Epidemiology: Principles and Methods.* Boston: Little, Brown and Company. A general textbook on epidemiology in which are described most of the measures used in summarizing epidemiological data.

Nie N. H., Hull C. H., Jenkins J. G., Steinbrenner K. & Bent D. H. (1975) *SPSS: Statistical Package for the Social Sciences.* New York: McGraw-Hill Book Company. The manual for a very comprehensive statistical package for data analysis available in most large computing centres. The description of each computer program is preceded by a good discussion of the background to the statistical procedure involved. Many additions to the package have been made since the publication of this book, and well over 90 per cent of the analytic techniques required to analyse medical studies are now implemented. Contact your local computer centre for more details.

Peto R., Pike M. C., Armitage P., Breslow N. E., Cox D. R., Howard S. V., Mantel N., McPherson K., Peto J. & Smith P. G. (1976) Design and analysis of randomized clinical trials requiring prolonged observation of each patient. I. Introduction and design. *British Journal of Cancer* **34**, 585–612.

Peto R., Pike M. C., Armitage P., Breslow N. E., Cox D. R., Howard S. V., Mantel N., McPherson K., Peto, J. & Smith P. G. (1977) Design and analysis of randomized clinical trials requiring prolonged observation of each patient. II. Analysis and examples. *British Journal of Cancer* **35**, 1–39. Two articles on the design and analysis of clinical trials with particular emphasis on survival as an end-point. This article describes life tables and the logrank test in a readily understandable manner and is required reading for those interest in this area. A computer program to implement life table analysis is available from the authors.

Remington R. D. & Schork M. A. (1970) *Statistics with Applications to the Biological and Health Sciences.* New Jersey: Prentice-Hall Inc. A very readable textbook which goes into somewhat more mathematical detail than the present text.

Sackett D. L. (1979) Bias in analytic research. *Journal of Chronic Disease* **32**, 51–63. A catalogue of biases in medical research with references to their occurrence in the literature.

Siegel S. (1956) *Nonparametric Statistics for the Behavioural Sciences.* Tokyo: McGraw-Hill Kogakusha, Ltd. A textbook describing most of the non-parametric statistical tests in a readable comprehensible manner.

Smoking and Health (1964) A report of the advisory committee to the Surgeon General of the Public Health Service. Washington D.C.: U.S. Department of Health, Education and Welfare. A report including a description of the criteria for judging the causal significance of an association.

SOKAL R. R. & ROHLF F. J. (1981) *Biometry.* San Francisco: W. H. Freeman and Company. A large and detailed text with emphasis on statistics in biological applications. Many complex techniques are covered but the application of each is explained in a simple step-by-step manner. Much more advanced than this book but a useful book to have available. Statistical tables are unfortunately published in a separate volume.

SWINSCOW D. V. (1976) *Statistics at Square One.* London: British Medical Association. A short book which outlines the computations required for some of the simpler statistical tests.

ZELEN M. (1979) A new design for randomized clinical trials. *New England Journal of Medicine* **300**, 1242–46. A paper describing a particular design for a clinical trial which avoids some of the ethical problems caused by the demands of informed consent.

References

DALY L. E., MULCAHY R., GRAHAM I. & HICKEY N. (1983) Long term effect on mortality of stopping smoking after unstable angina and myocardial infarction. *British Medical Journal* **287**, 324–6.

DAWBER T. R. (1980) The Framingham Study: The Epidemiology of Atherosclerotic Disease. Cambridge (Mass.): Harvard University Press.

DOLL R. & PETO R. (1976) Mortality in relation to smoking: 20 years' observations on male British doctors. *British Medical Journal* **2**, 1525–36.

GREEN T. P., THOMPSON T. R., JOHNSON D. E. & LOCK J. E. (1983) Furosemide promotes patent ductus arteriosus in premature infants with the respiratory-distress syndrome. *New England Journal of Medicine* **308**, 743–8.

GREGG N. M. (1941) Congenital cataract following German measles in the mother. *Transactions of the Ophthalmological Society of Australia* **III**, 35–46.

HAYES A., DALY L., O'BRIEN N. G. & MACDONALD D. (1983) Anthropometric standards for Irish newborn. *Irish Medical Journal* **76**, 60–70.

HICKEY N., MULCAHY R., DALY L., BOURKE G. & MORIARTY J. (1979) The relationship between blood glucose and prevalence of coronary heart disease: A study in the Republic of Ireland. *Journal of Chronic Diseases* **32**, 767–72.

HERITY B., MORIARTY M., BOURKE G. J. & DALY L. (1981) A case-control study of head and neck cancer in the Republic of Ireland. *British Journal of Cancer* **43**, 177–82.

HORGAN J. M., DALY L., BOURKE G. J. & WILSON-DAVIS K. (1978) University entrance performance and pre-medical examination results. *Irish Medical Journal* **71**, 428–33.

IRISH STATISTICAL BULLETIN (1976) Vol. **L1**, No. 1. Dublin: Stationery Office.

LAGOS P., LAGONA E., KATTAMIS C. & MATSANIOTIS N. (1980) Serum ferritin in β-thalassaemia intermedia. *Lancet* **1**, 204–5.

LOWES J. A., WILLIAMS G., TABAQCHALI S., HILL I. M., HAMER J., HOUANG E., SHAW E. J., & REES G. M. (1980) 10 years of infective endocarditis at St. Bartholomew's Hospital: analysis of clinical features and treatment in relation to prognosis and mortality. *Lancet* **1**, 133–36.

MITCHELL J. R. A. (1981) Timolol after myocardial infarction: an answer or a new set of questions? *British Medical Journal* **282**, 1565–70.

O'CONNOR J., & DALY M. (1983) *Smoking and drinking behaviour.* Vol. 1. Dublin: Health Education Bureau.

OFFICE OF POPULATION CENSUSES AND SURVEYS (1974) *The Registrar General's Statistical Review of England and Wales for the year 1972*, Part I, Tables Medical. London: HMSO.

OFFICE OF POPULATION CENSUSES AND SURVEYS (1983) *Population Trends* 33, Autumn 1983. London: HMSO.

PALMERI S. T., HARRISON D. G., COBB F. R., MORRIS K. G., HARRELL F. E., IDEKER R. E., SELVESTER R. H. & WAGNER G. S. (1982) A QRS scoring system for assessing left ventricular function after myocardial infarction. *New England Journal of Medicine* 306, 4–9.

PARKS J. H., COE F. L. & STRAUSS A. L. (1982) Calcium nephrolithiasis and medullary sponge kidney in women. *New England Journal of Medicine* 306, 1088–91.

PILLOCK E., WINES W. & HALL D. (1981) A survey of blood pressure in 10-year-old children of a health district together with a consideration of screening policy for hypertension. *Community Medicine* 3, 199–204.

REGISTRAR GENERAL SCOTLAND (1983) *Annual Report 1982.* Edinburgh: HMSO.

SALONEN J. T. & VOHLONEN I. (1982) Longitudinal cross-national analysis of coronary mortality. *International Journal of Epidemiology* 11, 229–38.

THE NORWEGIAN MULTICENTRE STUDY GROUP. (1981) Timolol-induced reduction in mortality and reinfarction in patients surviving acute myocardial infarction. *New England Journal of Medicine* 304, 801–7.

UNITED NATIONS (1984) *Demographic Yearbook 1982.* New York: United Nations.

Index